■ Clinical Electrocardiography for Nurses

Hannelore M. Sweetwood, R.N., M.S.

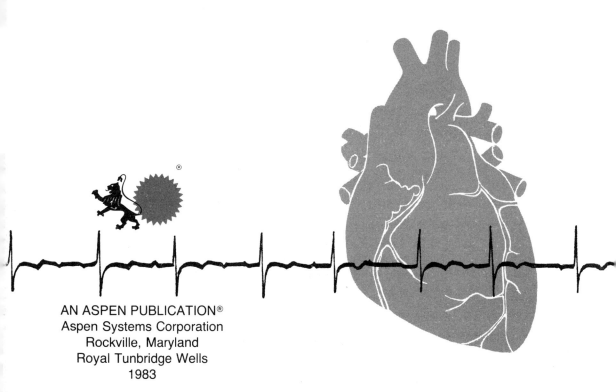

AN ASPEN PUBLICATION®
Aspen Systems Corporation
Rockville, Maryland
Royal Tunbridge Wells
1983

Library of Congress Cataloging in Publication Data

Sweetwood, Hannelore M.
Clinical electrocardiography for nurses.

Bibliography: p. 499
Includes index.
1. Electrocardiography. 2. Cardiovascular
disease nursing. I. Title [DNLM: 1. Cardiovascular diseases—Nursing. 2. Coronary care
units—Nursing texts. 3. Electrocardiography—
Nursing texts. WY 152.5 S974c]
RC683.5 E5S84 1983 616.1'207547 82-25282
ISBN: 0-89443-846-8

Publisher: John Marozsan
Editorial Director: Darlene Como
Executive Managing Editor: Margot Raphael
Printing and Manufacturing: Debbie Collins

The author and publisher have made an effort to ensure that drug
selection and dosage agree with recommendations and practice
current at the time of publication. However, it remains the
responsibility of every practitioner to consult appropriate
information sources and to evaluate the appropriateness of a
particular opinion in the context of the actual clinical situation and
with due consideration to any new developments in the field.

Library of Congress Catalog Card Number: 82-25282
ISBN: 0-89443-846-8
Printed in the United States of America
3 4 5

To the critical care nurses, cardiologists, and ECG technicians
of Jersey Shore Medical Center

Table of Contents

Foreword

It has been more than two decades since nurses began interpreting dysrhythmias and acting upon their interpretations. Initially, nursing practice was a dynamic state, altered as patients' needs dictated. The rapid increase in the body of knowledge developed by practicing nurses, as well as the explosive technological revolution, lead to the birth of critical-care nursing. And the roots of critical-care nursing are found in the 1960s beginning with cardiovascular nursing.

A basic foundation found in every curriculum for critical care education is dysrhythmia identification, intervention, and evaluation. Time spent learning and expanding this knowledge base of cardiac function is time well spent, and will be returned in benefits to our patients many times over. So, when a master teacher puts pen to paper and records for us her methods of teaching this specific topic, we are indeed enriched.

Hannelore Sweetwood has done that for us. This book has evolved from her years of experience teaching ECG interpretation to her students. The book contains many patient case studies, as well as many "pearls" that practitioners seek. Only a clinical educator such as Hannelore Sweetwood could have provided the book that you are about to read and study. She has remained close to patients and nurses and, therefore, has never lost her clinical relevance for the reality of the practice setting.

It has been my pleasure to participate, even in this small way, to the making of such a fine book.

Diane C. Adler, M.A., C.C.R.N., R.R.T.
Clinical Director
Critical Care Department
Hospital of the University of Pennsylvania

Foreword

The establishment of Coronary Care Units resulted in a significant decrease in in-hospital mortality primarily from deaths due to cardiac arrhythmias. Nurses have played an important role in maintaining this decrease in mortality. However, the nurse's role in caring for critically ill patients has been expanding and will continue to expand. We have come to expect nurses to be expert in many areas (electrocardiographic interpretation, cardiovascular pharmacology, hemodynamic monitoring, etc.) while maintaining high standards in their traditional role of providing patient care. The achievement of these formidable goals begins with education and training by dedicated educators within the medical profession. Hannelore Sweetwood is a dedicated educator. In this 14 chapter book she has succinctly and clearly presented the essentials for the beginning of mastering this subject.

Anthony N. Damato, MD

Preface

Few professional groups have expanded the scope of their knowledge and responsibilities as widely and rapidly as critical care nurses have during the last decade. This book was written to provide these nurses with the full use of an extremely sensitive diagnostic tool, the 12-lead ECG. It is my hope that they will have as much interest, and occasionally fun, in acquiring and using this knowledge, as I do.

This text does not explain "all there is to know" about electrocardiography. Perfect and complete knowledge is a goal we may never attain, but in striving toward it, we advance and grow.

Hannelore Sweetwood, R.N., M.S.

## Chapter 1

The 12-Lead Electrocardiogram

Diagnostic Use

There are several approaches to diagnostic ECG interpretation. One method is to carefully commit all possible patterns and criteria to memory and then to examine each ECG for the presence of these patterns. If one has a perfect memory and is always presented with textbook ECGs, this technique will prove successful. Another method is to keep in mind some basic facts of anatomy, electrophysiology, and pathophysiology and to interpret deviations from the norm in light of such knowledge. This approach may seem more complicated at first, but it is preferable because it helps to reveal existing abnormalities even if a specific pattern is forgotten or, more likely, the patient does not have a classic ECG.

Anatomical Considerations

Although most anatomical diagrams depict the heart as a more or less symmetrically placed organ, the apex of the heart actually points forward and to the left, and the heart is rotated on its vertical axis so that the right ventricle extends beyond the left sternal border. It is necessary to remember this position when reading an ECG.

Another important factor is that the left ventricle of the adult heart normally has about three times as much muscle mass as the right, so the greater share of current is generated by depolarization of left ventricular myocardium.

Electrophysiological Factors

What are you actually looking at when you inspect a 12-lead ECG? You see a record of currents moving through the heart from 12 different vantage points, namely, the positive poles of 12 leads. The ECG gives three major pieces of information about this current: duration, magnitude, and direction.

The duration is the time required to depolarize various structures; it is measured in milliseconds on the horizontal markings of the ECG paper. Abnormal duration may indicate impairment or irregularities of current propagation.

The magnitude of the currents is expressed in millivolts and is measured by the vertical markings of the ECG paper: 10 mm = 1 mV, when the ECG machine is set at "standard." Voltage is determined in part by the size of the cardiac chambers but is also affected by body structure and various pathological conditions.

The direction of currents indicates their point of origin and course through the chambers of the heart. A great variety of abnormalities affect the direction of currents produced by depolarization as well as repolarization.

All ECG recording devices are built so that an upstroke is produced when currents move toward the positive pole of a lead, while movement away from it produces a negative deflection. When currents move perpendicularly to a given lead, an equiphasic wave is created, that is, a complex in which the space occupied by the positive deflection equals that of the negative deflection. To interpret current direction correctly, therefore, one must remember the placement of the positive pole (electrode) of each lead.

Frontal Plane Leads

These leads reflect currents moving in the frontal plane, that is, toward the head or feet and toward the right or left side of the body. They are also called limb leads, because originally the electrodes were placed on the arms and legs, as is still customary when an ECG is taken. From an electrophysiological point of view, however, the same effect can be achieved by placing the electrodes on the chest, as is generally done for continuous monitoring.

Standard Limb Leads

Einthoven designed his apparatus with three leads, which form a triangle around the heart, as shown by imaginary lines drawn to connect the positive and negative poles of each lead (Fig 1-1).

Lead I connects positive left arm (LA) electrode and negative right arm (RA) electrode. In lead II, negative pole is at RA, and positive pole is at the left leg (LL). In lead III, LA is negative and LL is positive.

When an ECG machine is used, the polarity of the electrodes is automatically adjusted as current is switched from one lead to the next. With most monitoring systems it is necessary to move the positive and negative electrodes as indicated in Figure 1-1, to obtain the desired lead. In each instance, the third electrode is electrically neutral and acts as a ground.

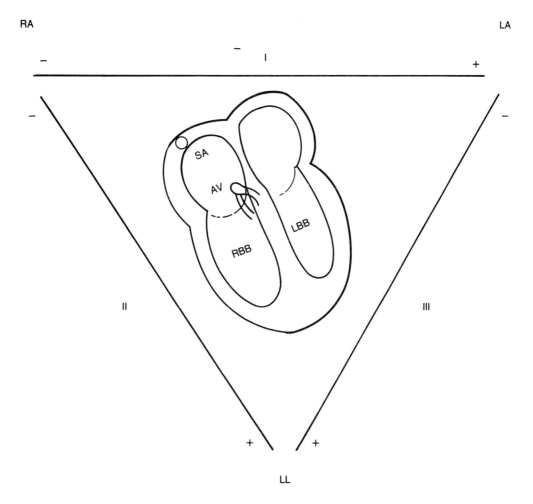

Fig 1-1.—Standard limb leads (Einthoven's triangle). SA = sinoatrial node, AV = atrioventricular node; RBB = right bundle branch, LBB = left bundle branch; I, II, and III = limb leads; and RA = right arm, LA = left arm, LL = left leg electrodes.

Augmented Voltage Leads

In leads aVR, aVL, and aVF, the positive electrode is at the limb named (AVR, right arm; AVL, left arm; and AVF, left leg), while the negative pole is at an imaginary electrical center (Fig 1-2). The necessary adjustment in electrical polarity is made by the ECG machine, as the lead selector switch is turned.

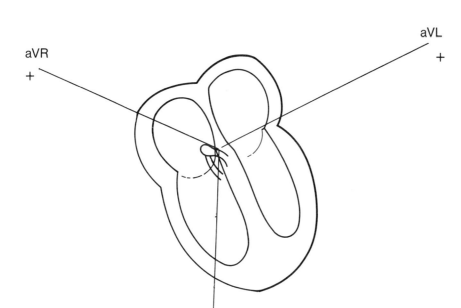

Fig. 1-2.—Augmented voltage leads. In aVR, aVL, and aVF, positive poles are at right arm, left arm, and left leg, respectively.

Inscription of Frontal Plane ECG

Vectors

The term vector is used to describe a force such as an electric current. A vector has a given direction, magnitude, and sense and is usually represented by an arrow (Fig 1-3).

The length of the arrow represents the magnitude of the force. The sense of the vector indicates the angle at which it lies, and the point of the arrow shows its direction. The sense and direction of the QRS vector are also referred to as the axis.

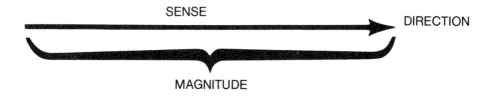

Fig 1-3.—Diagrammatic representation of a vector.

When the ventricles depolarize, innumerable simultaneous vectors move in different directions, since ventricular myocardium is depolarized from endocardium toward epicardium.

A summation of all of these simultaneous vectors represents the main QRS vector, and it is this summation vector that is seen on the ECG. The main vectors of P and T waves are produced in a similar manner.

Reflection of Vectors on ECG

In Figure 1-4, the main atrial vector (long arrow, top left) points toward the positive poles of leads I, II, III, and aVF, producing a positive P wave in these leads. Generally, the atrial axis is nearly perpendicular to lead aVL, so the P wave in this lead usually looks somewhat flat or biphasic. The main vector of atrial depolarization moves directly away from the positive pole of aVR, and the normal P wave in aVR is, therefore, negative.

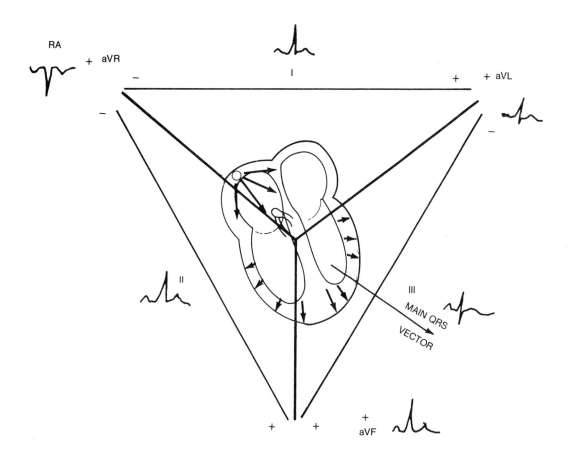

Fig. 1-4.—Reflection of vectors on frontal plane ECG P waves. I, II, and III = limb leads. In augmented voltage leads aVR, aVL, and aVF, positive poles are at right arm, left arm, and left leg, respectively.

QRS Complexes

The ventricular vector normally points toward the positive poles of leads I, II, aVL, and aVF, so the QRS complexes in these leads are predominantly positive. It points directly away from the positive pole of aVR, and consequently, the QRS in this lead is negative. In Figure 1-4, the vector is perpendicular to lead III, so it first approaches the positive pole of that lead and then moves past it. For this reason the QRS complex in lead III appears to be equiphasic.

To appreciate the effect of the position and/or pathology of the heart on the ECG, note the changes that occur in the patient with a condition that causes hypertrophy of the right ventricle (Fig 1-5). The shift of the QRS vector to the right has changed the configuration of QRS complexes in most leads.

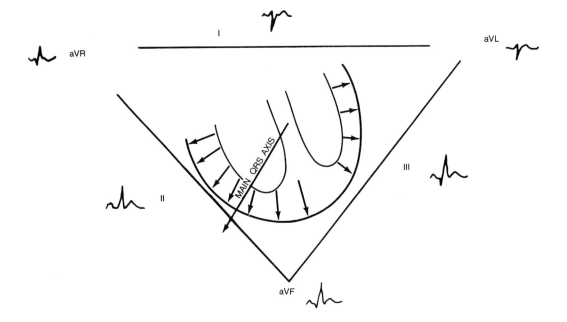

Fig. 1-5.—Effect of right ventricular hypertrophy on QRS vector and I, II, and III = limb leads. In augmented voltage leads aVR, aVL, and aVF, positive poles are at right arm, left arm, and left leg, respectively.

Determination of QRS Axis

Since a number of pathological conditions produce characteristic changes in the direction of the main QRS vector, it is useful to be able to identify the axis with precise numerical values. For this reason the six limb leads were used to construct a reference diagram, the hexaxial system. Leads I, II, and III were moved so that they intersect at a common center, and the resulting diagram is superimposed on the augmented limb leads as shown in Figure 1-6.

Numbers, given in degrees, are assigned to each pole of each lead. If the axis falls into the quadrant between +90° and 0°, it is called normal. If the axis points between 0° and − 90°, there is left axis deviation. The area from + 90° to + 180° indicates right axis deviation, and the quadrant between + 180° and − 90° is called indeterminate, since there could be either extreme right or extreme left axis deviation.

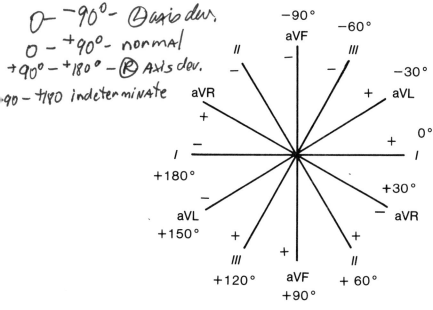

0 − −90° − ⊕ axis dev.
0 − +90° − normal
+90° − +180° − ⓡ Axis dev.
-90 − +180 indeterminate

Fig 1-6.—The hexaxial reference system.

The electrical axis is affected by many factors other than disease, notably the height, weight, and especially the age of the subject. An axis of + 128° to + 137° is normally seen in the ECG of a healthy infant.[1] With increasing age the axis shifts toward the left,[2] and an axis of − 30° is not necessarily a sign of cardiac disorder, especially in the older adult. On the other hand, if the axis is + 90° or less in the newborn or + 75° or less at age 3 months, it is considered to represent left axis deviation.[3]

The following three steps are generally used to determine the QRS axis in the frontal plane.

1. Find the most nearly equiphasic lead; the QRS vector is perpendicular to the equiphasic lead.
2. Check the diagram to see which lead is perpendicular to the equiphasic lead; this will indicate the sense of the QRS vector.
3. Determine whether the lead showing the sense of the QRS vector has a positive or negative QRS; this will give the direction of the vector.

In Figure 1-7, the following axis determination can be made.

- Lead III is equiphasic; therefore, the axis must be perpendicular to lead III.
- In the hexaxial reference system (Fig 1-6), lead aVR is perpendicular to lead III; therefore, the axis lies at the same angle as aVR.

- The QRS complex in lead aVR is negative; therefore, the vector is directed toward the negative pole of aVR.
- The negative pole of aVR is designated as +30° in the reference system.

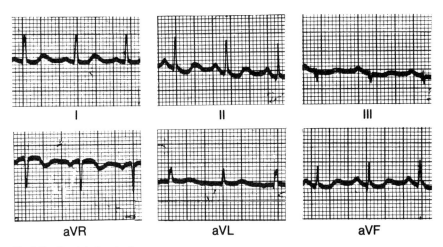

Fig 1-7.—Frontal plane leads.

Thus, the axis of the ECG shown is +30°.
Another example is shown in Figure 1-8:

- The equiphasic lead is II.
- Lead aVL is perpendicular to II.
- The QRS complex in lead aVL is positive in the tracing shown.
- The positive pole of aVL is −30°.

Thus, the axis is −30°.
The axes for the P and T waves are determined in the same manner.

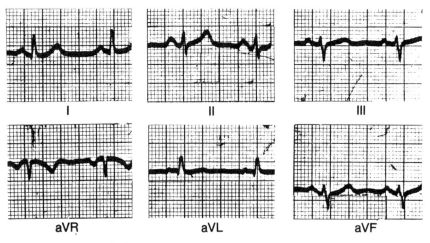

Fig 1-8.—Frontal plane leads.

Precordial Leads

Leads V_1 through V_6 are placed across the anterior and left lateral chest as shown in Figure 1-9. They reflect currents moving in the horizontal plane, that is, toward or away from the anterior and left surface of the chest. The recording electrode placed on the chest wall represents the positive pole.

To interpret precordial leads, the anatomical structures underlying each lead must be considered. The approximate electrode positions with reference to the normal adult heart are shown in Figures 1-9 and 1-10.

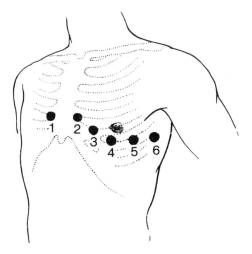

Fig 1-9.—Positions of precordial electrodes: V_1, fourth intercostal space to right of sternum, usually over junction of right atrium and right ventricle; V_2, fourth intercostal space to left of sternum, usually over right ventricle; V_3, halfway between V_2 and V_4, usually over septum or left ventricle; V_4, fifth intercostal space in midclavicular line, usually over septum or left ventricle; V_5, fifth intercostal space in anterior axillary line, usually over left ventricle; V_6, fifth intercostal space in midaxillary line, usually over left ventricle (from Goldman[4(p10)]).

The positions of anatomical structures with reference to the customary electrode sites are affected by age, body build, and disease processes. For example, in a tall, thin person the heart may be vertically placed, whereas it may be more horizontally placed in a short, obese person or in a pregnant woman.

Right Precordial Leads

Since lead V_1 is placed in close proximity to the right atrium, it generally shows a very distinct P wave. The currents produced by right atrial depolarization move directly toward V_1, producing an initial upright component of the P wave. Left atrial depolarization occurs a fraction of a second later and may produce a small negative deflection.

Unipolar Chest Leads

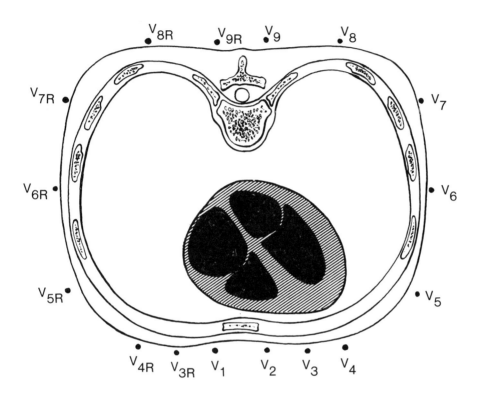

Fig 1-10.—Transverse section of thorax illustrating positions of unipolar chest leads. Leads V_{3R} through V_{9R} are right-sided chest leads (from Goldman[4(p12)]).

The first ventricular structure depolarized is the septum (Fig 1-11). Normally this structure is depolarized from left to right, producing a small initial R wave in leads V_1 and V_2 (Fig 1-11). This is followed immediately by the depolarization of the free walls of the ventricles. Since the left ventricle has by far the greater muscle mass, more current is generated on the left side. For this reason the main QRS vector points toward the left, producing a deep S wave in V_1 and V_2.

Midprecordial Leads

The P wave is generally upright. Depending on the position of the septum with reference to leads V_2 through V_4, a nearly equiphasic QRS complex may be seen in

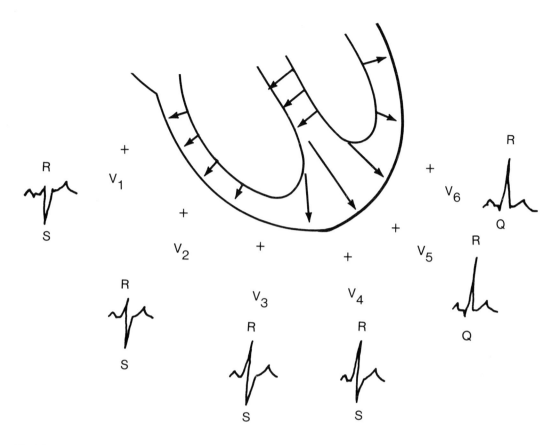

Fig 1-11.—Depolarization of ventricles as seen in precordial leads.

one of these leads, indicating transition from right to left ventricle. At other times transition may occur quite abruptly, with V_3 or V_4 predominantly positive.

Left Precordial Leads

The P wave is upright but may appear flat at times. Left to right septal depolarization is indicated in leads V_5 and V_6 by a very small "septal Q wave." Then the main QRS vector moving toward the left produces a tall R wave in V_5 and V_6, with the R in V_5 generally taller than that in V_6. The increasing height of the R wave from V_1 to V_5 is referred to as the normal R wave progression.

Age, body build, and disease processes may affect this progression of the R waves. The continuation of small R waves and the persistence of S waves to lead V_5 or V_6 is called clockwise rotation of the precordial leads. The appearance of tall R waves in V_2, with early disappearance of the S waves, on the other hand, is called counterclockwise rotation.

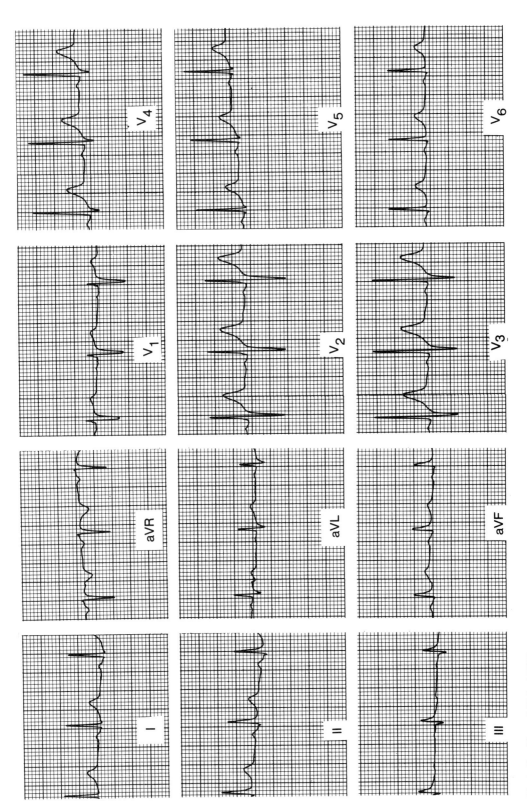

Fig 1-12.—Normal 12-lead ECG.

Additional Leads

Right Chest Leads

Leads may be placed over the right chest to discover abnormalities, especially when congenital defects are suspected. These leads, V_{3R} through V_{6R}, are shown in Figure 1-10. Their placement corresponds to that of V_3 to V_6.

Posterior Leads

Leads V_7 through V_9 may be placed to find abnormalities of the posterior wall of the left ventricle, such as posterior wall infarction. The placement of the electrodes is indicated in Figure 1-10. They are positioned in the fifth interspace in the posterior axillary, scapular, and paravertebral line.

MCl₁ Lead

Marriott[5] and others have demonstrated the usefulness of precordial leads, especially V_1, in determining the origin of premature beats, as well as other abnormalities. Unfortunately, most monitoring systems do not provide precordial leads. For this reason, an arrangement that closely resembles V_1 is frequently used in monitoring. This modified chest lead, MCl₁, is obtained by placing the negative electrode in the left subclavicular area and the positive electrode in the fourth interspace to the right of the sternum (Fig 1-13). The ground electrode is generally placed in the right subclavicular area.

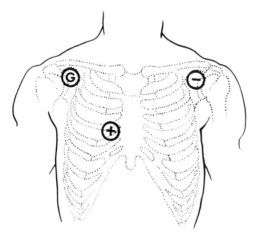

Fig 1-13.—Placement of electrodes for lead MCl₁ (from Marriott[6]).

Application

Once the few technical details discussed in this chapter have been mastered, one can actually visualize currents moving through the heart; determine their origin, magnitude, and direction; find where they are blocked; and discover the electrical "holes" where no current is moving—the necrotic tissues of infarcted areas.

REFERENCES

1. Friedman HH: *Diagnostic Electrocardiography and Vectorcardiography,* ed 2. New York: McGraw-Hill Book Co, 1977, p 362.

2. Bachman S, Sparrow D, Smith KL: Effect of aging on the electrocardiogram. *Am J Cardiol* 1981; 48:513.

3. Perloff JK, Roberts NK, Cabeen WR: Left axis deviation. *Circulation* 1979; 60:12.

4. Goldman MJ: *Principles of Clinical Electrocardiography,* ed 7. Los Altos, Calif, Lange Medical Publications, 1970. Reprinted by permission.

5. Marriott HJL, Fogg E: Constant monitoring for cardiac dysrhythmias and blocks. *Mod Concepts Cardiovasc Dis* 1979;6:103.

6. Marriott HJL: *Workshop in Electrocardiography.* Tarpon Springs, Fla, Tampa Tracings, 1972, p 18. Reprinted by permission.

## Chapter 2

The Electrophysiology of Cardiac Arrhythmias

Since the invention of the ECG, researchers have studied the origin and mechanisms of arrhythmias, and many theories have been advanced to account for abnormalities of cardiac rhythm. Some of these theories will be discussed in this chapter.

To understand the electrophysiological disturbances that may cause arrhythmias, a basic knowledge of the normal electrical activity of cardiac cells is necessary.

Normal Electrical Activity of Cardiac Cells

Non-Pacemaking Cells

Resting State and Depolarization

The cell membrane of the resting cardiac fiber is impermeable to sodium but permits the passage of potassium ions.[1] These tend to move from an area of high concentration (150 mEq) within the cell to an area of lower concentration (4 mEq) in the surrounding interstitium. The loss of positively charged ions causes the inside of the myocardial cell to become negative with respect to the outside of the cell. This electrical difference is known as the *transmembrane resting potential* (TRP); it usually measures about -90 mV. When such a cell is stimulated, its membrane becomes permeable to sodium, and positively charged sodium ions rush into the cell from the interstitium. This influx occurs because the concentration of sodium is much higher in the interstitium than within the cell, and electrolytes always strive to move from an area of high concentration to an area of lower concentration.

The influx of ions carrying a positive charge causes the inside of the cell to become electrically positive.[2] This sudden change in electrical charge is called depolarization and is reflected in the steep, rapid *phase 0* of the action potential (Fig 2-1). Depolarization of ventricular myocardium produces the QRS complex on the ECG.

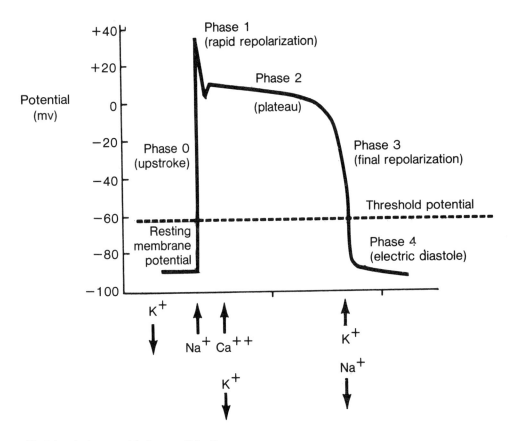

Fig 2-1.—Action potential of myocardial cell.

Repolarization

As soon as the inside of the cell has reached a potential of about +30 mV ("overshoot"), the fast sodium channels close, and sodium influx ceases abruptly. At the same time, the slow channels open and permit calcium ions to enter the cell. This inward movement of calcium is thought to continue throughout *phase 2*, the plateau phase.[3,4] Potassium ions leave the cell at the same time, so that the intracellular level of electricity remains relatively stable during phase 2. Repolarization occurs rapidly during *phase 3*, due to continued efflux of potassium ions. The repolarization of ventricular myocardium is represented by the T wave on the surface ECG.

The resting ionic balance must be restored to enable the cell to function again. This is accomplished by the sodium pump, which removes sodium from the interior of the cell and permits potassium to reenter. Energy in the form of adenosine triphosphate is required for this purpose, since the sodium must move to an area of higher concentration. This process takes place during *phase 4* of the action potential and during diastole of the ventricles.

The non-pacemaking cell requires an outside stimulus to raise the action potential to a level from which depolarization will continue spontaneously. This level is called the *threshold potential* (TP); it usually measures about −60 mV.

po
old
stronger

The *exc*
bring it to th
and TP is smal
therefore, more ex

The speed of phase
Reduced phase 0 velocity
strong to act as stimuli to a
fails. The rate of phase 0 depol
TRP. The lower (more negative)
rapid is the upstroke of phase 0.

This aspect of impulse conduction is
myocardial conductivity. An excess of ser
it less negative), the rate of phase 0 is decre
slowed.[2]

Refractoriness

During the various phases of repolarization, the respons
stimulation undergoes changes known as stages of refractorin
is totally incapable of responding to any stimulus; this is know
refractory period. During the next stage, the cell may respond
potential that is not of sufficient magnitude to stimulate neighboring
period, together with the absolute refractory period, is known as the
refractory period. It is followed by the *relative refractory period*, during wh
stronger-than-normal stimulus produces an action potential that is propagated
adjacent cells, or a stimulus of normal strength may be conducted with some
delay.

Figure 2-2 shows the various periods of refractoriness in relation to the T wave.
The danger of ventricular stimulation during the relative refractory period, the
"vulnerable" portion of the T wave, has frequently been discussed.[5] The "supernormal" period of conduction is a postulated phenomenon. Impulses falling into
this period tend to be conducted in a nearly normal manner in individuals who
usually show an intraventricular conduction defect.

Pacemaking Cells

Sinus Node

The action potential of the sinoatrial (SA) node differs from that of the ordinary
myocardial cells.[6(p15)]

- Resting potential is less negative.
- Phase 0 velocity is somewhat slower.
- Phase 2 has a steeper decline, and there is no distinct plateau.
- There is spontaneous depolarization during phase 4.

A stimulus that is not strong enough to cause the TRP to rise to threshold ...tential will not cause depolarization of the cell and is referred to as a subthresh- ...timulus. The greater the electrical difference between TRP and TP, the ...the stimulus must be to effect depolarization.[2] ...*itability* of a cell is related to the strength of the stimulus required to ...eshold potential. Thus, cells in which the difference between TRP ...do not require a strong stimulus for depolarization and are, ...citable than cells in which this difference is greater. ...0 depolarization has an important effect on conduction. ...results in action potentials that may not be sufficiently ...diacent cells, so conduction of impulses is slowed or ...arization is directly related to the magnitude of the ...the TRP is at the time of stimulation, the more ...llustrated by the effect of hyperkalemia on ...m potassium reduces the TRP (makes ...sed, and myocardial conduction is

...e of the cell to outside ...ss. Initially the cell ...as the *absolute* ...ith an action ...cells. This ...*ffective* ...ich a ...to

...polarization has been completed, sodium and possibly calcium ions[4] begin to flow back into the cell until the cell's threshold potential is reached and the cell depolarizes spontaneously.

It is this capacity for *spontaneous phase 4 depolarization* that gives the SA node its inherent automaticity, that is, its ability to produce impulses that are transmitted to the rest of the heart without requiring any outside stimulation (Fig 2-3).

The factors that affect the rate of automatic discharge are the level of the TRP, the level of the TP, and the rate or slope of spontaneous diastolic depolarization (SDD). For example, the rate is slowed by lowering the TRP, raising the TP, or decreasing the slope of SDD.

Other Pacemaking Cells

Subsidiary pacemaking cells are found in the atria, the atrioventricular (AV) junctional area, and the His-Purkinje system. They have the same inherent capacity for spontaneous phase 4 depolarization as the SA node. However, since the rate of depolarization of these cells is slower in descending order (Fig 2-4), they are normally depolarized by impulses coming from above, before they have a chance to reach threshold.

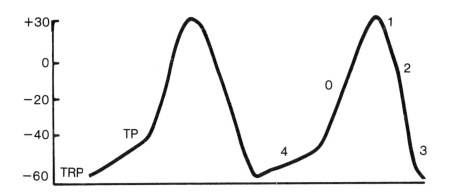

Fig 2-3.—Action potential of the sinoatrial node. TRP = transmembrane resting potential; and TP = threshold potential.

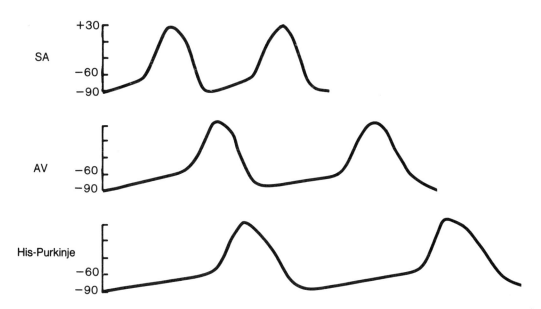

Fig 2-4.—Comparison of slope of spontaneous diastolic depolarization of sinoatrial (SA) node, atrioventricular (AV) junction, and His-Purkinje cells.

It is clear, therefore, that subsidiary (ectopic) pacemaking cells have the opportunity to depolarize spontaneously and produce impulses that will be propagated to the rest of the heart in two sets of circumstances:

1. When sinus impulses are delayed or blocked, a lower pacemaker has time to depolarize spontaneously and produce an escape beat.
2. When the rate of spontaneous diastolic depolarization of an ectopic pacemaking cell is enhanced, the cell depolarizes spontaneously before arrival of a sinus impulse and produces a premature beat or extrasystole. If the cell continues to depolarize at this enhanced rate, an ectopic tachycardia results.

Variations in the three components (TRP, TP, and slope of SDD) affecting spontaneous depolarization explain the origin of many arrhythmias and are also responsible for the effects of many drugs (Fig 2-5).

THREEFOLD EFFECT OF ACETYLCHOLINE

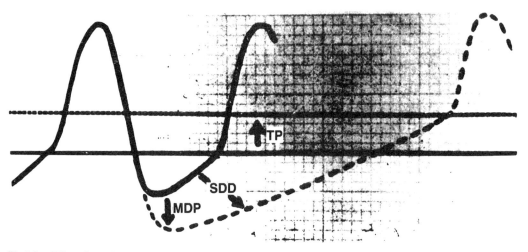

Fig 2-5.—Effect of acetylcholine on action potential. TP = threshold potential; SDD = spontaneous diastolic depolarization; MDP = maximal diastolic potential (from Marriott[7(p30)]).

Origin and Mechanisms of Arrhythmias

All arrhythmias are due to disturbances of impulse formation, impulse conduction, or a combination thereof.

Abnormalities of Impulse Formation

Abnormalities of impulse formation are either due to disturbances of the sinus rhythm or are caused by impulses produced by a focus other than the SA node, that is, by an ectopic focus.

Disturbances of Sinus Rhythm

Various physiological factors and pharmacological agents may affect the rate of discharge of the sinus node by altering the slope of spontaneous diastolic depolarization. Some of these are listed in Figure 2-6.

Ectopic Impulse Formation

Impulses arising from foci other than the SA node may be broadly divided into two groups: escape beats and extrasystoles.

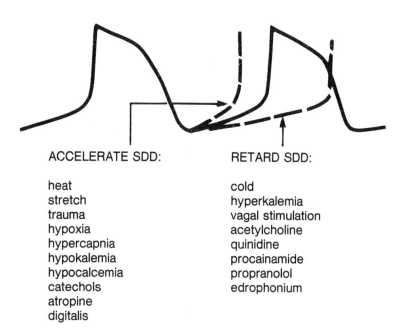

ACCELERATE SDD: RETARD SDD:

heat   cold
stretch   hyperkalemia
trauma   vagal stimulation
hypoxia   acetylcholine
hypercapnia   quinidine
hypokalemia   procainamide
hypocalcemia   propranolol
catechols   edrophonium
atropine
digitalis

Fig 2-6.—Factors affecting spontaneous diastolic depolarization (SDD) (from Marriott[7(p31)]).

Escape beats

When the formation or conduction of sinus impulses is delayed or blocked due to any cause, a subsidiary pacemaker is able to "escape" and produce an impulse that is conducted and depolarizes the myocardium (Fig 2-7). This escape mechanism is made possible by the inherent automaticity of cells in various portions of the conduction system.

Extrasystoles

Although any impulse that does not arise from the SA node may be classified as an extrasystole, the term is generally reserved for ectopic impulses that are produced early, that is, before the next sinus beat is due (Fig 2-8).

There are many theories to explain the origin of extrasystoles. The final answer has not been found, and it is likely that several mechanisms are responsible for the occurrence of premature ectopic impulses.

Enhanced automaticity of ectopic pacemaking cells.—The same factors that enhance spontaneous phase 4 depolarization of the SA node (Fig 2-6) may also be responsible for enhanced automaticity of ectopic foci. This seems to correlate with clinical findings, since we observe many ectopic beats in patients who are hypoxic or hypokalemic, as well as in digitalis toxicity and as a result of endogenous or exogenous catecholamines. On the other hand, drugs listed for use in decreasing SDD, such as quinidine and procainamide, are used to abolish extrasystoles.

Reentry.—Many authorities state that there must be a relationship between the preceding normal beat and the extrasystole when the extrasystole occurs with a constant coupling interval. A theory that would explain this apparent relationship is reentry.[8(p11)]

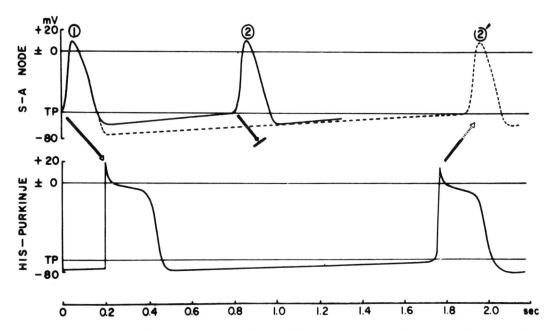

Fig 2-7.—Schematic representation of escape beat. SA = sinoatrial, TP = threshold potential. First sinus beat (1) is conducted to ventricles and depolarizes idioventricular pacemakers. Second sinus beat (2) is blocked; permitting slow, spontaneous depolarization of pacemaker in His-Purkinje system, which finally fires and depolarizes ventricles (2'). Reprinted by permission from Watanabe Y, Dreifus LS: Arrhythmias: Mechanisms and pathogenesis, in Dreifus LS, Watanabe Y (eds): *Cardiac Arrhythmias,* New York, Grune & Stratton, Inc. 1973, p 36.

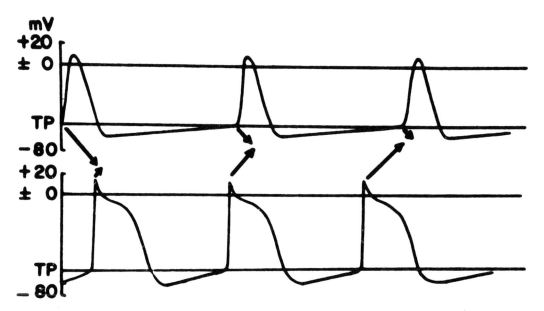

Fig 2-8.—Schematic representation of extrasystole. TP = threshold potential. First beat is sinus beat that depolarizes entire heart. Second beat originates in ventricle and is due to increased rate of SDD of pacemaking cell in His-Purkinje system. Reprinted by permission from Watanabe Y, Dreifus LS: Arrhythmias: Mechanisms and pathogenesis, in Dreifus LS, Watanabe Y (eds): *Cardiac Arrhythmias,* New York, Grune & Stratton, Inc, 1973, p 37.

Unidirectional block and reentry is believed to occur most commonly in the AV node (Fig 2-9), which is composed of numerous interconnected conducting pathways. Some of these are thought to be capable of conducting more rapidly than others. This makes it possible for an impulse to travel down a fast pathway, while others are still refractory. By the time an impulse has traveled down the fast pathway, it may find the previously blocked path open and return through it to its point of origin, to start all over again. In this manner, unidirectional block and reentry in the AV junction may give rise to reciprocating tachycardias.

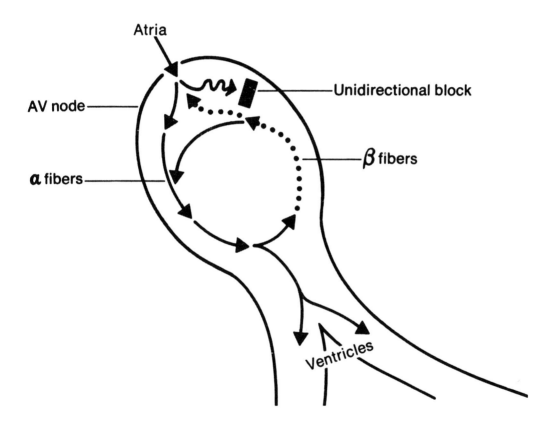

Fig 2-9.—Schematic illustration of atrioventricular (AV) node reentry (from Singh[8(p20)]).

Localized block and microreentry (Fig 2-10) are thought to be the cause of many coupled extrasystoles, ectopic tachycardia, and possibly, atrial and ventricular fibrillation.

Myocardial ischemia and infarction favor the appearance of reentry arrhythmias by causing nonuniform conduction of impulses. This mechanism can be illustrated in the epicardial border zone overlying a transmural infarct and may be responsible for the occurrence of ventricular arrhythmias several days after infarction.[9]

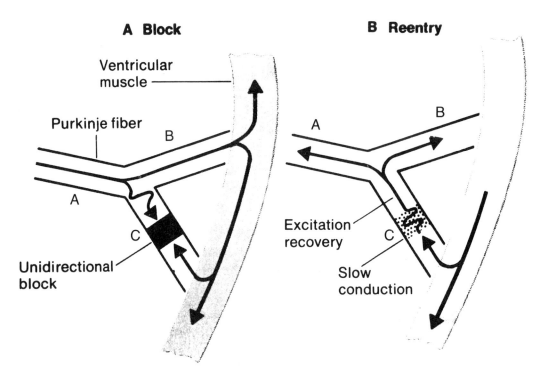

A Block

B Reentry

Ventricular muscle

Purkinje fiber

B

B

A

A

Excitation recovery

C

C

Unidirectional block

Slow conduction

Fig 2-10.—Schematic illustration of microreentry. Impulse on pathway A finds path B open, while C is still refractory. By the time impulse has traveled down B and spread throughout myocardium, pathway C is no longer blocked and conducts impulse back to point x. If timing is right, excitation can once again be conducted through B, producing a reciprocal or reentry beat (from Singh[8(p13)]).

The reentry mechanism can be clearly demonstrated by electrographic surface mapping, as shown in Figure 2-11. The ECG (top) shows the premature pacer impulse. The striped area of the subsequent ventricular complex reflects the first 80 ms of depolarization; the stippled area represents the next 40 ms. The premature beat is followed by a short run of ventricular tachycardia. The impulse is initially conducted around the area over the infarction (left panel). Then the wave front is propagated in retrograde over the affected area and reenters the normal myocardium (right panel), setting up a reentry ventricular tachycardia.

Wedensky effect and Wedensky facilitation.—These theories have been used to explain the constant coupling interval between normal beats and following ectopic beats.[6(p154)]

Wedensky postulated that an impulse of subthreshold strength could depolarize adjacent cells if the preceding impulse was strong. For example, if an ectopic focus is producing small action potentials that cannot affect neighboring cells, the occurrence of a strong stimulus, such as a sinus beat, might enable a subthreshold stimulus to depolarize adjacent cells and produce an extrasystole.

In Wedensky facilitation, a strong impulse exerts some effect on a blocked zone without actually entering and depolarizing the zone. If an ectopic focus is producing subthreshold stimuli within the blocked zone, the effect of the remote strong stimulus allows depolarization of the adjacent myocardium by the ectopic stimulus, producing an ectopic beat.

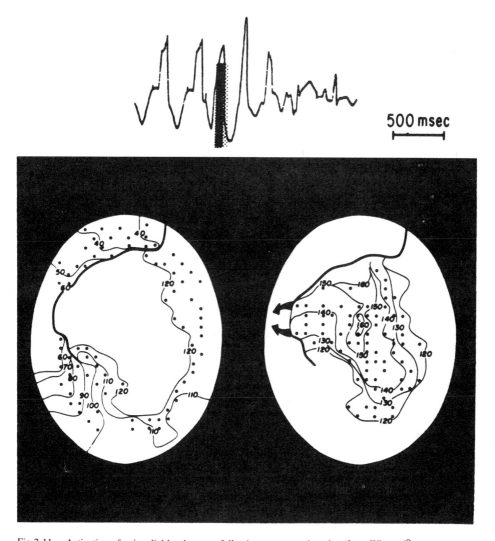

Fig 2-11.—Activation of epicardial border zone following premature impulse (from Wit et al[9]).

Both of these hypotheses are interesting but difficult to prove in a living individual, although they can be demonstrated in laboratory preparations.

Slow rates and the rule of bigeminy.—Slow rates frequently give rise to premature ventricular contractions (PVCs). For example, PVCs frequently occur in healthy individuals at rest and disappear when the heart rate is increased by exercise.

According to the rule of bigeminy, once a ventricular extrasystole occurs, the subsequent prolongation of the R-R interval caused by the compensatory pause favors the occurrence of further PVCs, resulting in bigeminy.

This phenomenon may be due to the theory of temporal dispersion of recovery, as stated by Moe (Marriott[7(p38)]), who discovered that, with slower rates, the state of repolarization in adjacent cells is not uniform (Fig 2-12). Rapid rates, on the other hand, cause neighboring fibers to repolarize at more nearly the same rate.

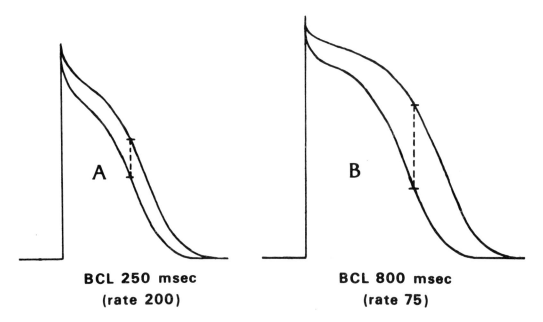

Fig 2-12.—Schematic illustration of changes in dispersion of recovery with change in rate. Repolarization of adjacent fibers is similar when rate is rapid (A) but becomes uneven at slow rates (B) (from Marriott[7(p38)]).

Such uneven recovery may facilitate reentry, or the difference in electrical potential of two neighboring cells may be sufficient to produce an electrical impulse that is propagated.

The administration of digitalis is said to favor uneven recovery; this may be one of the causes of the ventricular extrasystoles seen in digitalis toxicity.

Abnormalities of Impulse Conduction

Refractoriness

The action potential, and with it, refractoriness, becomes progressively prolonged from atrial cells, to junctional tissues, to cells in the His-Purkinje system. It is therefore entirely possible for a stimulus to arrive from above and find conducting fibers still in a refractory state. This will cause either a delay or failure of conduction. For example, a premature supraventricular impulse may arrive in the common bundle of His and find the right bundle branch still refractory; the impulse is then conducted with a right bundle branch block pattern. This accounts for the frequent aberrant conduction of supraventricular premature beats (chap. 5).

Decremental Conduction

An impulse may be propagated from cell to cell with decreasing effectiveness due to a progressive decrease in the magnitude of action potentials. Finally, an action potential may be too weak to stimulate the next cell, and propagation of the impulse ceases.

The AV node is considered to be more susceptible to such decremental conduction than other portions of the conduction system. Decremental conduction is enhanced in the AV junctional area by acetylcholine, cardiac glycosides (digitalis), and ischemia. Decremental conduction may cause concealed conduction.

Concealed Conduction

When an impulse partially penetrates a structure such as the AV junction, it may cause partial depolarization and subsequent refractoriness that prevents depolarization of the structure by the next impulse that arrives. Since evidence of such partial depolarization is not visible on the surface ECG, it is called concealed conduction. For example, a premature impulse from an ectopic atrial focus may penetrate and depolarize the SA node as well as the rest of the atrium. This depolarization of the SA node generally does not produce a visible sinus P wave, but it does produce a pause that occurs because the SA node must repolarize before it can produce the next impulse.

It is believed that the totally irregular ventricular response to atrial fibrillation is due to the concealed conduction of many atrial impulses into the AV node.

Exit Block

At times an impulse is produced but is prevented from stimulating adjacent fibers, due to a surrounding condition that prevents the exit of the stimulus. An example of this problem is sinus block, in which sinus impulses are produced at a regular rate but occasionally fail to be propagated to the atria. This may be due to increased vagal tone, or occasionally, to the administration of digitalis, quinidine, or potassium salts. It has also been attributed to inflammatory and degenerative processes and acute ischemia surrounding the area of the SA node.

Blocks in General

Propagation of impulses through any portion of the conduction system may be slowed or blocked entirely by a variety of well-known factors, including administration of certain drugs, ischemia, inflammation, necrosis, or degenerative disease of conducting fibers (chap. 4).

Combination of Abnormal Impulse Formation and Conduction

Disturbances of impulse formation and conduction often coexist and give rise to various types of arrhythmias. It is important to determine whether more than one abnormality is present and to be aware that one disturbance may be caused by another. The simplest example of this condition is probably the escape beat.

The inexperienced individual observing the ECG in Figure 2-13 might notice only the grossly abnormal QRS complex and might be tempted to attack it with lidocaine. The more knowledgeable practitioner would immediately recognize that this beat represents a ventricular escape, since it is preceded by a long pause, due to the nonconducted premature atrial contraction (PAC). It is likely that this PAC caused concealed conduction into the SA node, since the sinus cycle has been interrupted.

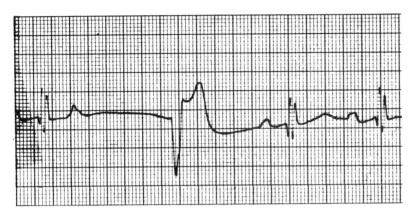

Fig 2-13.—Ventricular escape beat.

Parasystole

Parasystole is a combination of abnormal impulse formation and conduction. The term parasystole implies that two independent rhythms, coming from two different foci, are depolarizing the ventricles. Most commonly, one pacemaker is the SA node, while another is in the Purkinje system, although other foci are possible. The ectopic rhythm is generally thought to be due to enhanced automaticity of an ectopic pacemaking cell.

What is the conduction defect? Some investigators believe that the ectopic focus is protected by an entrance block, since it is not depolarized, and thereby prevented from depolarizing spontaneously, by impulses coming from the SA node. In addition, many authorities feel that the rate of discharge of the ectopic focus may be very rapid at times and that there is an exit block preventing the majority of ectopic impulses from stimulating neighboring cells, since the rate of the ectopic rhythm in parasystole is usually quite slow.

AV Dissociation

The term AV dissociation is sometimes used as a synonym for complete heart block. Obviously, AV dissociation occurs in complete heart block with an idioventricular pacemaker, but it also usually occurs in ventricular tachycardia.

Chung[10] lists 23 causes of AV dissociation; therefore, this term alone cannot be used to describe an arrhythmia; other features must also be described, eg, AV dissociation due to complete heart block.

Specifically, the term AV dissociation implies any rhythm in which the atria and the ventricles are depolarized by different pacemakers, each of which has its own independent rate and rhythm. This situation also requires a block or barrier that prevents the faster pacemaker from depolarizing the domain of the slower one. In complete heart block, an antegrade conduction barrier prevents the sinus impulses from reaching the ventricles, which are depolarized by the slower junctional or ventricular pacemaker. In ventricular tachycardia there is frequently a retrograde block that prevents the rapidly occurring ventricular impulses from penetrating the atria, which may continue to be activated at a slower rate by the sinus node.

Supraventricular Tachycardias With AV Block

Fortunately, the AV node exercises its physiological function of protecting the ventricles in cases of atrial fibrillation and flutter, since ventricular rates of 300 to 600 beats/min would certainly not be well tolerated. Due to its inherent refractoriness, the AV node blocks many of these excess impulses.

To emphasize the physiological role of this type of block, it is best to describe the resulting rhythm in terms of atrial rate and ventricular response. For example, atrial tachycardia with 2:1 conduction is not the same as 2:1 AV block. Inexact nomenclature can lead to misunderstandings and should be avoided.

REFERENCES

1. *Calcium in Cardiac Metabolism*. Whippany, NJ, Knoll Pharmaceutical Co, 1981.

2. Fish C: Electrophysiologic basis of arrhythmias. *Heart Lung* 1974;3:51.

3. Bailey JC: The electrophysiologic basis for cardiac electrical activity: Normal and abnormal. *Heart Lung* 1981;10:455.

4. Hummelgard AB, Esrig BC: Calcium and calcium slow channel blockers: An overview. *Crit Care Quart* 1981;4:17.

5. Fiol M, Ibañez J, DeLuna RR, et al: Significance of the prematurity index and sinus rate in warning arrhythmias of ventricular fibrillation. *Crit Care Med* 1981;9:229.

6. Schamroth L: *The Disorders of Cardiac Rhythm*. Oxford, England, Blackwell Scientific Publications, 1971.

7. Marriott HJL: *Workshop in Electrocardiography*. Tarpon Springs, Fla, Tampa Tracings, 1972. Reprinted by permission.

8. Singh BN: The genesis of arrhythmias, in *Cornell Postgraduate Course on Cardiac Arrhythmias*. New York, Medcom, Inc; 1979. Reprinted by permission.

9. Wit AL, Allessie MA, Fenoglio JJ, et al: Significance of the endocardial and epicardial border zones in the genesis of myocardial infarction arrhythmias, in Harrison DC (ed): *Cardiac Arrhythmias, A Decade of Progress*. Boston, GK Hall Medical Publishers, 1981, p 58. Reprinted by permission.

10. Chung EK: Diagnosis and clinical significance of atrioventricular (AV) dissociation, in Sandoe E, Jensen EF, Olesen KH (eds): *Cardiac Arrhythmias*. Södertälje, Sweden, AB Astra, 1970, p 172.

## Chapter 3

ECG Analysis of Cardiac Arrhythmias

I am assuming that readers of this book have considerable experience in identifying cardiac arrhythmias. For this reason I shall barely mention the more commonly seen arrhythmias, and concentrate instead upon some of the more complex and unusual rhythm disturbances.

Disturbances of Sinus Rhythm

Sinus Tachycardia

The rate limits for sinus tachycardia are generally set somewhat arbitrarily at 100 to 150 beats/min, but exceptions are frequently seen. For example, a sinus rate of 120 beats/min is normal in the infant, and the healthy young adult has sinus rates of 180 beats/min and more with vigorous exercise.

The tracing in Figure 3-1a shows a P wave that is not normal, compared to the tracing from the same patient in normal sinus rhythm (Fig 3-1b). The arrhythmia is atrial tachycardia, although the rate is unusually slow for this dysrhythmia. The shape and axis of the P wave, as well as the P-R interval, must be considered in determining the origin of supraventricular tachycardias.

Sinus Bradycardia

Sinus bradycardia may be normal in young, athletic individuals, may be caused by the administration of a great variety of drugs, or may be due to cardiac as well as extracardiac pathology. It may permit the escape of ectopic pacemakers.

Escape-Capture Bigeminy

Disturbances that cause slowing of the sinus rate may give rise to escape-capture bigeminy. In many instances the precise mechanism of slowing of the sinus node cannot be identified.

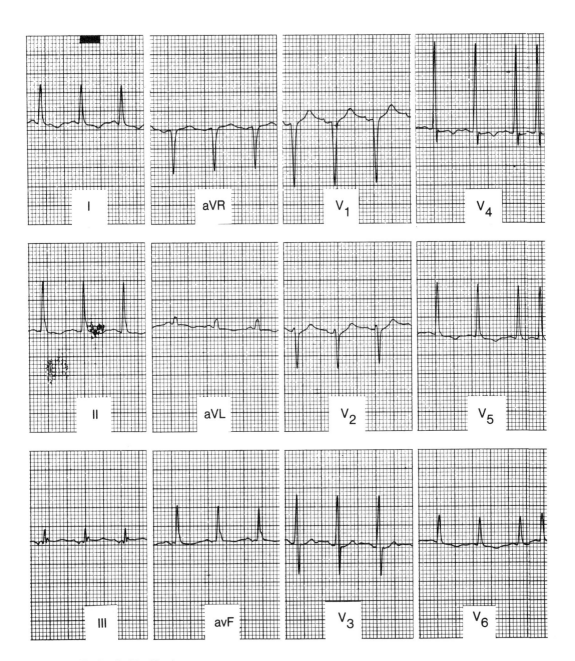

Fig 3-1a.—Tracing for identification.

ECG characteristics

- alternating sinus and ectopic beats
- sinus beat following ectopic beat
- R-R interval between ectopic beat and following sinus beat shorter than R-R interval from sinus beat to following ectopic beat

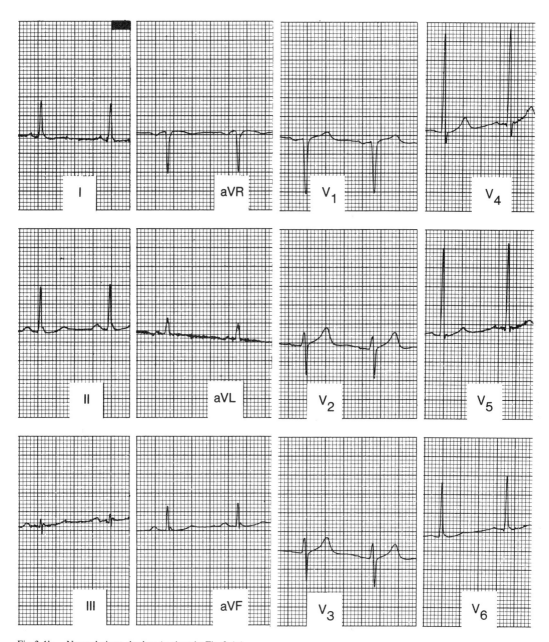

Fig 3-1b.—Normal sinus rhythm (patient in Fig 3-1a).

Cause

- mechanism often unidentified

Figure 3-2 shows junctional escape beats followed by sinus beats. The junctional to sinus R-R interval is 800 ms, while the sinus to junctional beat R-R interval is 1,060 ms. From this tracing it is not clear whether the slow sinus rate is due to an extreme sinus bradycardia or a sinus rhythm with 2:1 exit block.

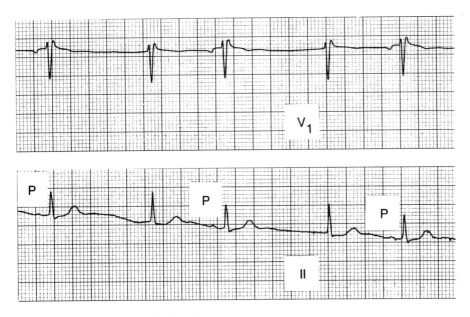

Fig 3-2.—Escape-capture bigeminy. P = P wave.

Sinus Arrhythmia

The most common form of sinus arrhythmia is the "respiratory" arrhythmia, in which the rate increases with inhalation and decreases with exhalation. This rhythm is normal in infants and children and may also be seen in healthy adults.

Cause

- may be caused by factors that increase vagal tone, such as administration of morphine, digitalis, or neostigmine (Prostigmin)

At times the R-R interval in the slow phase may be sufficiently prolonged to permit the appearance of escape beats, which may be atrial, junctional, or ventricular in origin. The arrhythmia becomes more complicated when waxing and waning vagal influences also affect the rate of AV conduction. Figure 3-3 shows an unusual and exaggerated example of this mechanism.

Sinus Premature Beats

Sinus premature beats are thought to arise in the sinus node, although not necessarily in the same pacemaking cell or focus that is providing the regular sinus rhythm.[1(p30)]

ECG characteristics

- premature P wave identical to normal sinus P waves in all leads
- constant coupling interval followed by incomplete compensatory pause

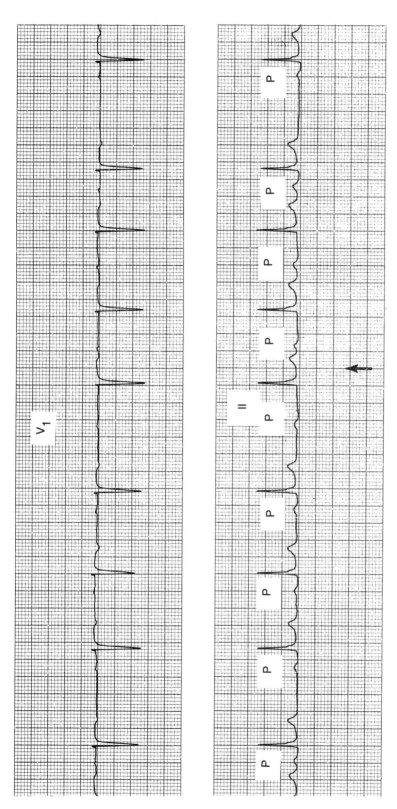

Fig 3-3.—Vagotonia affecting sinus rate and atrioventricular conduction. P = P wave.

There is one premature beat in the tracing in Figure 3-4. The P wave configuration is identical to that of the regular sinus P waves in the three simultaneous leads shown, so this early beat probably represents a sinus premature beat, which is rare and difficult to distinguish from an atrial premature beat.

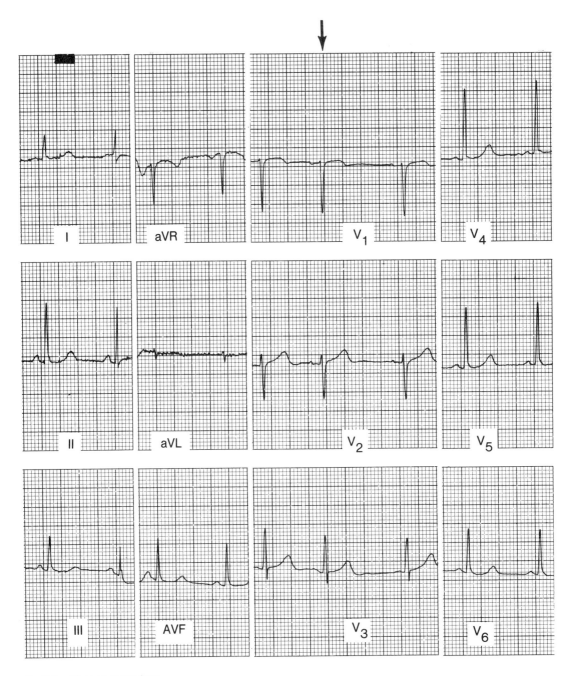

Fig 3-4.—Sinus premature beat.

Sinus Arrest

In sinus arrest (sinus pause), the sinus node fails to fire for one or more beats. The resulting standstill is generally relieved by return of the sinus mechanism or the appearance of an escape rhythm.

ECG characteristics

- regular sinus rhythm interrupted by a pause of variable length
- pause bears no mathematical relationship to previous P-P intervals
- resumption of sinus activity or occurrence of escape rhythm

Causes

- vagal influences
- digitalis toxicity
- carotid sinus syncope

Figure 3-5 shows a regular sinus rhythm at the rate of 70 beats/min, interrupted by a pause. The pause measuring 1,240 ms bears no mathematical relationship to the regular P-P interval of 840 ms.

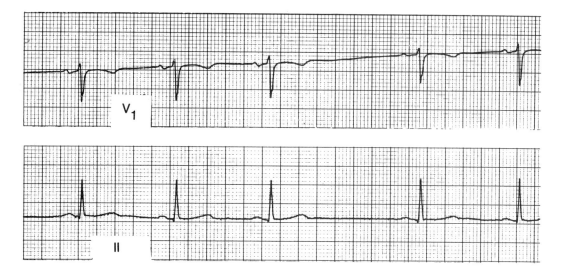

Fig 3-5.—Sinus pause.

Carotid Sinus Syncope

Carotid sinus syncope is a rare problem. In the cardioinhibitory type, the sinus rate slows or ceases entirely when the carotid sinus is stimulated. In patients with this disorder, such everyday actions as sudden head motion, wearing a tight collar, or shaving in the neck area may precipitate cardiac standstill.[2]

Causes

- hyperirritability of carotid sinus
- neoplasm or inflammatory masses in neck

Figure 3-6, an unusual tracing, shows a sinus arrest lasting 9 seconds as a result of carotid sinus pressure. Note that no escape mechanism appears until carotid sinus pressure is released.

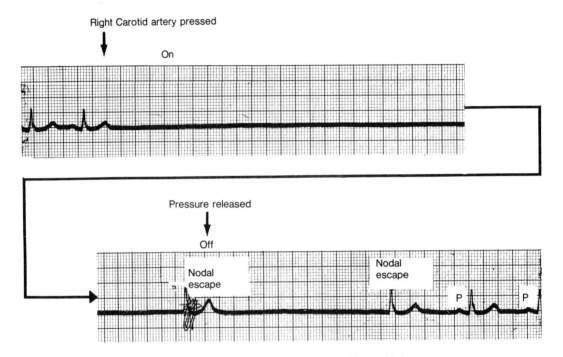

Fig 3-6.—Cardiac standstill due to carotid sinus pressure (arrow) in patient with carotid sinus syncope.

Other Pauses

Not all pauses that interrupt sinus rhythm are due to sinus arrest. The tracing in Figure 3-7 shows one of the most common causes of such pauses. Careful inspection of the tracing reveals very premature, nonconducted P′ waves superimposed on the T wave preceding the pause.

ECG characteristics

- premature, ectopic wave
- pause in sinus rhythm

Cause

- premature, nonconducted, ectopic P waves

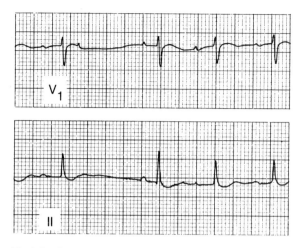

Fig 3-7.—Tracing for identification.

Sick Sinus Syndrome

Sick sinus syndrome (Fig 3-8) is also called tachybradyarrhythmia. At times this term is more accurate, since the tachycardia associated with this syndrome does not always arise from the sinus node.[3,4]

ECG characteristics

- supraventricular tachycardia followed by pronounced sinus bradycardia or periods of sinus arrest
- escape beats may occur during slow phase
- discrepancy between rapid and slow phases much more marked than in sinus arrhythmia

Causes

- disease or ischemia of SA node
- sinus arrest following tachycardia may be due to overdrive-suppression of sinus pacemaker

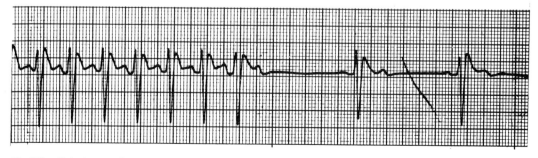

Fig 3-8.—Sick sinus syndrome.

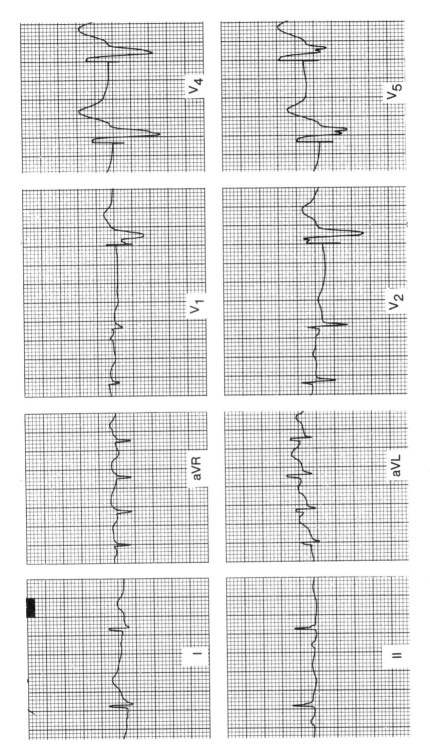

Fig 3-9.—Sick sinus syndrome with ventricular-inhibited pacing.

In Figure 3-9, sinus rhythm at a rate of 72 beats/min is followed by a burst of supraventricular tachycardia at a rate of 150 beats/min. Then there is a sudden cessation of supraventricular impulses. Ventricular depolarization is provided by mechanical pacing at a rate of 70 beats/min. In persistent sick sinus syndrome, mechanical pacing, together with antiarrhythmic therapy, usually constitutes the treatment of choice.

Atrial Arrhythmias

Atrial Escape Rhythm

Atrial escape beats may occur whenever the sinus rate drops below the spontaneous depolarization rate of an atrial pacemaking cell. Such beats may occur occasionally if there is intermittent slowing of the sinus rate, or they may appear as an idioatrial rhythm (Fig 3-10) at a rate of about 50 beats/min. If the sinus rate is irregular, escapes from various atrial as well as junctional foci may be seen. This may produce a "wandering atrial pacemaker" (Fig 3-11).

ECG characteristics of idioatrial rhythm

- P′ waves differ from sinus P waves
- Atrial beats occur later in cycle or at any rate slower than preceding sinus rhythm

In Figure 3-10, the early beats are of sinus origin, since they exhibit an upright P wave in lead II. The beats occurring at a rate of about 75 beats/min represent an idioatrial mechanism.

ECG characteristics of wandering atrial pacemaker

- P′ waves of various configurations
- P-P intervals usually slightly irregular, with P-P′ and P′-P′ intervals somewhat longer than sinus P-P intervals

Cause

- slowing of sinus rhythm due to any cause

The precise location of the atrial pacemaker is difficult to determine from the surface ECG, and at times it is impossible to distinguish between atrial and junctional escapes. This fact is really of no particular importance, since the clinical significance of the arrhythmia depends on the cause of slowing of the sinus rhythm, rather than the precise location of the escape pacemaker.

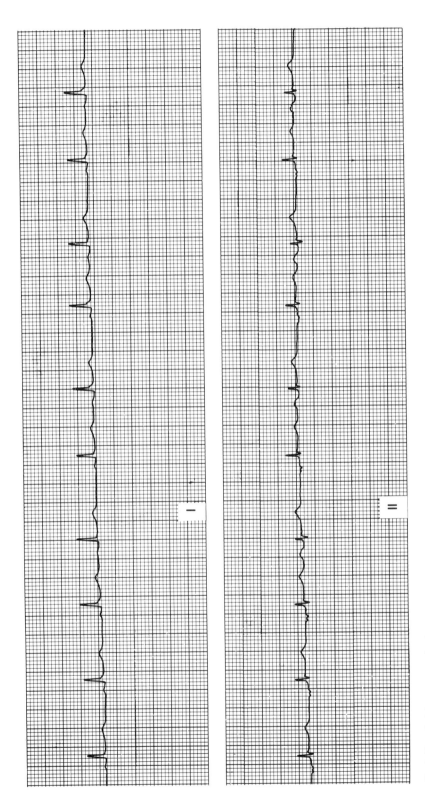

Fig 3-10.—Atrial escape mechanism.

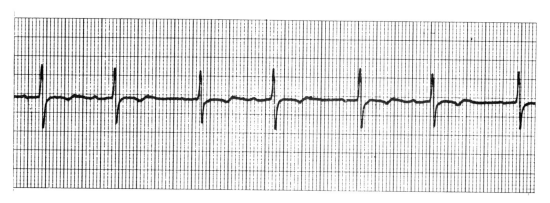

Fig 3-11.—Wandering atrial pacemaker.

Atrial Extrasystole

An atrial extrasystole (PAC) is produced by premature atrial depolarization due either to enhanced automaticity of an atrial pacemaker or to a reentry phenomenon. Premature atrial depolarization may be followed by ventricular depolarization. PACs may occur singly, in a bigeminal pattern, or in salvoes.

ECG characteristics

- P' wave with different shape from normal sinus P wave
- ventricular depolarization may be normal, slow, blocked, or aberrant (chap 5)
- premature P' wave with P-P' interval shorter than patient's usual P-P interval
- coupling interval usually constant
- compensatory pause generally incomplete

The following series of tracings (Figures 3-12a through c) shows various patterns of PACs obtained within a period of 20 minutes from a 2-year-old boy recovering from halothane (Fluothane) anesthesia. The child had been previously healthy and made an excellent recovery. The ECG is normal for the age, with the exception of the arrhythmias shown. Fluothane is known to increase myocardial sensitivity to endogenous and exogenous catecholamines, and arrhythmias are frequently seen during induction and anesthesia.[5]

The tracing in Figure 3-12a might be interpreted as ventricular bigeminy. Careful inspection, however, reveals that each of the wide, early QRS complexes is preceded by a premature, abnormally shaped P' wave (chap 5).

There are triplets in Figure 3-12b. The first beat in each set is a sinus beat with normal ventricular conduction. The P wave of the second beat is early and slightly different and is followed by a slightly different QRS complex. The third P' wave is even earlier, and both the P' wave and the QRS complex are abnormal. This tracing represents atrial trigeminy.

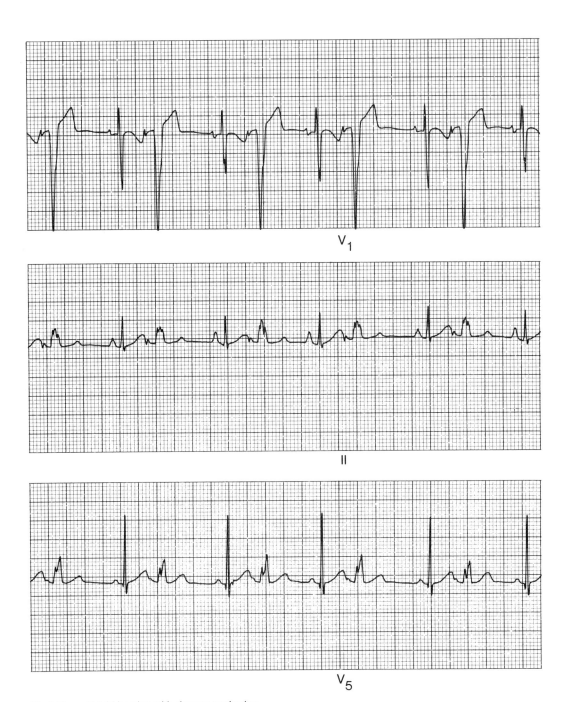

Fig 3-12a.—Atrial bigeminy with aberrant conduction.

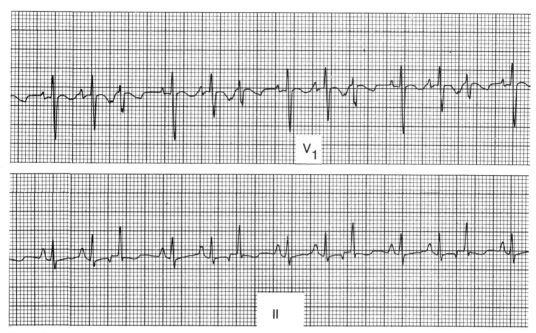

Fig 3-12b.—Atrial trigeminy with aberrant conduction.

In Figure 3-12c, the premature P′ wave arrives so early in the cycle that it cannot be conducted to the ventricles, so the ventricular rate drops to 60 beats/min. Again, the tracing must be examined carefully to see the P′ waves superimposed on the T waves.

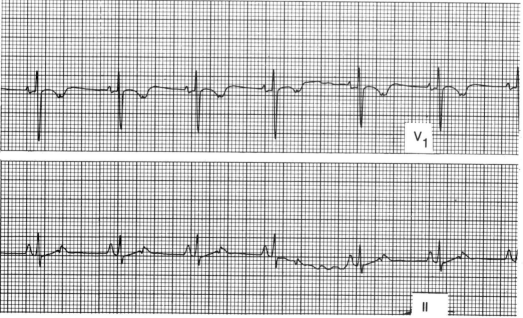

Fig 3-12c.—Atrial bigeminy with 2:1 ventricular conduction.

Location of Ectopic Atrial Foci

Attempts have been made to determine the approximate location of ectopic atrial foci by the morphology of the P' waves. Terms such as coronary sinus rhythm, low atrial rhythm, and left atrial rhythm have been used to describe the probable origin of atrial beats, and criteria have been developed to assist in their identification.

ECG characteristics of left atrial impulses[1(p38)]

- negative P' wave in lead V_6
- dominantly positive and sharply pointed P' in V_1 or "dome and dart" deflection in V_1
- negative P' in standard leads II, III, and aVF

In Figure 3-13, the beats marked with an arrow show the criteria for left atrial beats.

Figure 3-14 shows a P' wave that is inverted in leads II, III, and aVF, indicating its ectopic atrial origin. The normal P-R interval of 0.13 second indicates that the origin is not junctional, since nodal beats generally show a shorter P-R interval.

Many authorities agree that such precise localization of ectopic supraventricular pacemakers cannot be accomplished with a surface ECG. At times it is nearly impossible to distinguish between atrial and junctional premature beats.[6]

Causes of PACs

- may occur in healthy individuals
- may be enhanced by social drugs such as coffee, nicotine, amphetamines, and marijuana
- may be due to drugs such as catecholamines or anesthetic agents
- may be associated with disease of heart or lungs or with hyperthyroidism

Atrial Echoes

Atrial echoes represent premature atrial depolarization due to an impulse that reenters that atrium from the AV junction after having been propagated through the ventricles. They may be the precipitant factor in reentrant supraventricular tachycardias. Atrial echoes are rare and difficult to distinguish from blocked PACs.

ECG characteristics

- P-R interval of preceding beat is prolonged
- P' wave that follows closely on QRS complex
- P' wave that shows different configuration from normal P wave
- P' wave that may not be conducted to ventricles

Causes

- delayed AV conduction
- pathways with different conduction velocities within AV node

Figure 3-15 shows normal sinus rhythm with frequent nonconducted PACs. Where the sinus P-R interval is 0.20 second or more, the QRS is immediately followed by an abnormally shaped P′ wave. In several instances the atrial mechanism continues for several beats in a manner resembling atrial flutter. When this apparent flutter mechanism is seen, conduction to the ventricles occurs after each third P′ wave with a prolonged P-R interval.

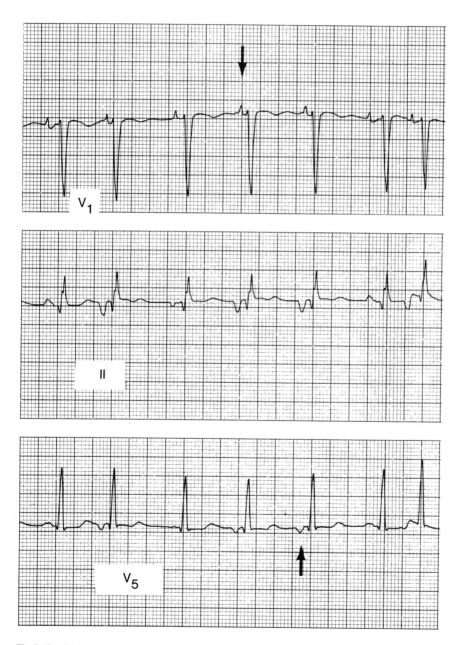

Fig 3-13.—Multifocal PACs (simultaneous leads V_1, II, and V_5). Left atrial beats (arrows).

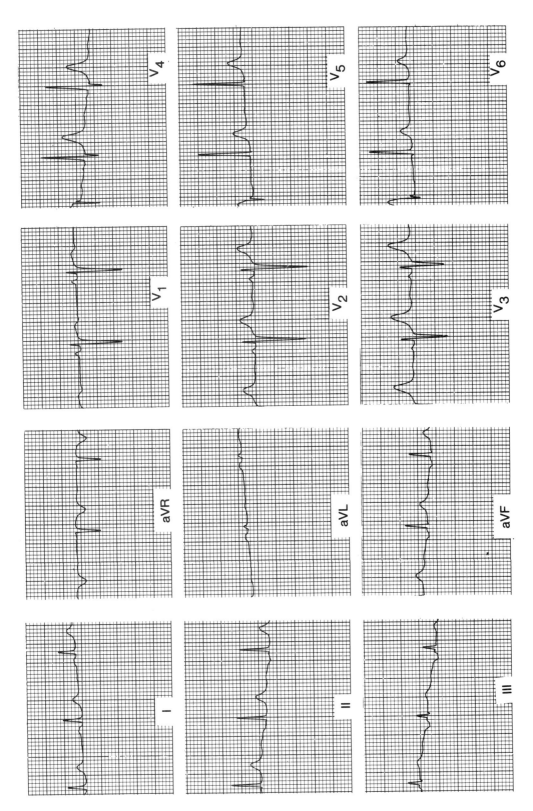

Fig 3-14.—Low atrial beats.

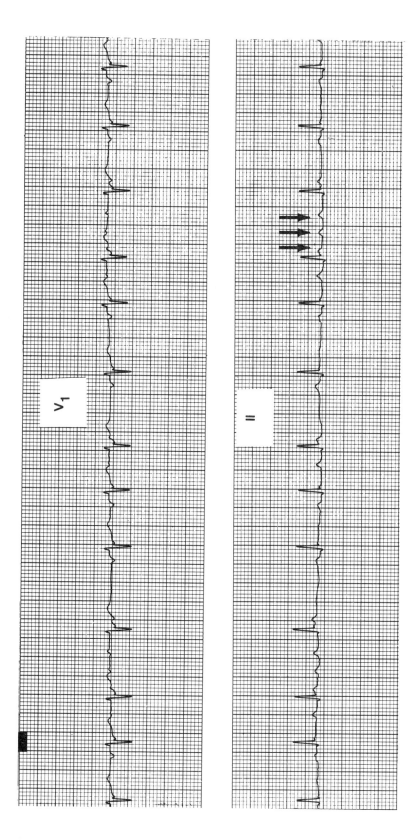

Fig 3-15.—Atrial echoes.

Atrial Parasystole

In atrial parasystole, two independent rhythms coexist and depolarize the atria and ventricles; one has its origin in the sinus node and the other in an ectopic atrial focus. The ectopic focus is protected by an entrance block against depolarization by the sinus impulses.[7]

ECG characteristics

- abnormal P′ wave
- irregular coupling interval to preceding sinus beat
- all interectopic intervals bear precise mathematical relationship to shortest interectopic interval

Causes

- may appear in patients with normal hearts
- may be related to heart disease and/or digitalis therapy

At first glance, Figure 3-16 seems to demonstrate atrial bigeminy. Closer examination reveals that the coupling intervals between sinus and ectopic beats vary from 460 to 660 ms. Measurement of the distance between the premature beats shows a constant interectopic interval of 1,460 ms.

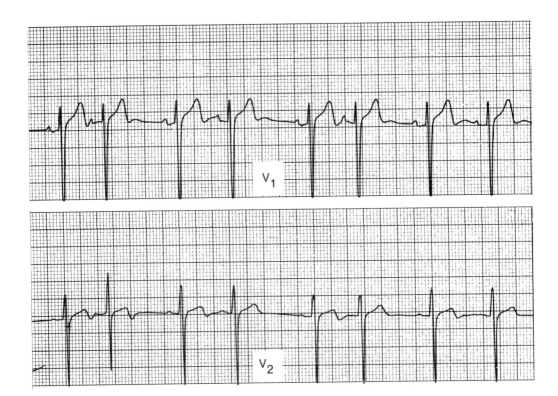

Fig 3-16.—Atrial parasystole.

Atrial Tachycardia

Atrial tachycardia is generally due to the very rapid spontaneous depolarization of an ectopic atrial pacemaker or to reentry. Usually, atrial and ventricular rates ranging from 160 to 220 beats/min are seen. There are two forms of atrial tachycardia that deserve special attention: atrial tachycardia with block and multi-focal atrial tachycardia.

Atrial Tachycardia with Block

A rapid ectopic atrial rhythm is conducted to the ventricles with varying degrees of block. This block is generally of the 2:1 type but may also show Wenckebach periods.

ECG characteristics

- rapid atrial rate, generally greater than 200 beats/min
- abnormal configuration of P′ waves
- ventricular response shows 2:1 or Wenckebach conduction

Cause

- digitalis toxicity

Since this arrhythmia is frequently related to digitalis toxicity, particular care must be taken to identify it. For example, cursory inspection of leads I to aVF in Figure 3-17 may lead to an interpretation of sinus tachycardia. Close scrutiny of the tracing, especially lead V_1, indicates that the "bump" on the T wave is another P′ wave.

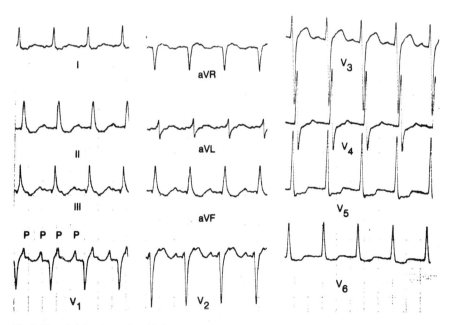

Fig 3-17.—Atrial tachycardia with 2:1 conduction. P = P wave.

This tracing points out the importance of looking at several leads, especially V_1, whenever the rhythm is in doubt.

The top tracing in Figure 3-18 shows an irregular supraventricular tachycardia in which P waves cannot be seen. At first glance this rhythm might be identified as atrial fibrillation, but closer inspection shows the grouped QRS complexes that suggest Wenckebach conduction. The bottom tracing in Figure 3-18 (lead V_1 in the same patient) shows atrial tachycardia with Wenckebach conduction.

This again points out the importance of not making the first diagnosis that comes to mind. Take a second look, and if possible, inspect several leads before you reach a conclusion.

In the presence of very rapid atrial rates the 2° block represents the normal protective physiological function of the AV node. Second-degree block at normal atrial rates, on the other hand, is generally due to pathology of the AV node or the lower conduction system. Atrial tachycardia with 2:1 block is, therefore, not the same thing as 2° AV block. It is probably better to speak of atrial tachycardia with 2:1 conduction, to avoid misunderstandings.

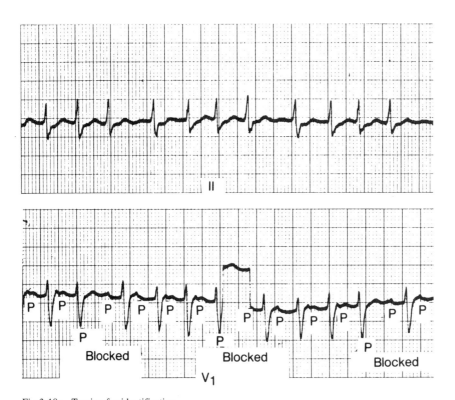

Fig 3-18.—Tracing for identification.

Multifocal Atrial Tachycardia

When several atrial foci initiate impulses that depolarize the atria at short intervals, an arrhythmia known as multifocal or chaotic atrial tachycardia is produced.[8]

ECG characteristics

- at least three differently shaped P′ waves
- at least three different P-R intervals
- overall rate above 100 beats/min
- frequent nonconducted PACs
- very irregular rhythm

Causes

- most frequently, chronic obstructive lung disease and cor pulmonale
- other causes mentioned for PACs

In Figure 3-19, at least three different types of P′ waves, three different P-R intervals, and several blocked PACs can be identified. The overall rate is 160 beats/min.

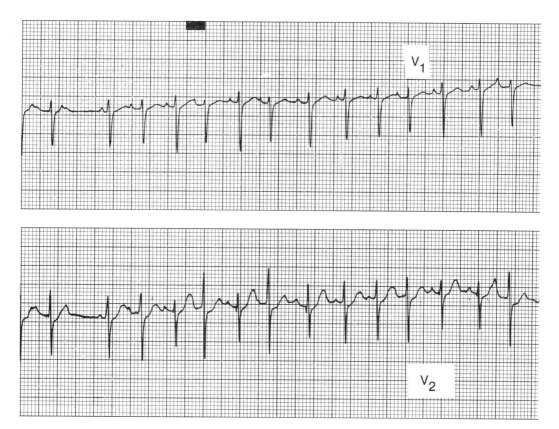

Fig 3-19.—Multifocal atrial tachycardia.

When the rate of discharge of the atrial ectopic foci becomes very rapid and irregular, the arrhythmia closely resembles atrial fibrillation (Fig 3-20, precordial leads). Multifocal atrial tachycardia is often the forerunner of atrial fibrillation.

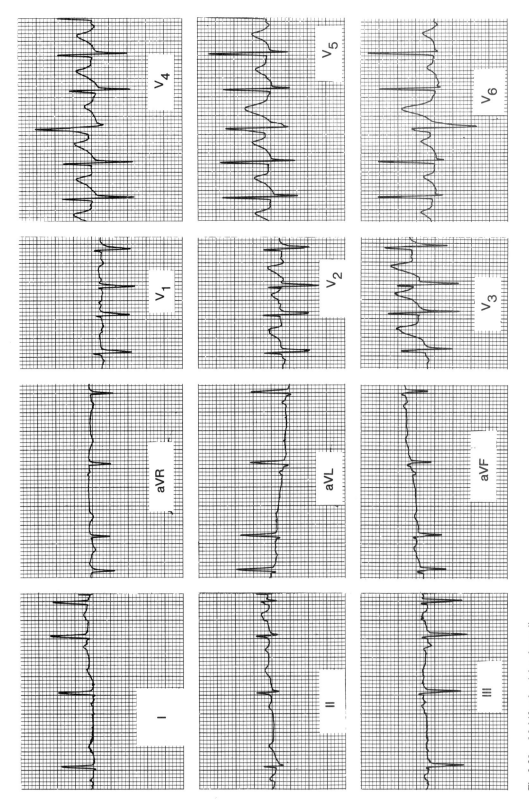

Fig 3-20.—Multifocal atrial tachycardia.

Atrial Flutter

The causes and appearance of atrial flutter, a common arrhythmia, are familiar to all nurses who have attended a basic ECG course. A few words of caution should be included concerning 2:1 flutter, however, since this arrhythmia is too often missed; its presence should be suspected whenever the ventricular rate is 150 beats/min.

ECG characteristics

- atrial rate about 300 beats/min
- abnormal P′ waves produce sawtooth pattern
- ventricular response usually regular and 2:1, 3:1, or 4:1

Causes

- congestive heart failure
- pulmonary disease
- thyroid toxicosis
- arteriosclerotic or rheumatic heart disease

The top tracing in Figure 3-21 could easily be mistaken for sinus tachycardia at a rate of 140 beats/min. When the sweep is changed to 50 mm/s, the bump on the S-T segment becomes more apparent, and measurements can be made to confirm that this represents a second P′ wave superimposed on the T wave. Sometimes a look at previous tracings is helpful. The bottom strip in Figure 3-21 had been obtained from the same patient on the preceding day and clearly shows flutter waves.

Vagal stimulation through the Valsalva maneuver or carotid sinus pressure is frequently helpful in identifying the underlying flutter, since it results in a decrease in AV conductivity and causes 2:1 flutter to become 4:1 flutter (Fig 3-22).

As the tracings in Figures 3-23 and 3-24 show, vagal maneuvers must be initiated with a certain amount of forethought, since they are not without danger. The patient must be monitored, and emergency equipment must be readily available.

In Figure 3-23, carotid sinus pressure greatly facilitated the identification of the atrial flutter mechanism, but at the same time it inhibited conduction to the ventricles for 6 seconds.

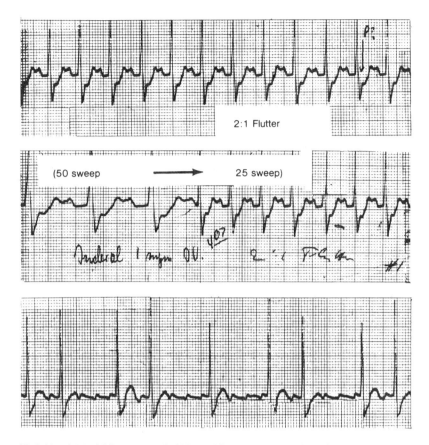

Fig 3-21.—2:1 Atrial flutter (top and middle) and flutter waves shown in tracing taken on preceding day (bottom). P = P wave.

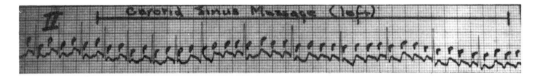

Fig 3-22.—2:1 Flutter changed to 4:1 flutter by carotid sinus pressure.

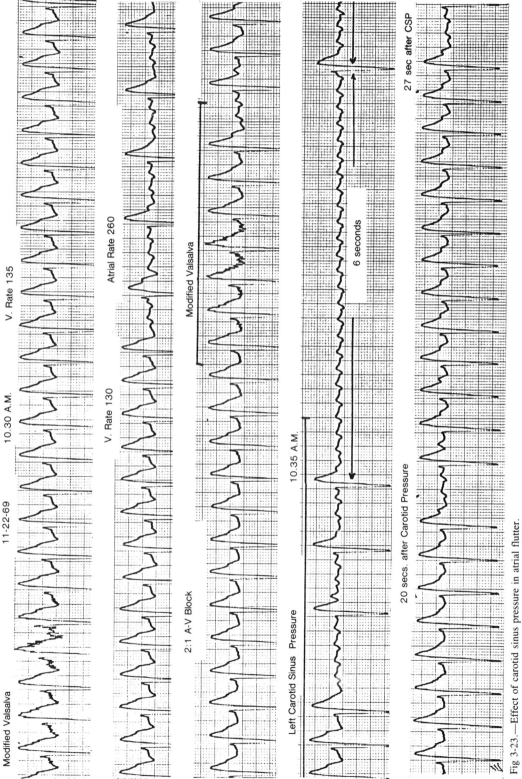

Fig 3-23.—Effect of carotid sinus pressure in atrial flutter.

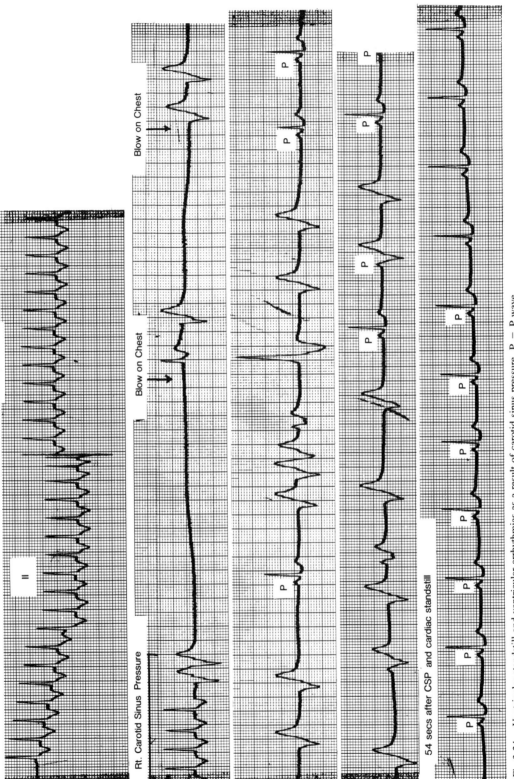

Fig 3-24.—Ventricular standstill and ventricular arrhythmias as a result of carotid sinus pressure. P = P wave.

The consecutive tracings shown in Figure 3-24 represent an even more alarming result of carotid sinus pressure, which had been applied in an attempt to terminate paroxysmal atrial tachycardia. The effort was successful; after 54 seconds the patient had normal sinus rhythm. To those who were present, those 54 seconds seemed awfully long.

The application of carotid sinus pressure is not generally considered a nursing procedure. The patient is usually asked to take a deep breath, hold it, and bear down (a Valsalva maneuver). However, even this "harmless" procedure may have occasional unpleasant consequences. It is not unusual to see transient slowing of sinus rhythm or the appearance of ventricular extrasystole whenever a very rapid supraventricular rhythm is suddenly terminated. No intervention is generally required, since the sinus rhythm usually "settles down," as shown in Figure 3-25.

Atrial Fibrillation

The reader is no doubt thoroughly familiar with atrial fibrillation, which is characterized by fine, irregular f waves and an "irregularly irregular" ventricular response. When the ventricular response to atrial fibrillation becomes totally regular, complete AV block is present, and the pacemaker for the ventricles is either a junctional or ventricular focus.

ECG characteristics

- fine, irregular f waves
- a regular, usually slow, ventricular rhythm
- ventricular complexes may be either normal or wide

Causes

- frequently due to digitalis toxicity
- disease of AV node or lower conduction system
- administration of verapamil

In Figure 3-26a the fine, irregular f waves of atrial fibrillation can be seen. The wide QRS complexes and slow ventricular rate suggest the presence of an idioventricular rhythm.

Figure 3-26b shows results of isoproterenol, given to the patient as an emergency measure. The resulting ventricular tachycardia demonstrates the effectiveness of this drug in enhancing the automaticity of the idioventricular pacemaker. The arrhythmia in this 96-year-old woman was corrected by mechanical pacing.

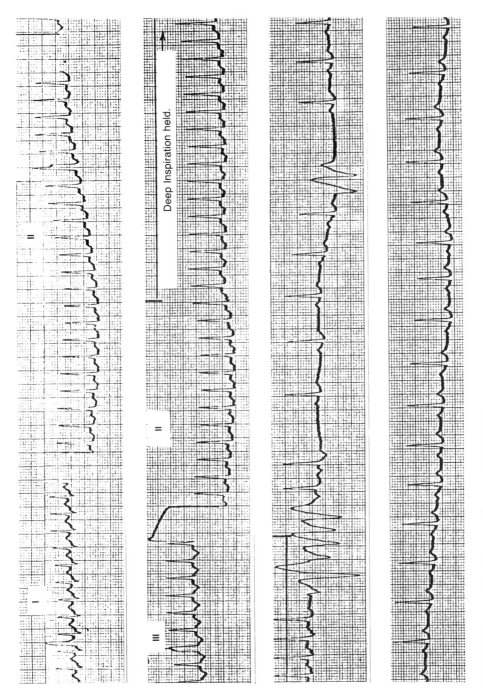

Fig 3-25.—Paroxysmal atrial tachycardia converted by Valsalva maneuver.

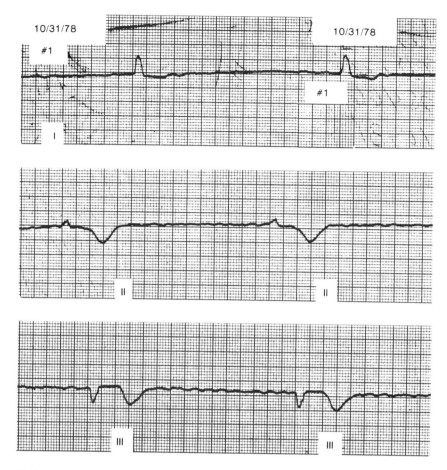

Fig 3-26a.—Atrial fibrillation with complete atrioventricular block and an idioventricular rhythm at a rate of 20 beats/min (consecutive tracing, leads I to III).

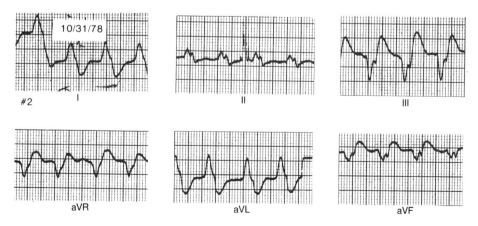

Fig 3-26b.—Ventricular tachycardia.

Junctional Rhythms

Strictly speaking, the term nodal rhythms is probably not correct, since pace-making cells are apparently not located within the AV node. The previously used terms high nodal, midnodal, and low nodal probably do not correspond to actual anatomical locations, but they will be used where they may be of help in identifying a rhythm.

Junctional beats that show an inverted P′ wave before the QRS may be difficult to distinguish from the left atrial or low atrial beats. The only differentiating factor may be the P-R interval, which is generally less than 0.12 second in high nodal beats. The configuration of the P′ wave may also be similar to that described for coronary sinus or coronary nodal rhythm by some authors.

There is no general agreement on criteria for the identification of these beats. Fortunately, knowledge of the precise location of such ectopic pacemakers is not essential for the appropriate care of the patient.

Idionodal Rhythm

An inherent junctional pacemaker fires at a rate of 40 to 60 beats/min, providing a mechanism for ventricular depolarization when the arrival of sinus impulses is slowed or prevented for some reason. This rhythm is not necessarily a sign of disease and is frequently encountered in healthy athletes at rest.

ECG characteristics

- P′ waves are negative and preceding QRS, with short P-R interval; negative and behind QRS; or not seen
- generally normal QRS complexes may differ slightly from those seen with sinus beats
- junctional rhythm corresponds to rate of 40 to 60 beats/min

There are only two sinus beats in the tracing in Figure 3-27; the dominant rhythm consists of normal QRS complexes that occur at a rate of 48 beats/min. No P waves can be identified.

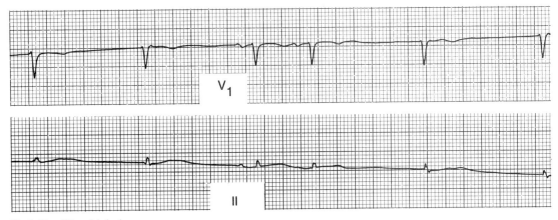

Fig 3-27.—Idionodal rhythm.

Accelerated Idionodal Rhythm

Since the inherent rate of junctional pacemakers is usually about 40 to 60 beats/min, nodal rhythms with rates ranging from 70 to 90 beats/min are generally referred to as accelerated idionodal rhythms. This may occasionally be seen when the nodal rhythm represents an escape mechanism but may also be a form of nonparoxysmal nodal tachycardia.[9]

The tracing shown in Figure 3-28 was obtained from a 4-year-old boy. It shows an accelerated idionodal rhythm that varies with respirations in the same manner as is usually observed in sinus arrhythmia in children. The youngster is the brother of the patient with Wolff-Parkinson-White syndrome in Figure 6-12.

Junctional escape rhythms may be fairly rapid, especially in young persons. This is shown in the tracing in Figure 3-29, which was obtained from a woman in her 20s and shows sinus tachycardia alternating with an accelerated idionodal rhythm.

Nonparoxysmal Nodal Tachycardia

ECG characteristic

- junctional rhythm with rates ranging from 70 to 150 beats/min (idionodal tachycardia)

Cause

- disease such as rheumatic carditis, acute inferior wall infarction, and digitalis toxicity

Junctional Extrasystole

In junctional extrasystole, the occasional premature discharge of a junctional pacemaker produces an early beat with the characteristics previously described.

Causes

- may occur in normal individuals
- may be associated with heart disease

Junctional Parasystole

Similar to atrial and ventricular pacemaking cells, a junctional focus may be protected against impulses coming from the dominant pacemaker. It may, therefore, spontaneously discharge at regular intervals and depolarize the ventricles; this is junctional parasystole.

The tracing in Figure 3-30 shows frequent premature junctional beats and demonstrates some of the characteristics of parasystole. A longer tracing would be necessary to prove or disprove the presence of a junctional parasystole.

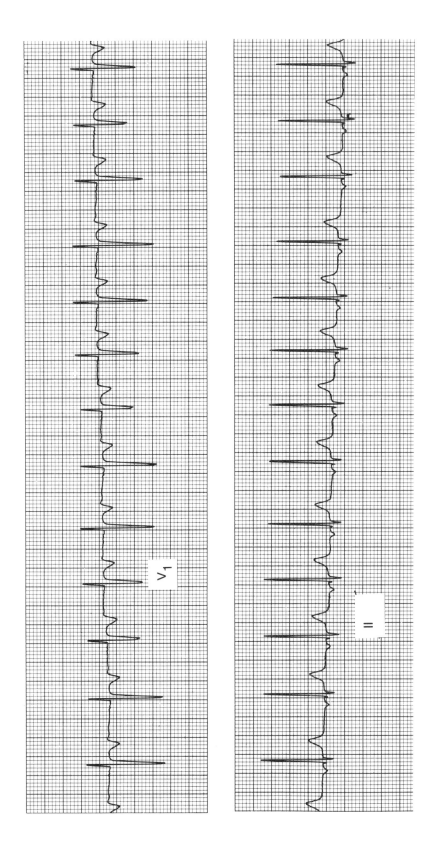

Fig 3-28.—Accelerated idionodal rhythm.

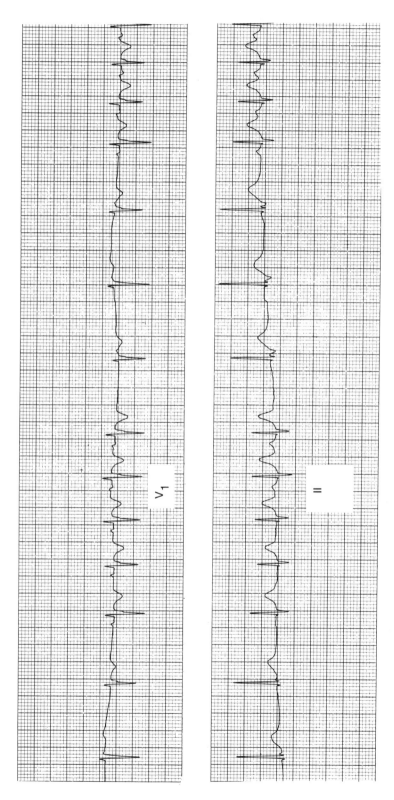

Fig 3-29.—Sinus tachycardia alternating with accelerated idionodal rhythm.

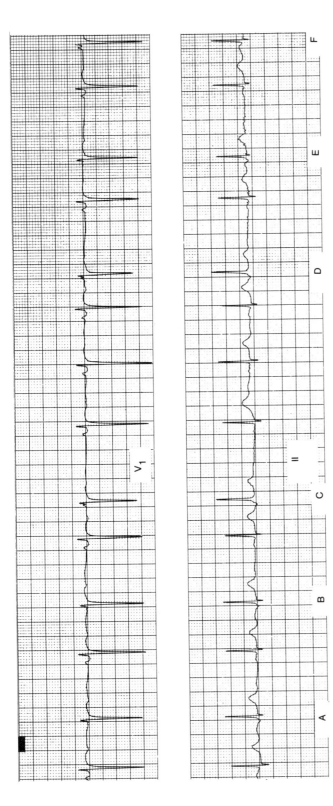

Fig 3-30.—Junctional parasystole. Coupling intervals are variable and interectopic intervals appear to have mathematical relationship. Distance from A to B is 1,600 ms; from C to D measures double, that is 3,200 ms; from E to F is again 1,600 ms. Only interval that does not fit pattern is from B to C.

Junctional Tachycardia

To distinguish junctional tachycardia from nonparoxysmal or idionodal tachycardia, it is often called paroxysmal or extrasystolic junctional tachycardia.

ECG characteristics

- 150 to 200 beats/min
- onset and cessation usually abrupt

Causes

- similar to those of paroxysmal atrial tachycardia
- dysrhythmia may be due to a reciprocating (reentry) mechanism

Consecutive tracings (Fig 3-31a through f) show first a slowing of the rate from 140 beats/min in Figure 3-31a to 105 beats/min in Figure 3-31d, as a result of administration of propranolol (Inderal). In Figure 3-31f, a lengthening of the R-P interval becomes noticeable as retrograde conduction to the atria is slowed. Carotid sinus pressure applied at this point is successful in restoring sinus rhythm.

Isorhythmic AV Dissociation

In isorhythmic AV dissociation, the sinus node initiates atrial depolarization, while the ventricles are depolarized by impulses coming from the AV junctional area at a slightly faster rate. For this dissociation to occur, retrograde conduction from the junction to the atria must be blocked. Without such a block, retrograde impulses from the junction would prevent at least some of the sinus impulses from depolarizing the atria.

In Figure 3-32, the sinus rhythm is regular but very slow, with a cycle length of 1,440 ms and a rate of about 43 beats/min. The ventricular rate is minimally faster at 44 beats/min and a cycle length of about 1,400 ms. There is no fixed relationship between the P waves and the QRS complexes.

Isorhythmic AV Dissociation with Interference

In isorhythmic AV dissociation with interference, which is uncommon, the coexisting sinus and junctional rhythms tend to disrupt or influence each other, as an occasional sinus impulse "sneaks through" and "captures" the ventricles.

A ladder diagram is used to illustrate the rather complex rhythm shown in Figure 3-33. The continuation of the rhythm can be understood by following the diagram. This tracing not only shows a fine example of interference dissociation but also demonstrates the utility of ladder diagrams in interpreting and explaining complicated arrhythmias.

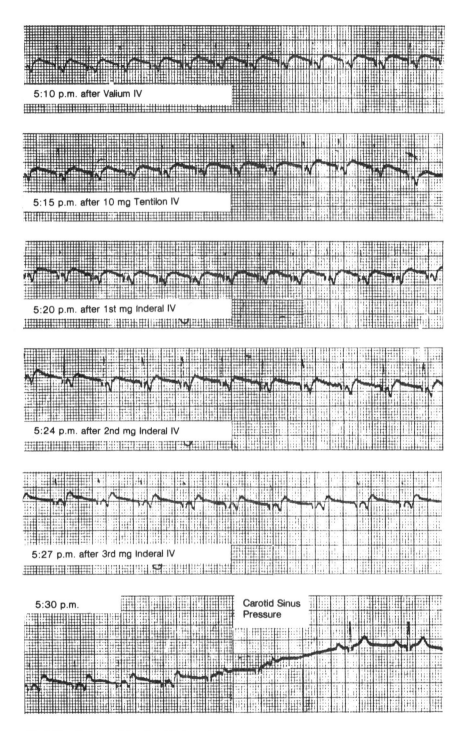

5:10 p.m. after Valium IV

5:15 p.m. after 10 mg Tentilon IV

5:20 p.m. after 1st mg Inderal IV

5:24 p.m. after 2nd mg Inderal IV

5:27 p.m. after 3rd mg Inderal IV

5:30 p.m.

Carotid Sinus Pressure

Fig 3-31.—Paroxysmal junctional tachycardia.

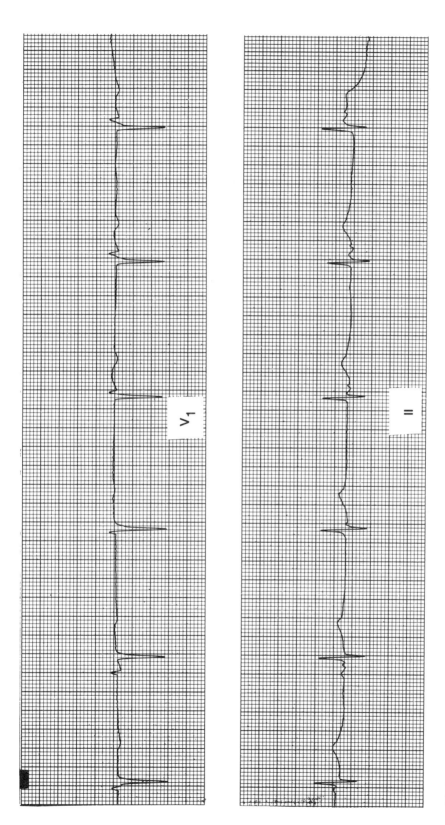

Fig 3-32.—Isorhythmic atrioventricular dissociation.

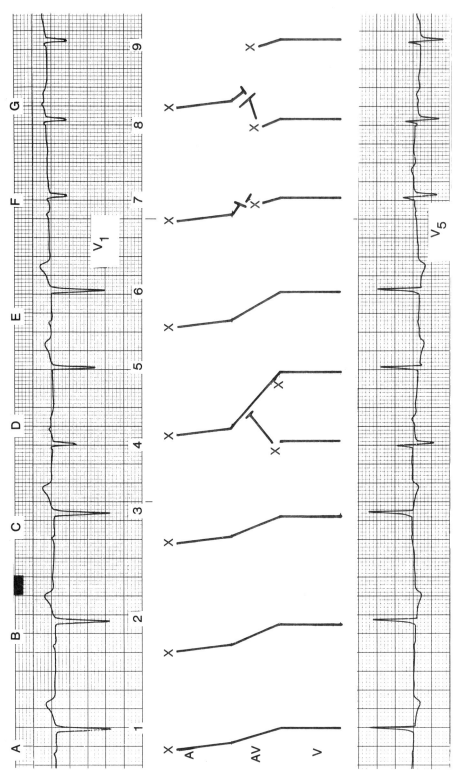

Fig 3-33.—Isorhythmic atrioventricular dissociation with interference. QRS complexes are numbered; P waves are identified by letters. Ventricular complexes 1 to 3 originate in sinus node and are conducted with prolonged P-R interval. QRS 4, which is narrow but somewhat different from previous QRS complexes, originates in junctional area. Atrial depolarization by a sinus impulse (D) prevents junctional beat from penetrating to atria. At the same time, partial depolarization of the atrioventricular (AV) node by junctional beat (4) causes prolongation of P-R interval preceding QRS 5. Thus, the two pacemakers interfere with each other. QRS 5 probably represents a fusion beat produced by both sinus and junctional pacemaker.

Here is one more case of isorhythmic AV dissociation (Fig 3-34). During the first six beats the sinus rate is 110 beats/min, while the ventricular rate is 118 beats/min. This produces an ECG peculiarity often associated with this arrhythmia, reverse Wenckebach phenomenon, as the P-R intervals become shorter and shorter. This is merely an interesting phenomenon, since there is no relationship between the atrial and ventricular rhythms.

The seventh beat is a premature ventricular contraction that disrupts the rhythm and allows the sinus pacemaker to take over.

Isorhythmic AV dissociation is a relatively rare arrhythmia that is usually due to digitalis toxicity.

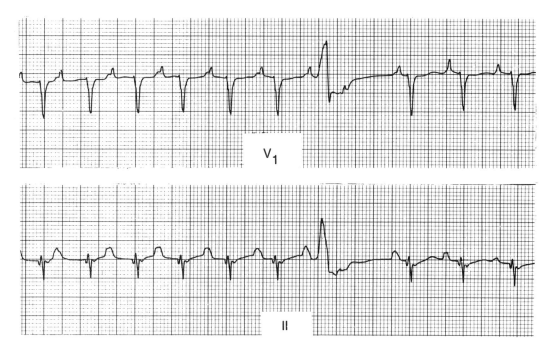

Fig 3-34.—Isorhythmic atrioventricular dissociation changing to normal sinus rhythm.

Ventricular Arrhythmias

Idioventricular Rhythm

ECG characteristic

- wide, bizarre QRS complexes occurring regularly at a rate of about 30 beats/min

Idioventricular rhythm may be seen when supraventricular impulses are greatly slowed or are prevented from reaching the ventricles. This rhythm is produced through the inherent automaticity of a pacemaking cell in the His-Purkinje system.

The idioventricular rhythm in Figure 3-35 was recorded in a young man dying from the results of an automobile accident. Usually you will see idioventricular rhythms in cases of 3° (complete) heart block (Fig. 3-36).

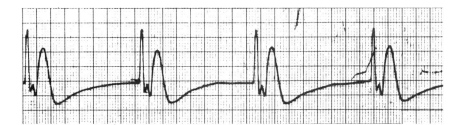

Fig 3-35.—Idioventricular rhythm.

Figure 3-36 shows that idioventricular pacemakers often tend to be unstable, especially in patients with acute infarction. In these patients, mechanical pacing is the only safe method of increasing the heart rate.

Accelerated Idioventricular Rhythm

Idioventricular rhythm at rates ranging from 60 to 90 beats/min are frequently seen in patients with acute myocardial infarction.[10]

The term slow ventricular tachycardia should be assiduously avoided when describing this rhythm, since such terminology tends to bring out the "lidocaine reflex." Idioventricular rhythm is an escape mechanism due to slowing of the sinus rate. For example, in Figure 3-37 there is alternating sinus and idioventricular rhythm. The latter sets in whenever the sinus rate slows. The distance between the sinus beats and the following ventricular escape beats is clearly greater than the R-R interval of the sinus beats.

In true ventricular tachycardia, the first ventricular ectopic complex is always premature.[11] To describe ventricular tachycardia with a slower than usual ventricular rate (about 100 to 120 beats/min), it is probably better just to mention the ventricular rate, to avoid the paradox of calling it a "slow-fast."

Ventricular Extrasystole

Efforts have recently been made to achieve more precise nomenclature of beats that are caused by premature depolarization of ventricular ectopic foci. It has been stated that the term premature ventricular contraction is incorrect, since the ECG complex reflects electrical rather than muscular activity.[12] The same can, however, be said for the term ventricular premature beat, which has been suggested by some. It is hoped that a heart beat will follow ventricular depolarization, but again, the term implies muscular activity. More recently the term premature ventricular depolarization has come into use. I shall continue to use premature ventricular contraction since this term is familiar to all.

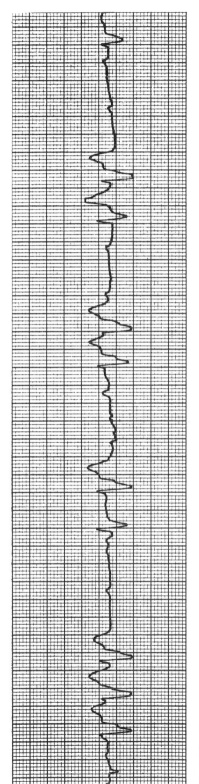

Fig 3-36.—Complete heart block with idioventricular rhythm.

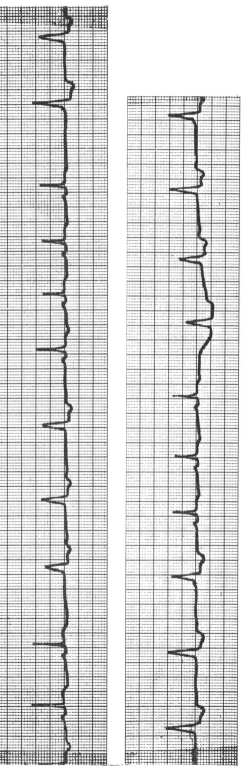

Fig 3-37.—Consecutive tracing showing alternating normal sinus rhythm and accelerated idioventricular rhythm.

A PVC, as the name implies, must be premature in the cycle. Wide, bizarre-looking beats that occur after the regular sinus interval has passed are escape beats. In addition, for practical purposes, beats that are initiated by ventricular foci are abnormal in configuration and width (greater than or equal to 0.12 second). Some authors have, indeed, described narrow PVCs arising from the bundle branch system; however, such beats are very difficult to distinguish from junctional beats on the surface ECG. We shall return to their consideration during the discussion of hemiblocks.

Location of Ventricular Ectopic Foci

At times it may be useful to discover whether a PVC originates from the left or right ventricle. This is especially true if there is reason to suspect that PVCs may be due to a misplaced Swan-Ganz catheter or pacing electrode. In many instances, this determination can be made easily, providing there are PVCs in lead V_1 and/or V_6.

When a PVC originates in the right ventricle, the main depolarizing wave front moves from right to left, that is, away from V_1 and toward V_6. Therefore, V_1 shows a negative complex, while the PVC is positive in V_6 (Fig 3-38). When the ectopic focus is located in the left ventricle, the current will move mainly from left to right, producing a positive QRS in V_1 and a negative ventricular complex in V_5 and V_6.

Ventricular Bigeminy

The occurrence of a prolonged R-R interval favors the occurrence of ventricular extrasystole, and the compensatory pause following a PVC facilitates the onset of a bigeminal rhythm. This arrhythmia is not necessarily a sign of disease. For example, Figure 3-39 shows ventricular bigeminy recorded from a healthy young man at rest. The sinus rate becomes so slow that the supraventricular rhythm is provided primarily by a junctional pacemaker. This dysrhythmia is simply due to the vagotonia of youth and disappears when the sinus rate is increased by exercise. More frequently, however, ventricular bigeminy is caused by digitalis toxicity or cardiac pathology.

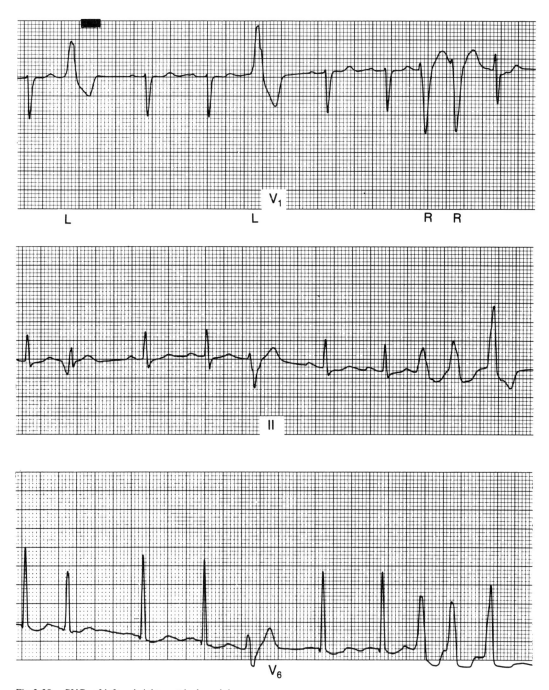

Fig 3-38.—PVCs of left and right ventricular origin.

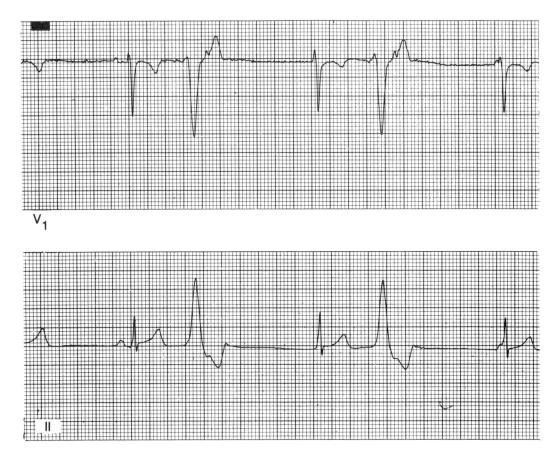

Fig 3-39.—Ventricular bigeminy.

Ventricular Parasystole

The characteristics of ventricular parasystole are those previously discussed for other parasystolic rhythms.

Figure 3-40 shows an example of ventricular parasystole that demonstrates a possible reason for the intermittent appearance of these ectopic beats.

Figure 3-41a again demonstrates the characteristics of ventricular parasystole. The shortest interectopic interval appears to be 2 seconds.

Some authorities believe that at times the parasystolic focus may depolarize at very rapid rates, but most of the impulses fail to be propagated to the ventricles due to exit block. They postulate that this must be a very high degree of exit block (for example, 4:1) to account for the slow rate of most parasystolic rhythms. It is also thought that the parasystolic rate may suddenly become much faster if the exit block is diminished or removed.

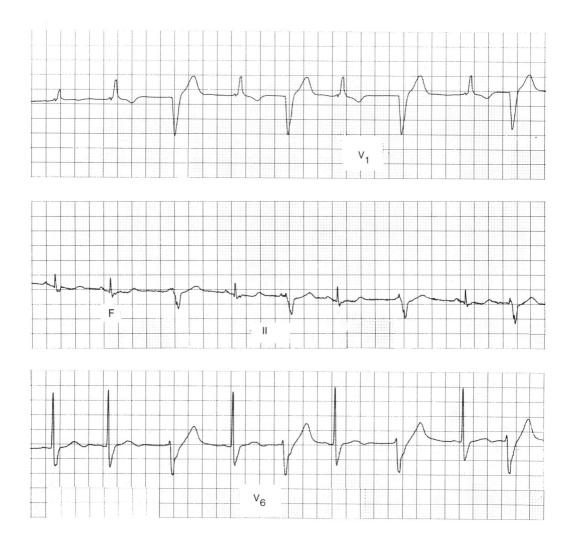

Fig 3-40.—Ventricular parasystole. If calipers are set for interectopic interval and measurement is made either forward or backward from an ectopic beat, it can be observed that parasystolic focus may have depolarized during the absolute refractory period of the ventricles that follows sinus beats. For this reason, the ectopic impulses cannot be propagated. The one exception is QRS complex marked F. This beat corresponds precisely to the interectopic interval. Since it is very slightly different from other sinus beats, it may represent a fusion beat produced by ventricular depolarization through impulses originating from sinus and parasystolic pacemakers.

Figures 3-41a through c were obtained from the same patient within the same hour. The configuration of the QRS complexes in the burst of ventricular tachycardia appears to be the same as that of the parasystolic beats. It is, therefore, possible that this represents an example of a rapidly discharging parasystolic focus with sudden, intermittent changes in the degree of exit block.

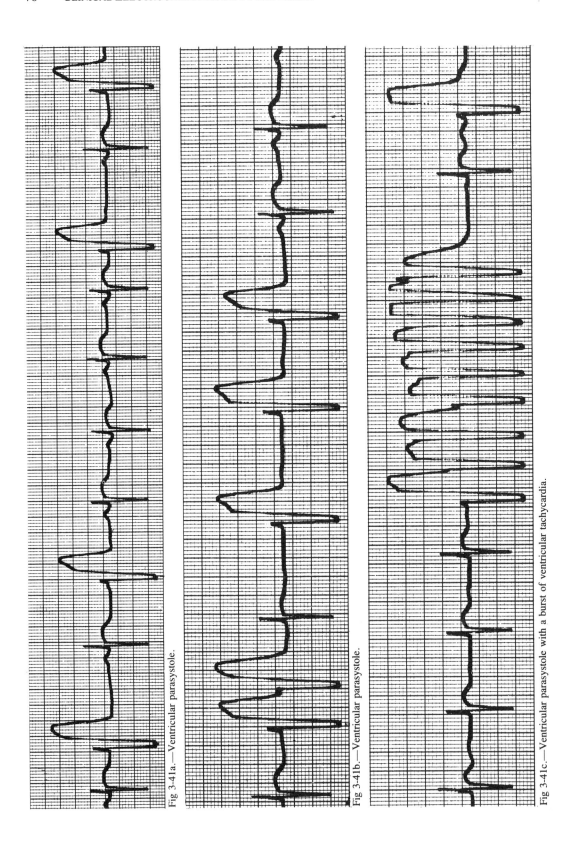

Fig 3-41a.—Ventricular parasystole.

Fig 3-41b.—Ventricular parasystole.

Fig 3-41c.—Ventricular parasystole with a burst of ventricular tachycardia.

Ventricular Tachycardia

The characteristics of ventricular tachycardia will be discussed in great detail in the chapter on aberrant conduction. At this time I will confine myself to introducing the subject by showing you an unusual example (Fig 3-42) of ventricular tachycardia. It may be misread as a supraventricular tachycardia with aberrant conduction (chap 5).

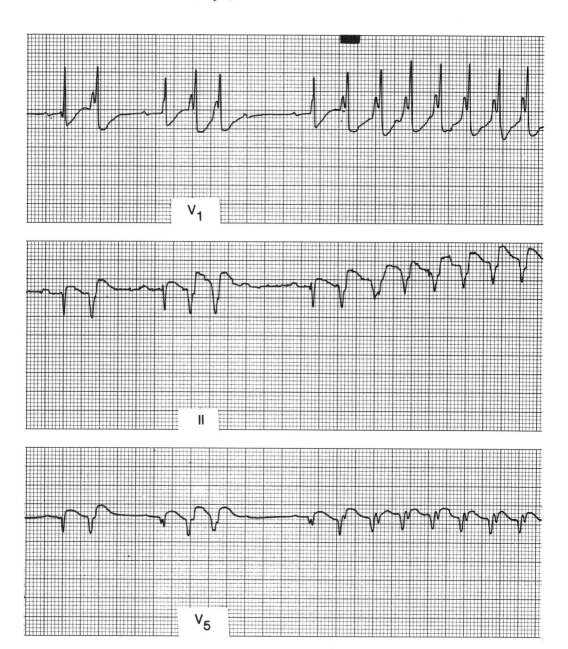

Fig 3-42.—Ventricular trigeminy, bigeminy, and run of ventricular tachycardia.

Bidirectional Tachycardia

ECG characteristics

- abnormal ventricular complexes inscribed in directly opposite directions in an alternating manner (Fig 3-43)
- equal distances between the QRS complexes, with neither identifiable as a sinus beat

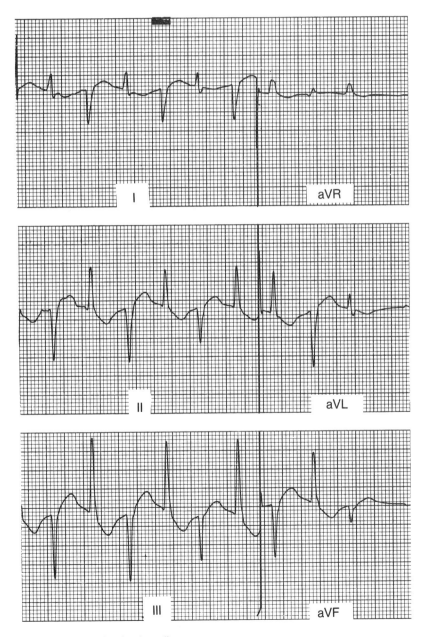

Fig 3-43.—Bidirectional tachycardia.

Bidirectional tachycardia has been described as both ventricular and supraventricular.[1(p106)] If it is ventricular in origin, there must be two ventricular foci firing independently and alternately. The more likely explanation is that the beats originate from a supraventricular focus and are conducted with alternating hemiblock; this explanation is generally accepted.[13(p685)]

Torsades de Pointes

Torsades de pointes is a ventricular tachyarrhythmia that must be distinguished from the more common ventricular tachycardia because the drugs usually used in the treatment of ventricular arrhythmias may be ineffective or may aggravate the arrhythmia.

The term torsades de pointes (twisting of the points) was given to this arrhythmia by Dessertenne[14] because the ventricular complexes appear to twist or spiral around the isoelectric line so that the QRS complexes show changing electrical polarity. In this respect, the arrhythmia resembles the "swinging pattern" described by Marriott.[13(p228)]

ECG characteristics[15]

- prolonged Q-T interval
- prominent U wave may be present
- arrhythmia starting with PVC that falls on summit of prolonged T-U wave
- amplitude of successive ventricular complexes may vary in sinusoidal manner
- usual ventricular rate of 200 to 240 beats/min (maximum range, 160-280)
- sinus rhythm resuming spontaneously or tachycardia deteriorating to ventricular fibrillation

Torsades de pointes is thought to be caused by a reentry mechanism that is facilitated by temporal dispersion of recovery due to delayed ventricular repolarization. The arrhythmia may be caused by any condition associated with an abnormally long Q-T interval.

Causes

- congenital (Romano-Ward, Jervell, or Lange-Nielsen syndrome)
- acquired

Causes of Acquired Torsades de Pointes

1. Drugs
2. Antiarrhythmics—amiodarone,[16] disopyramide (Norpace), quinidine, procainamide (Pronestyl), or a combination of these[17]
3. Psychotropics—phenothiazines or tricyclic antidepressants[15]
4. Coronary vasodilators—phenylamine, lidoflazin[15,16]
5. Electrolyte imbalance—hypokalemia,[18] hypocalcemia,[15] hypomagnesemia,[15] or liquid protein diet[18]
6. Heart disease—myocardial infarction, myocarditis, variant angina, bradycardia, or complete heart block[15]
7. Neurological problems—cerebrovascular accident or subarachnoid hemorrhage
8. Hypothermia
9. Mechanical pacing—pacing artifact falling on T wave (Fig 9-41)

Because of the potentially fatal outcome of this arrhythmia, vigorous steps are necessary to prevent and treat it.

Treatment

- elimination of precipitating factors
- mechanical pacing (preferably atrial)
- isoproterenol infusion
- lidocaine, propranolol, or bretylium sometimes successful[15]
- phenytoin sodium[18]
- tocainide[19]

Case Study

The tracing shown in Figure 3-44a was obtained in a 70-year-old woman who was admitted for severe congestive failure. She was treated with digitalis and diuretics to control the failure, and procainamide was administered because of frequent ventricular ectopic beats.

The Q-T interval of 0.44 second is greatly prolonged; the normal interval for her rate of 90 beats/min is 0.33 to 0.36 second. Prominent U waves can be seen in a number of leads.

During the next day she had frequent, short bursts of a very rapid ventricular arrhythmia (Fig 3-44b). The PVC that initiates the tachyarrhythmia is not especially early but does fall on the prolonged T-U wave. This finding is characteristic of torsades de pointes.

The arrhythmia did not respond to the administration of lidocaine in the usual manner, and further doses of Pronestyl were given. A very rapid ventricular tachycardia ensued (Fig 3-44c) that was terminated with electrical countershock. The characteristic waxing and waning of QRS amplitude can readily be seen.

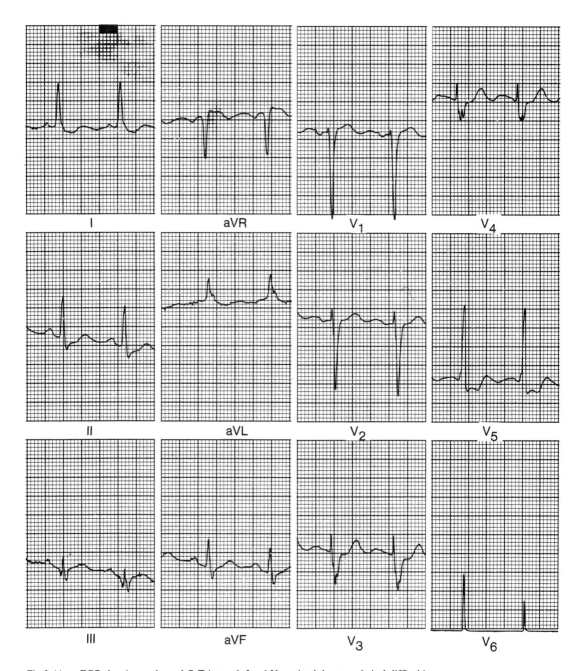

Fig 3-44a.—ECG showing prolonged Q-T interval. Lead V_6 omitted due to technical difficulties.

Procainamide was discontinued, and mechanical pacing at a rate of 110 pulses/minute was started in an effort to overdrive the arrhythmia. Since the Q-T interval varies directly with the ventricular rate, faster rates shorten the Q-T interval and may thus favor more uniform ventricular repolarization.

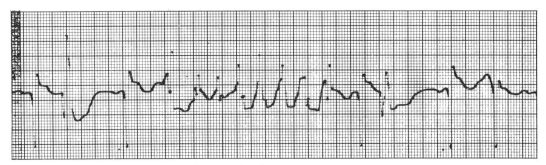

Fig 3-44b.—Rhythm strip showing burst of torsades de pointes.

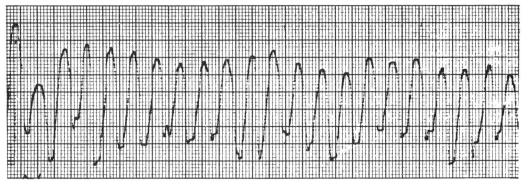

Fig 3-44c.—Rhythm strip showing rapid ventricular tachycardia.

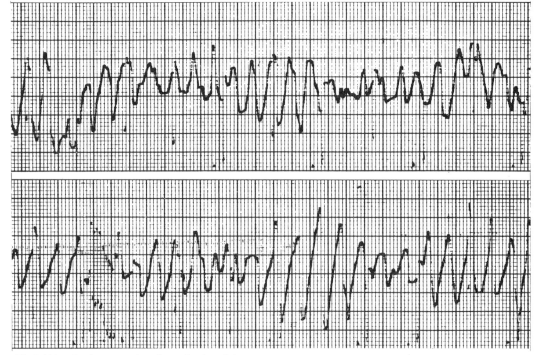

Fig 3-44d.—Continuous tracing of torsades de pointes.

The last tracing in this series (Fig 3-44d) shows the terminal ventricular arrhythmia that could not be successfully terminated by any means. This tracing clearly shows many of the characteristics of torsades de pointes. The rate is very rapid (260 beats/min), the QRS amplitude changes in a sinusoidal manner, and at times the apex of the ventricular complexes appears to point upward, while at other times it points down. The arrhythmia closely resembles ventricular fibrillation and has the same hemodynamic effect. (Pacing artifacts can also be seen.)

REFERENCES

1. Schamroth L: *The Disorders of Cardiac Rhythm*. Oxford, England, Blackwell Scientific Publications, 1971.

2. Cohen FL, Fruehan CT, King RB: Carotid sinus syndrome. *J Neurosurg* 1976;45-78.

3. Chung EK: Sick sinus syndrome: Current views. *Mod Concepts Cardiovasc Dis* 1980;49:67.

4. Kaplan BM: Tachycardia-bradycardia syndrome (so-called sick sinus syndrome). *Am J Cardiol* 1973;31:497.

5. Collins VJ: *Principles of Anesthesiology*. Philadelphia, Lea & Febiger, 1978, p 1479.

6. Hecht HH, Kossman CE, Childers RW, et al: Atrioventricular and intraventricular conduction. *Am J Cardiol* 1973;31:232.

7. Chung EK: Reappraisal of parasystole. *Heart Lung* 1973;2:82.

8. Biggs FD, Lafrak SS, Kleiger RE, et al: Disturbances of rhythm in chronic lung disease. *Heart Lung* 1977;6:256.

9. Smart R, Schamroth L: A case of idionodal (non-paroxysmal) tachycardia. *Heart Lung* 1978;7:1053.

10. Hamer SS, Lemberg L: Accelerated idioventricular rhythm masquerading as complete AV block. *Heart Lung* 1978;7:505.

11. Sclarovsky S, Strasberg B, Martonovich G, et al: Ventricular rhythms with intermediate rates in acute myocardial infarction. *Chest* 1978;74:180.

12. Marriott HJL: *Workshop in Electrocardiography*. Tarpon Springs, Fla, Tampa Tracings, 1972, p 21.

13. Marriott HJL, Myerburg RJ: Recognition and treatment of cardiac arrhythmias and conduction disturbances, in Hurst JW (ed): *The Heart*. New York, McGraw-Hill Book Co, 1978.

14. Dessertenne F: La tachycardie ventriculaire à deux foyers opposés variable. *Arch Mal Coeur* 1966;59:263.

15. Smith WM, Gallagher JJ: Les torsades de pointes: An unusual ventricular arrhythmia. *Ann Intern Med* 1980;93:578.

16. Khan MM, Logan KR, McComb JM, et al: Management of recurrent ventricular tachyarrhythmias associated with Q-T prolongation. *Am J Cardiol* 1981;47:1301.

17. Ellrodt G, Singh BN: Adverse effects of disopyramide (Norpace): Toxic interactions with other antiarrhythmic agents. *Heart Lung* 1980;9:469.

18. Singh BN, Gaarder TD, Kanegae T, et al : Liquid protein diets and torsade de pointes. *JAMA* 1978;240:115.

19. Maloney JD, Nissen RG, McColgan JM: Chronic maintenance tocainide therapy in patients with recurrent sustained ventricular tachycardia, in Harrison DC (ed): *Cardiac Arrhythmias*. Boston, GK Hall Medical Publishers, 1981, p 271.

## Chapter 4

Heart Blocks

Impulses may be delayed or blocked anywhere in the conduction system due to ischemia or necrosis of conducting fibers, as a result of drug effects, or because of other pathological conditions. Some of these factors may also impair the transmission of impulses at the junction of conducting fibers and myocardium, as is thought to be the case in sinus exit block. Delay or block of impulse propagation may also occur in scarred areas of the ventricle, resulting in "peri-infarction" block.

Conduction System

Since blocks most commonly occur due to pathology of conducting fibers, knowledge of the conduction system (Fig 4-1) helps in the analysis of these disorders.[1]

Sinus Node

The sinus node is a crescent-shaped structure located at the crista terminalis near the entrance of the superior vena cava into the right atrium. It receives its blood supply from the SA nodal artery, a branch of the right coronary artery.

Internodal Tracts

These tracts are thought to consist of a combination of ordinary myocardial cells and Purkinje cells that form preferential pathways for impulse conduction.

Anterior Internodal Tract

Bachmann's bundle is one of the two branches of the anterior internodal tract. It courses to the left atrium and is responsible for depolarization of that chamber. It receives its blood supply from the artery of Condorelli.

The *descending branch* connects the SA node with the crest of the AV node. It lies anterior to the intra-atrial septum.

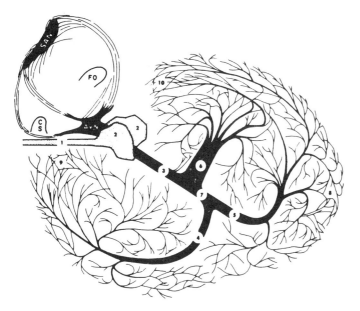

Fig 4-1.—The conduction system. SAN = sinoatrial node, AVN = atrioventricular (AV) node, FO = fossa ovalis, and CS = ostium of the coronary sinus. 1 = anulus fibrosus, 2 = right fibrous trigone, 3 = AV bundle, 4 = right bundle branch, 5 = anterior fascicle of left bundle, 6 = posterior fascicle of left bundle, 7 = terminal bifurcation of AV bundle, and 8 to 10 = Purkinje fiber arborization. Reprinted by permission from Truex RC: Anatomy of the specialized tissues of the heart, in Dreifus LS, Watanabe Y (eds): *Cardiac Arrhythmias*. New York, Grune & Stratton, Inc, 1973, p 2.

Middle Internodal Tract

The middle internodal tract (Wenckebach's bundle) descends posteriorly within the intra-atrial septum and enters the crest of the AV node.

Posterior Internodal Tract

The posterior internodal tract (Thorel's pathway) moves posterolaterally and enters the posterior margin of the AV node.

Bypass Tract

A bypass (James) tract has also been identified. This consists primarily of fibers of the posterior internodal tract, but it is also joined by fibers from the other two tracts. These fibers usually enter the distal portion of the AV node. They may, however, terminate in the common bundle of His. The fact that they thus may completely bypass the AV node accounts for their name, as well as their electrophysiological significance (chap 6).

Atrioventricular Node

The AV node is composed of a network of interconnected strands of cells. It lies in the inferior, posterior portion of the right atrium near the orifice of the coronary sinus and receives its blood supply from the AV nodal artery, a branch of the right coronary artery.

Bundle of His

This bundle is continuous with the AV node. It is composed of conducting fibers arranged in parallel. Its length of 1 to 2 cm is divided into penetrating and branching portions. The penetrating portion of the His bundle penetrates the central fibrous body from its superior, posterior aspect toward the membranous septum. In the branching portion, fibers leave the common bundle and penetrate to the left ventricle, where they form the left bundle branch (LBB) system. The remaining fibers form the right bundle branch (RBB).

Right Bundle Branch

The RBB is a long (45 to 50 mm), thin (1 to 2 mm), conducting fascicle that passes through the membranous septum and across the summit of the muscular septum and continues downward subendocardially along the interventricular septum. From there it crosses to the anterior papillary muscle, where it breaks up into Purkinje fibers. Because the distal portion has little muscular support as it crosses the free wall of the right ventricle, it is subject to strain.

The beginning portion of the RBB receives its blood supply from the AV nodal artery. The remaining length is supplied by penetrating branches of the left anterior descending coronary artery.

Left Bundle Branch

The fibers leaving the branching portion of the common bundle of His over a stretch of 4 to 6 mm initially form a common LBB that spreads out in a fan-shaped manner below the endocardium along the membranous septum. This main left bundle is supplied with blood by both the left and right coronary arteries. It divides almost immediately into two more or less distinct fascicles or divisions.

Posterior (Inferior) Division

The left posterior (inferior) division is formed by the first conducting fibers leaving the common bundle of His. These form a relatively short (20 mm), thick (6 mm) fascicle that passes down the posterior wall of the left ventricle to the posterior papillary muscle. Here it branches into a Purkinje system that supplies the posterior and inferior portions of the left ventricle. Septal depolarization, too, is thought to originate from this division.

The left posterior division receives its blood supply from both the right and left coronary arteries.

Anterior (Superior) Division

The left anterior (superior) division is somewhat longer (25 mm) and thinner (3 mm). It moves subendocardially across the left ventricular outflow tract and the floor of the left ventricle until it reaches the anterior papillary muscle. Its Purkinje system conducts impulses to the apex and the anterior portion of the left ventricle.

The left anterior division is dependent on branches of the left anterior descending coronary artery for its blood supply.

Other descriptions of the left ventricular conduction system have been provided by some authors. I have chosen the above description not only because it is the one that is most commonly used, but also because it relates well to clinical and ECG findings. The anatomy and blood supply of the parts of the conduction system have been discussed in some detail to help in the understanding and anticipation of conduction disturbances encountered in pathological conditions.

For example, inferior and posterior wall infarctions generally involve the right coronary artery. Since this artery supplies the SA and AV nodes, disturbances of impulse formation and conduction involving these structures are to be expected with that type of infarction. Similarly, the exposed position and relatively weak structure of the RBB may account for conduction disturbances in that fascicle when the right ventricle dilates. Other conduction disturbances can be clearly related to these anatomical considerations.

Blocks Involving the Atria

Sinus Exit Block

In sinus exit block (Figs 4-2, 4-3) the sinus pacemaker continues to fire at a regular rate, but conduction to the atria fails for one or more beats.[2]

ECG characteristics

- regular sinus rhythm interrupted by pause of variable length
- pause showing precise mathematical relationship to previous P-P intervals
- escape beats possible during pauses; usually of junctional origin
- may take form of Wenckebach or 2:1 block

Causes

- administration of digitalis, quinidine, or potassium salts
- inflammatory processes such as rheumatic fever
- degenerative processes such as atherosclerosis
- ischemia

The tracing in Figure 4-2 shows a regular sinus rhythm interrupted by two pauses. In each instance, the pause is relieved by a junctional escape beat. The P-P interval of the pause measures 2,460 ms, a multiple of the regular P-P interval of 820 ms.

Intra-atrial Block

The term intra-atrial block is generally used to describe a delay between activation of the right and left atria, rather than a complete block. It is thought to be due to a conduction delay in Bachmann's bundle or to left atrial enlargement.

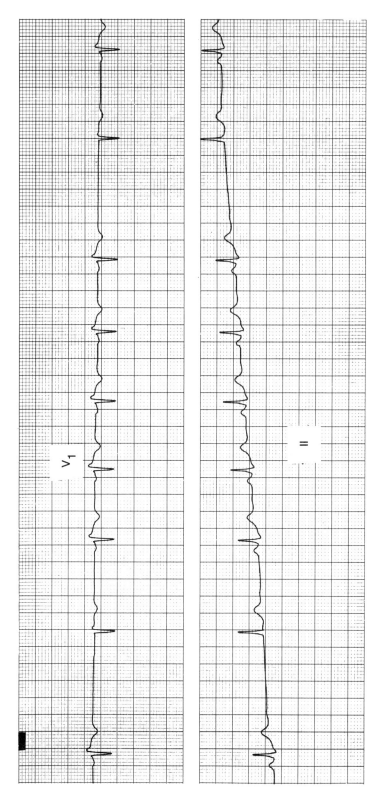

Fig 4-2.—Sinus exit block.

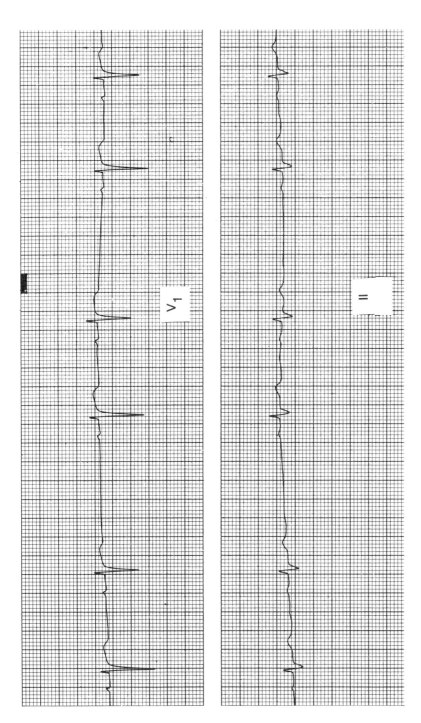

Fig 4.3.—3:2 sinus exit block. (Wenckebach)

ECG characteristics

- P wave that is 0.12 second in width (or more)
- double notching of P wave
- P-R interval may be prolonged

Causes

- digitalis or quinidine administration
- increased vagotonia
- left atrial enlargement
- coronary insufficiency

The diagnosis of intra-atrial block cannot be made with any degree of certainty, since the criteria mentioned above are equally valid for the diagnosis of left atrial abnormality. It is useful to consider this diagnosis when an ECG shows a long P-R interval. The prolonged P wave of intra-atrial block obviously tends to lengthen the P-R interval, as shown in Figure 4-4. When the P wave exhibits this abnormality, a slightly prolonged P-R interval does not necessarily mean that there is 1° AV block.

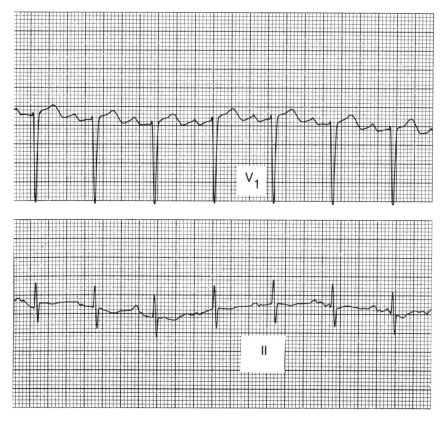

Fig 4-4.—Intra-atrial block.

Sinoventricular Conduction

Sinoventricular conduction represents a special version of intra-atrial block, in that no depolarization of the atria takes place. Impulses are conducted from the SA node to the AV node through the internodal tracts but are not propagated through the atrial myocardium. This conduction defect occurs in hyperkalemia, in which conductivity of the atrial myocardium is depressed by the potassium excess, before the SA node, AV node, and internodal tracts are affected (chap 12).

ECG characteristics

- No P waves
- QRS complexes regular and usually wide and abnormal

The diagnosis of sinoventricular conduction cannot be made from the surface ECG, but the concept does explain why, with increasing serum potassium levels, the P waves become flatter and finally disappear entirely (Fig 4-5).[3]

Atrioventricular Blocks

Although it is known that many of the AV blocks are due to block in the intraventricular conduction system, the term AV block is in general use and facilitates the identification of blocks.

1° Atrioventricular Block

The 1° AV block is a delay, rather than a complete block of conduction. This delay may occur in the atria or in the ventricular conduction system, but usually it is in the junctional area.

ECG characteristic

- P-R interval greater than 0.20 second (P-R interval normally does not exceed 0.40 seconds)

Causes

- may be seen in healthy individuals
- may occur due to physiological AV nodal refractoriness with very rapid supraventricular rates or early PACs
- vagotonia
- hypokalemia
- rheumatic fever
- coronary artery disease
- degenerative disease of conduction system

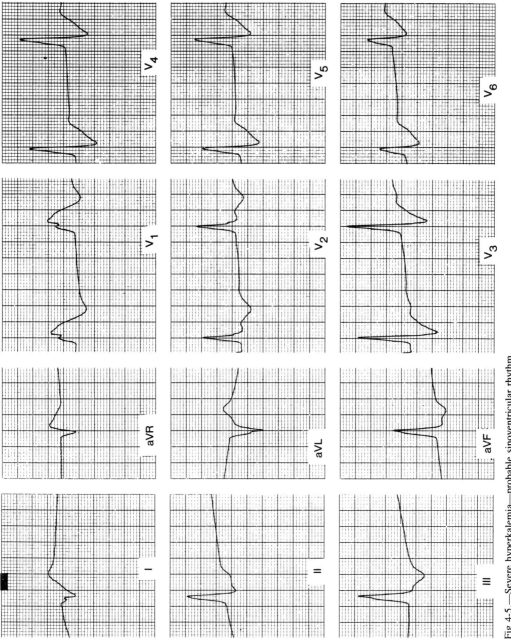

Fig 4-5.—Severe hyperkalemia—probable sinoventricular rhythm.

The example in Figure 4-6 shows an unusually long P-R interval of 480 ms. The irregularity of the rhythm is due to sinus arrhythmia. The notching of the P wave indicates that there is atrial abnormality as well, but the extreme length of the P-R interval makes it highly unlikely that the delay is due solely to intra-atrial block.

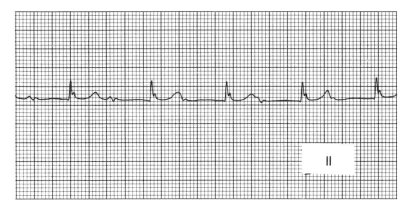

Fig 4-6.—1° atrioventricular block.

2° Atrioventricular Blocks

There are three categories of 2° AV blocks: Wenckebach block (Mobitz I), Mobitz II, and 2:1 blocks.

Wenckebach Block

The Wenckebach phenomenon may be observed in many types of blocks. For example, it may be seen in sinus exit block, where sinus impulses require increasing periods of time to penetrate into the atrium, until one sinus beat is not propagated to the atria at all. Ectopic pacemakers, too, may show a Wenckebach type of exit block. Most commonly, however, Wenckebach blocks are associated with AV conduction.[4]

ECG characteristics of atrioventricular Wenckebach block

- P-R interval progressively longer until one P wave is not conducted at all; then cycle resumes
- successive R-R intervals slightly shorter during each period
- overall pattern of grouped QRS complexes

Causes

- rarely seen in normal hearts
- may occur with rapid supraventricular rates
- digitalis toxicity
- coronary artery disease

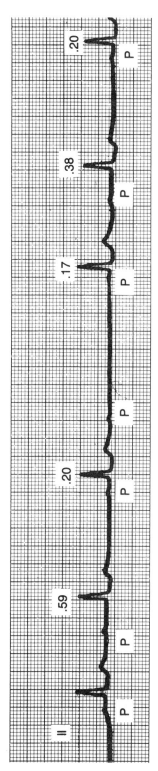

Fig 4-7.—Wenckebach block and 3:2 sinus exit block. P = P wave. Values = PR intervals in seconds.

- rheumatic fever
- degenerative disease of conduction system

In Figure 4-7, the AV Wenckebach periods can be clearly recognized. The conduction disturbance is complicated by the fact that every third P wave is missing, an example of 3:2 sinus exit block.

The tracing in Figure 4-8 might be mistaken for ventricular tachycardia. The grouped beats represent Wenckebach periods; the P waves represent an atrial rate of 175 beats/min.

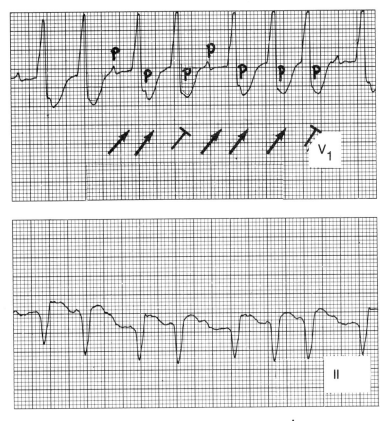

Fig 4-8.—Tracing for identification; ➤ = conducted and ⟍ = blocked.

Not all grouped beats necessarily represent Mobitz I. Although the P-R intervals in Figure 4-9 become longer, the nonconducted P wave is premature. It is possible that this would have turned into a Wenckebach block, if the premature P waves had not intervened. The premature P waves appear to meet the criteria for atrial echoes: their configuration differs from the normal P waves, they occur immediately after the QRS, and they follow beats that show prolonged P-R intervals. Conduction abnormalities within the AV node would explain the coexistence of these abnormalities.

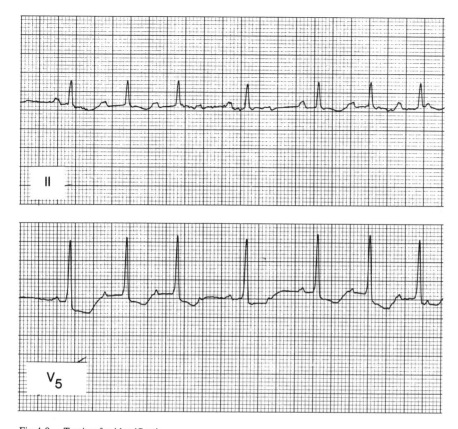

Fig 4-9.—Tracing for identification.

Mobitz II

The Mobitz II block is usually associated with disease of the ventricular conduction system.

ECG characteristics

- normal or prolonged but constant P-R interval
- occasional P wave not conducted to ventricles
- QRS complexes may be normal but are usually wide

Cause

- Usually associated with organic heart disease such as coronary artery disease or degenerative disease of ventricular conduction system

2:1 Block

Once 2:1 block is present Mobitz I cannot be distinguished from Mobitz II unless these can be identified on the same or previous tracings. If the QRS is narrow, it is more likely to be Mobitz I, whereas a wide QRS suggests Mobitz II; however, this is not always true.[5,6]

2° A-V Block 2:1 and 3:2 Wenckebach

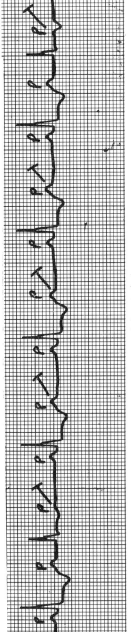

Fig 4-10.—Alternating Wenckebach and 2:1 block. P = P wave, ⌐ = block.

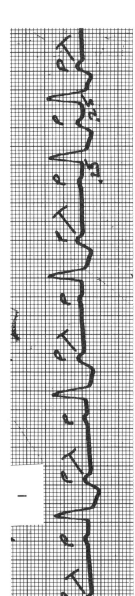

Fig 4-11.—2:1 block due to Mobitz II. P = P wave; ⌐ = block. Values = P-R intervals in seconds.

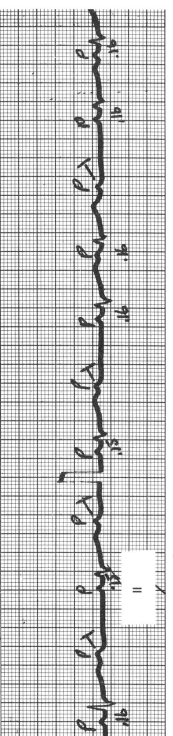

Fig 4-12.—Mobitz II. P = P wave, ⌐ = block. Values = P-R intervals in seconds.

ECG characteristics

- regular P waves, with every second wave nonconducted
- QRS complexes regular and normal or wide

Causes

- same as those listed for other 2° AV blocks
- in presence of very rapid atrial rates, cause is physiological refractoriness of AV node, rather than nodal malfunction

The tracing in Figure 4-10 indicates that the 2:1 block is due to Mobitz I.

In Figure 4-11, there is 2:1 block, except for the last two beats. The constant P-R interval indicates that it is a Mobitz II block. The wide QRS complex and prolonged P-R interval are often associated with Mobitz II.

Figure 4-12 is another example of 2:1 block alternating with Mobitz II.

The tracing in Figure 4-13 does not represent 2:1 block, although there are two P waves to each QRS complex. The nonconducted P′ wave is too premature to be propagated to the ventricles. This is an example of the very slow ventricular rate (40 beats/min) that can be caused by premature atrial beats.

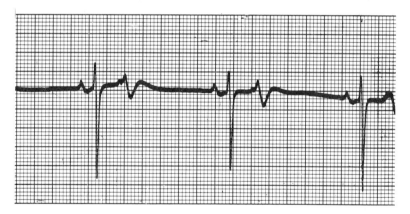

Fig 4-13.—Tracing for identification.

Blocks within the AV node are generally more likely to be transient than those in the ventricular conduction system. In the presence of myocardial infarction, intraventricular conduction defects are a grave prognostic sign, whereas AV blocks are not nearly as serious.[7,8] For these reasons it is useful to discover the likely location of the conduction defect.

First- and second-degree blocks associated with a normal QRS complex are in the junctional area. When the QRS is wide, the disturbance is more likely to be in the lower conduction system. If this type of arrhythmia is suddenly noticed in a monitored patient, it is best to obtain a 12-lead ECG, so that ventricular conduction can be evaluated.

High-Degree Atrioventricular Block

High-degree AV block is a term used to describe conduction defects that are more serious than those already discussed but are not quite complete heart block. It is usually employed when the majority of P waves are not conducted and a rare P wave captures the ventricles. This can readily be recognized when the regular, slow ventricular rate produced by a junctional or ventricular escape rhythm is interrupted by an early sinus beat (Fig 4-14). Some authorities regard 2:1 block as high-degree AV block (A. Damato, MD; written communication, 1981).

The top strip in Figure 4-15 shows the tracing of a patient who has normal sinus rhythm. The middle tracing shows a PVC followed by complete heart block with a very slow junctional escape rhythm. Not all of this patient's PVCs have such serious consequences (bottom), but many of them do, so this tracing probably shows a high degree of AV block.

3° Atrioventricular Block

In 3°, or complete heart block, no supraventricular beats are conducted to the ventricles. Ventricular depolarization is provided by a junctional or ventricular pacemaker. This complete block may occur in the junctional area; however, it is more frequently due to temporary or permanent conduction disturbances in the bundle branch system.

ECG characteristics

- independent, regular atrial rhythm bearing no relationship to ventricular complexes, which occur at slower rate
- narrow ventricular complexes producing regular rhythm at rate of 40 to 60 beats/min (junctional escape)
- wide and bizarre ventricular complexes producing regular rhythm of 30 to 40 beats/min (idioventricular escape rhythm)

Causes

- congenital (rare)
- surgical (rare)
- coronary artery disease
- degenerative disease of conduction system
- degenerative disease of structures surrounding or adjoining portions of conduction system

In Figure 4-16, there are two P waves to each QRS complex; this can be misleading. The changing distance between the P wave and the following QRS indicates that there is no fixed relationship between the two. The ventricular complexes are narrow and occur at a rate of 50 beats/min, indicating a junctional focus as the source of ventricular depolarization. The tracing was recorded in a 6-year-old child with congenital complete heart block.

Figure 4-17 represents the much more frequently seen complete heart block due to degenerative disease of the ventricular conduction system.

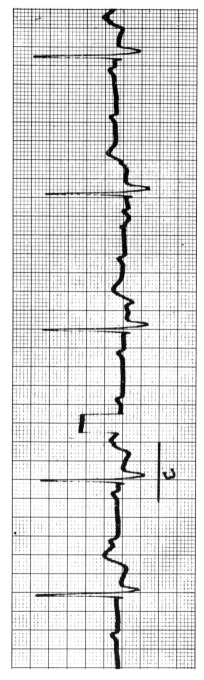

Fig 4-14.—High-degree AV block. Complex marked C probably represents a captured beat in this otherwise complete atrioventricular block.

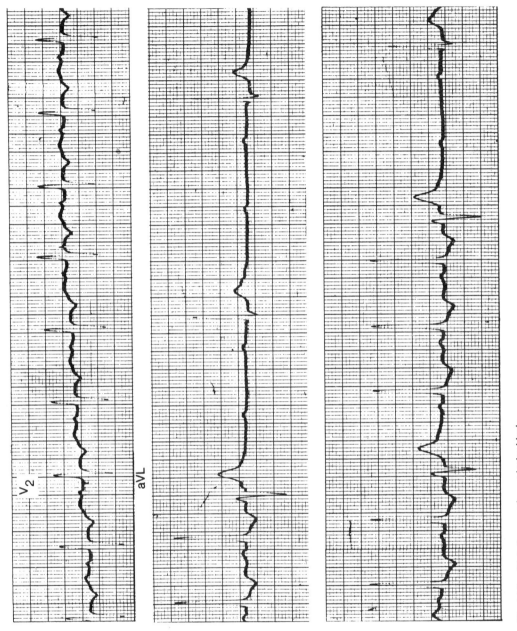

V$_2$

aVL

Fig 4-15. — High-degree atrioventricular block.

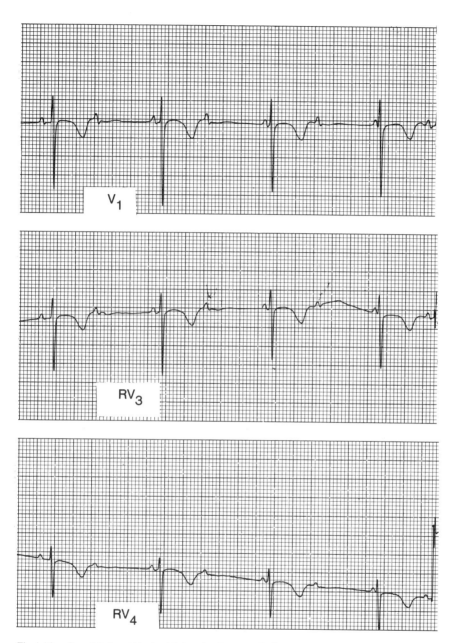

Fig 4-16.—Complete heart block with junctional escape rhythm.

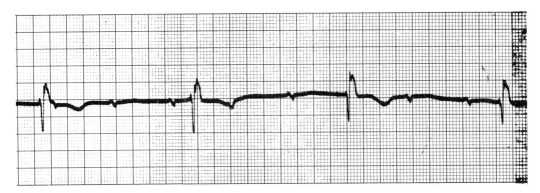

Fig 4-17.—Complete heart block with idioventricular escape rhythm.

Bundle Branch Blocks

When conduction through either the RBB or the LBB is impaired, bundle branch block ensues. The diagnosis of bundle branch block is made mainly from the precordial leads.

Right Bundle Branch Block

The RBB is very vulnerable due to its length, its single blood supply, and the unsupported position of its terminal portion. For this reason, right bundle branch block (RBBB) is frequently seen (Figs 4-18 and 4-19).

ECG characteristics

- QRS complex measuring 0.12 second or more in width
- QRS showing RSR′ configuration in lead V_1
- inverted T wave in V_1
- QRS showing late, prolonged S wave in left ventricular leads

Causes

- normal variant
- aberrant conduction (chap 5)
- congenital heart disease
- ventricular hypertrophy
- acute dilatation of right ventricle
- coronary artery disease
- degenerative disease of conduction system

Incomplete RBBB shows the same pattern, but the QRS complex measures less than 0.12 second in width.

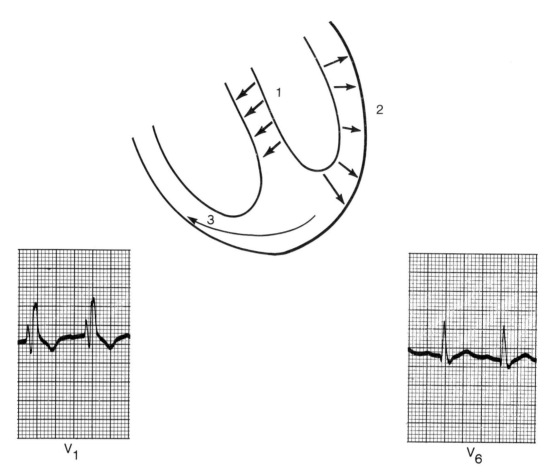

Fig 4-18.—Diagram of ventricular depolarization in right bundle branch block. (1) Septal depolarization proceeds normally from left to right, producing small R wave in lead V_1 and small Q wave in leads V_5 and V_6. (2) Depolarization of left ventricle is normal and is reflected in S wave in V_1 and R wave in left ventricular leads. (3) Late, slow propagation of impulses from left ventricle toward right ventricle produces tall, wide R′ wave in V_1 and late, wide S wave in V_5 and V_6.

Left Bundle Branch Block

ECG characteristics

- QRS complex measuring 0.12 second or more in width
- right precordial leads showing wide, deep S wave; QS configuration in lead V_1 at times
- transitional zone usually shifted toward left
- septal Q wave absent in V_5 and V_6
- wide, notched R wave in left ventricular leads V_5 and V_6 and usually in leads I and aVL
- leads with notched R waves also show inverted T waves

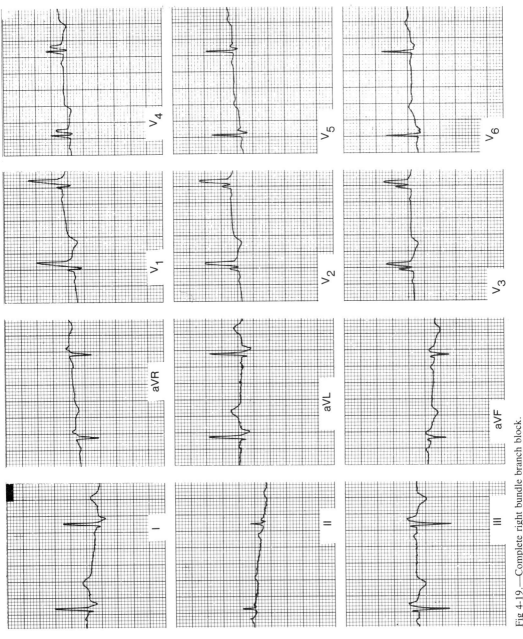

Fig 4-19.—Complete right bundle branch block.

Causes

- Usually due to organic heart disease such as hypertension or arteriosclerosis
- Congenital lesions (rare)

Figure 4-20 shows the conduction sequence in left bundle branch block (LBBB), and the tracing in Figure 4-21 shows LBBB.

Hemiblocks

If only one of the fascicles of the LBB system is impaired, the resultant conduction disturbance is called a hemiblock. The diagnosis of hemiblocks is based predominantly on the frontal plane leads.[1]

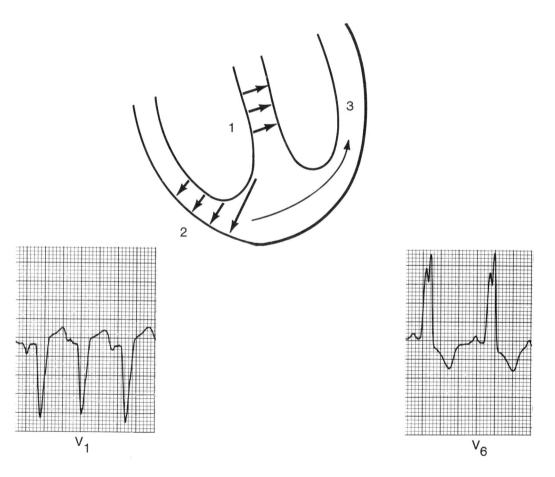

Fig 4-20.—Conduction sequence in left bundle branch block. (1) Septal depolarization must proceed from right to left, producing initial R wave in lead V_6 and occasionally contributing to QS complex in V_1. (2) Right ventricular impulse propagation is normal. It may produce very small R wave in V_1 and causes notching in QRS complex in V_5 and V_6.[1] Right ventricle normally produces only small amount of current. (3) Wave front then spreads from right to left, producing deep, wide S wave in V_1 and wide, tall R wave in left ventricular leads.

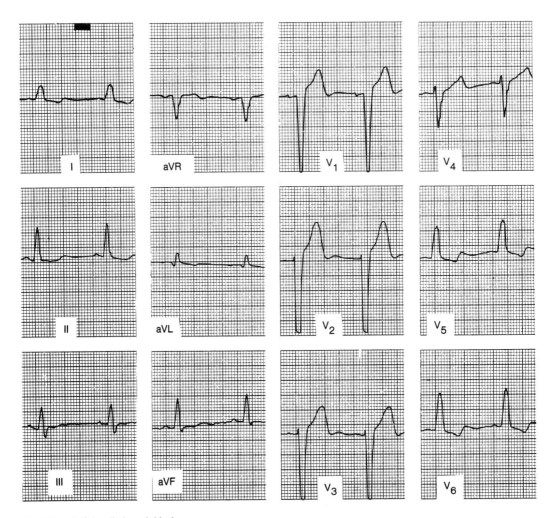

Fig 4-21.—Left bundle branch block.

Left Anterior Hemiblock

Conduction disturbances due to temporary or permanent pathology of the anterior (superior) division of the LBB results in left anterior hemiblock (LAH) (Figs 4-22 and 4-23).

ECG characteristics

- QRS axis in frontal plane is to left of $-45°$
- small Q and tall R waves in leads I and aVL
- small initial R wave followed by deep S wave in leads II, III, and aVF
- QRS complex generally not significantly widened
- septal Q wave in leads V_5 and V_6 generally disappears
- relatively deep S wave usually in V_5 and V_6

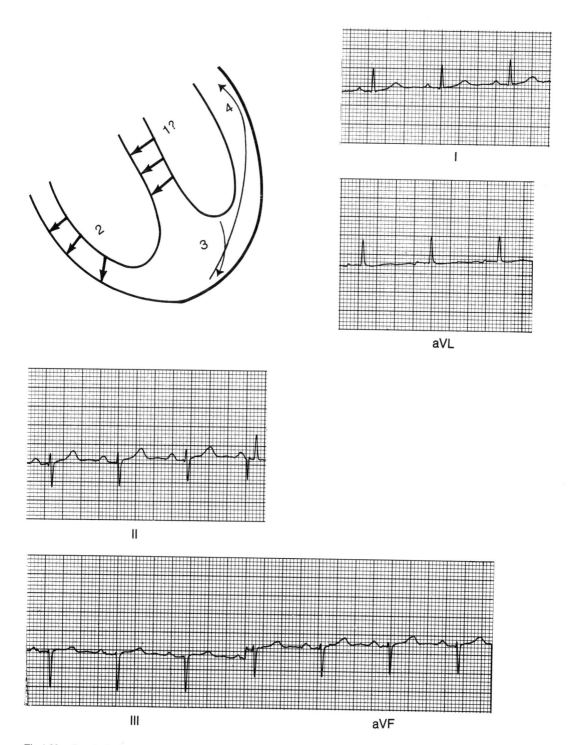

Fig 4-22.—Depolarization sequence in left anterior hemiblock. (1) Depolarization of septum is not entirely clear. (2,3) Right ventricle and posterior, inferior portion of left ventricle depolarize normally, producing small Q wave in leads I and aVL and initial R wave in II, III, and aVF. (4) Massive anterior and superior portions of left ventricle are depolarized last, producing tall R wave in leads I and aVL and deep S wave in II, III, and aVF.

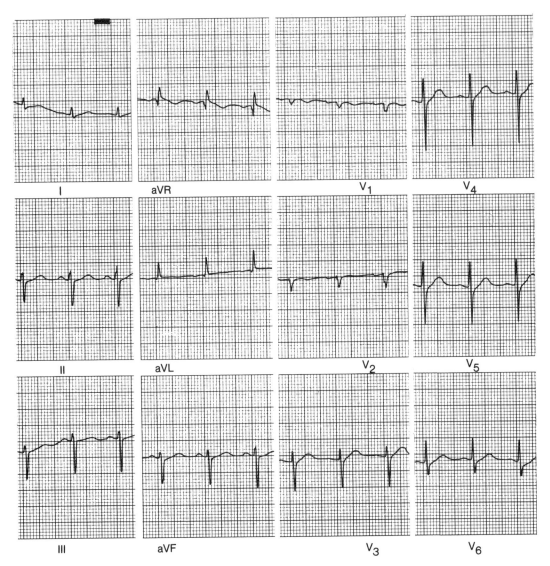

Fig 4-23.—Left anterior hemiblock.

Causes

- same as those listed for LBBB

The left anterior fascicle is very susceptible to damage due to its relatively fragile structure, its single blood supply, and its proximity to the left ventricular outflow tract and aortic valve.

Left Posterior Hemiblock

A conduction disturbance in the posterior (inferior) fascicle of the LBB is called a left posterior hemiblock (LPH). Figure 4-24 shows the depolarization sequence in LPH.

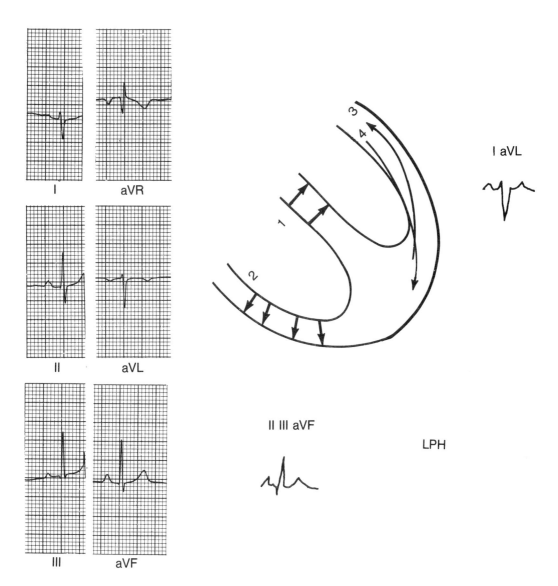

Fig 4-24.—Depolarization sequence in left posterior hemiblock. (1) Septal depolarization probably occurs from right to left. (2) Right ventricle is depolarized normally. (3) Initial left ventricular vector is directed superiorly and to the left, producing small R wave in leads I and aVL and Q wave in II, III, and aVF. (4) Posterior, inferior portion of left ventricle is depolarized late, producing vector that is directed downward and to right.

ECG characteristics

- mean and terminal QRS axes showing right axis deviation of about +120°
- Leads I and aVL showing small initial R wave followed by deep S wave
- Leads II, III, and aVF show small initial Q wave followed by tall R wave
- No septal Q wave in leads V_5 and V_6
- QRS complex may be slightly wider than normal

Causes

- same as those listed for LBBB
- Other causes of right axis deviation such as pulmonary diseases must be ruled out. A similar pattern may also be produced by clockwise rotation in people of slender build with a vertical heart. Left posterior hemiblock is not a pure ECG diagnosis.

The posterior fascicle is least susceptible to conduction disturbances due to its relatively sturdy construction, sheltered anatomical location, and double blood supply. For this reason, pure LPH is extremely rare.

The tracing in Figure 4-25 meets all of the criteria for LPH. It was taken in an apparently healthy 21-year-old man, and right ventricular hypertrophy and pulmonary disease could be ruled out as causative factors. It is likely, however, that the findings are due to clockwise rotation and a vertical heart. Pure LPH is extremely rare, and the diagnosis cannot be made solely on the basis of ECG findings.

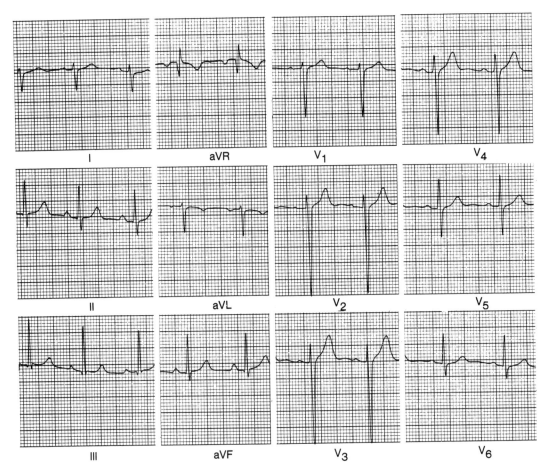

Fig 4-25.—Left posterior hemiblock.

It is possible that the pronounced right axis deviation shown in Figure 4-26 is due to an acute anterior wall myocardial infarction (AWMI), which may have extended to the lateral wall. There is, however, a small R wave in leads I and aVL, and the tracing meets the other criteria for LPH.

Bifascicular Block

The combination of RBB block with either LAH or LPH is referred to as bifascicular block.[9]

Right Bundle Branch Block with Left Anterior Hemiblock

The combination of RBBB with LAH (Fig 4-27) is seen frequently, since the two fascicles share a common blood supply and a common point of origin. The development of this conduction defect in an AWMI is an ominous sign.

ECG characteristics

- width of QRS complex measuring 0.12 second or more
- QRS complex showing characteristics of RBBB
- pronounced left axis deviation
- small Q wave, tall R wave in leads I and aVL
- small R wave, deep S wave in leads II, III, and aVF

Causes

- degenerative disease of conduction system
- myocardial infarction
- ischemia of conduction system
- causes listed for complete heart block

Right Bundle Branch Block with Left Posterior Hemiblock

The combination of RBBB with LPH (Figure 4-28) is not seen as frequently but does occur more often than pure LPH.

Trifascicular Block

When bifascicular block is seen in combination with 1° or 2° AV block, the conduction disturbance is usually not in the AV node but rather in the remaining conducting fascicle. Such blocks have a tendency to develop into complete heart block.[8]

This accounts for the warning usually issued to beginning coronary care unit nurses that 1° AV block with wide QRS complexes is more dangerous than that associated with narrow complexes (Fig 4-29). When such a conduction disturbance is observed, a 12-lead ECG should be obtained, since ECG of the precordial leads is necessary to diagnose bundle branch blocks and the frontal plane leads are necessary to discover hemiblocks.

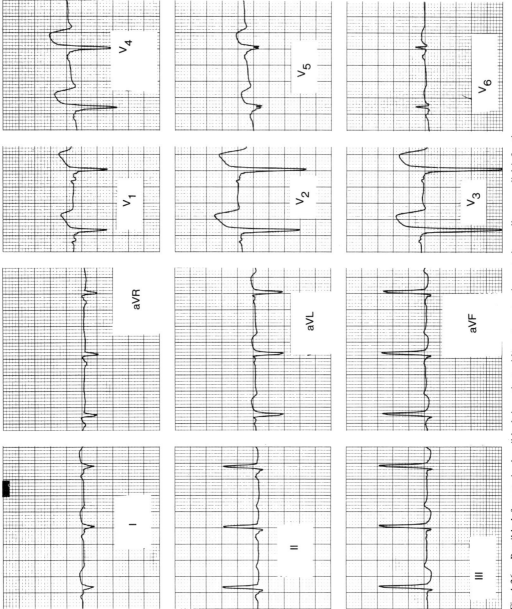

Fig 4-26.—Possible left posterior hemiblock in patient with acute, extensive anterior wall myocardial infarction.

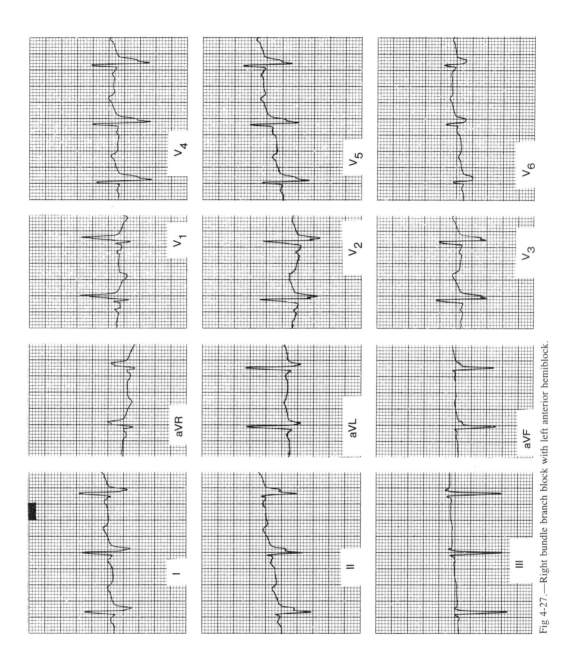

Fig 4-27.—Right bundle branch block with left anterior hemiblock.

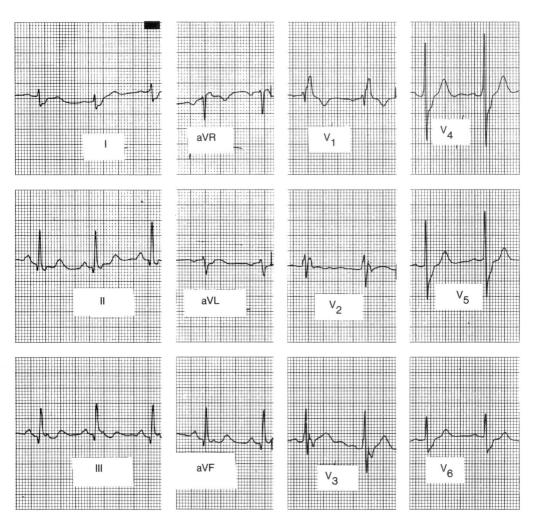

Fig 4-28.—Right bundle branch block with left posterior hemiblock.

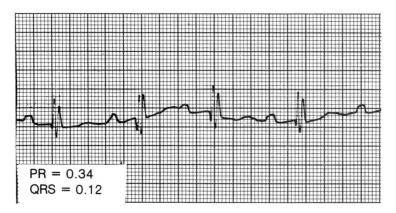

PR = 0.34
QRS = 0.12

Fig 4-29.—Monitoring lead showing 1° atrioventricular block and wide QRS complex.

In Figure 4-30, the first beat shows RBBB with LPH, the second shows RBBB with LAH, and the third P wave is not conducted. After that, the whole cycle resumes.

Whenever there is a 180° shift in the axis of the sinus beats on a monitoring lead, 12-lead ECG should be obtained; the problem is probably caused by the appearance of a hemiblock.

The tracings in Figures 4-31a and b were obtained in a 42-year-old woman who had dizzy spells. A stress test (Fig 4-31b) revealed the cause. After one minute of exercise she developed 3:1 block. The test was terminated immediately and the patient was placed in bed. By that time she had developed 7:1 block and lost consciousness. For the last 5 years she has led a very normal, active life with her demand pacemaker.

Figure 4-32 shows another example of trifascicular block.

The tracing in Figure 4-33 shows the rapid development of complete heart block in a patient with an acute inferior wall myocardial infarction (IWMI). Progress from first- to second- to third-degree block only took 15 minutes. It is likely that this block is in the AV node, since the second-degree block starts with a Wenckebach block and the QRS complexes remain normal in width. Heart blocks are frequently seen in IWMI, where they do not carry the same poor prognosis as in AWMI. The block in this patient disappeared spontaneously within a few days. This, too, is a frequent finding in IWMI.

Figure 4-34a shows a trifascicular block in a 73-year-old woman. When Figure 4-34b was obtained, she was age 75, with normal conduction. This proves once again that patients, and especially little old ladies, don't always "go by the book."

Nonspecific Intraventricular Conduction Defects

Peri-infarction Block

At times one will see QRS complexes that are wide, indicating a delay in intraventricular conduction, but they show none of the specific criteria discussed. When such blocks are seen in patients with myocardial infarction, they may be caused by the "detour" of currents around a necrotic area that is not able to conduct. Such blocks are often referred to as peri-infarction blocks (Fig 4-35).

Other Conduction Delays

Intraventricular conduction defects may also be caused by chamber enlargement, administration of certain drugs, or hyperkalemia.

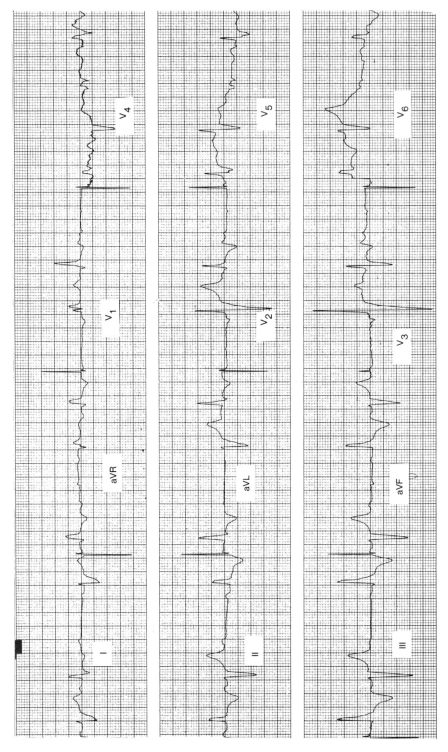

Fig 4-30.—Right bundle branch block with alternating left anterior hemiblock, left posterior hemiblock, and 3:2 atrioventricular block.

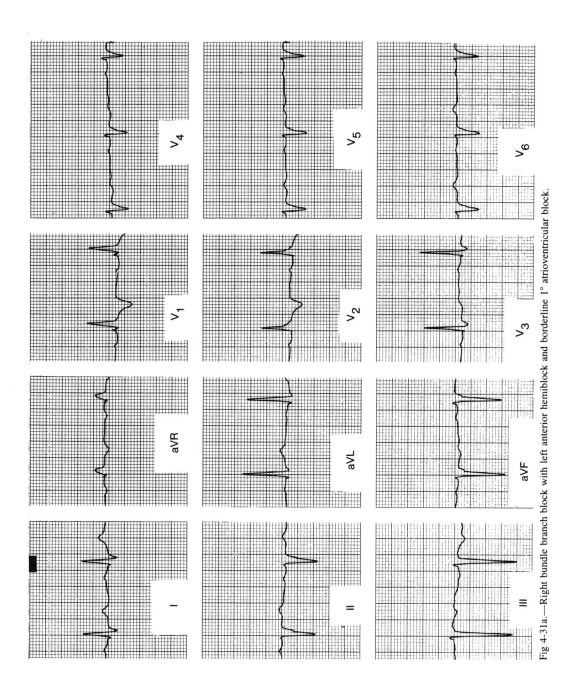

Fig 4·31a.—Right bundle branch block with left anterior hemiblock and borderline 1° atrioventricular block.

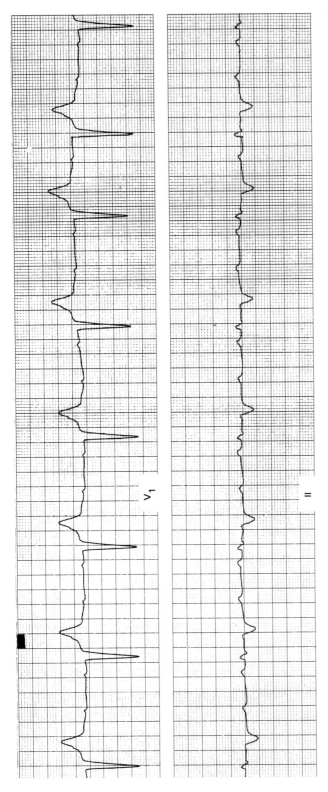

Fig 4-31b.—Stress test of same patient.

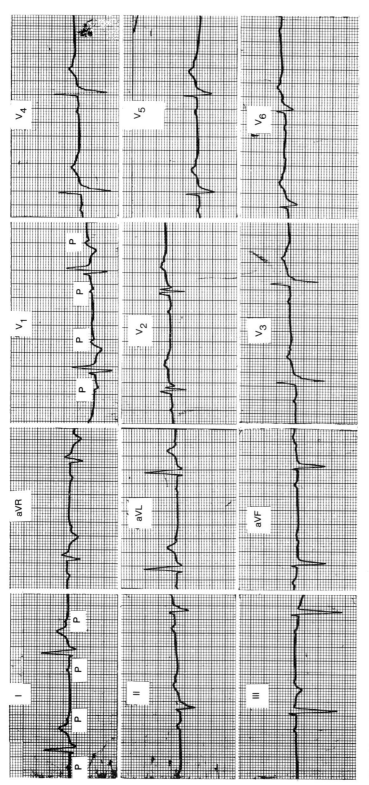

Fig 4-32.—Right bundle branch block and left anterior hemiblock with 2:1 block.

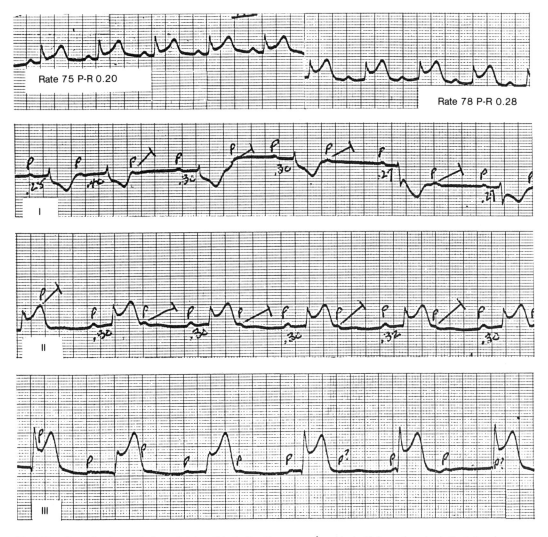

Fig 4-33.—Rapid development of complete heart block. P = P wave, ⟍ = block. Unless otherwise indicated, values = P-R intervals in seconds.

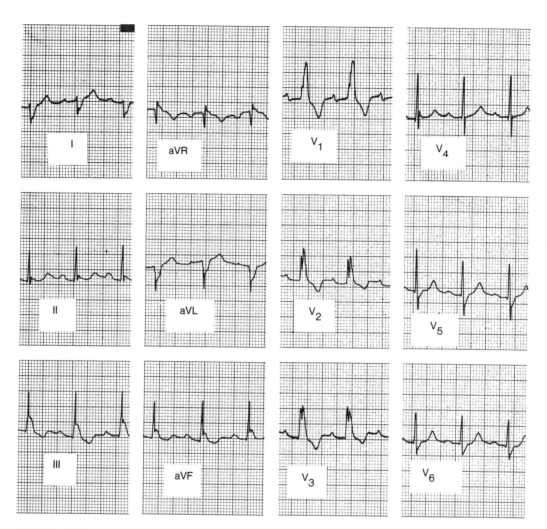

Fig 4-34a.—Right bundle branch block with left posterior hemiblock and borderline P-R interval.

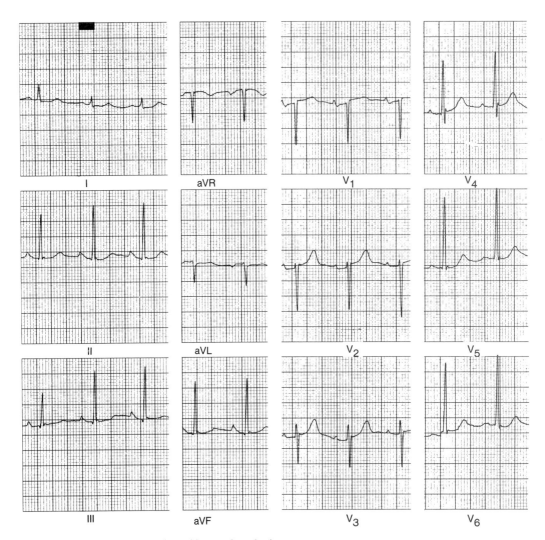

Fig 4-34b.—Tracing of secure patient with normal conduction.

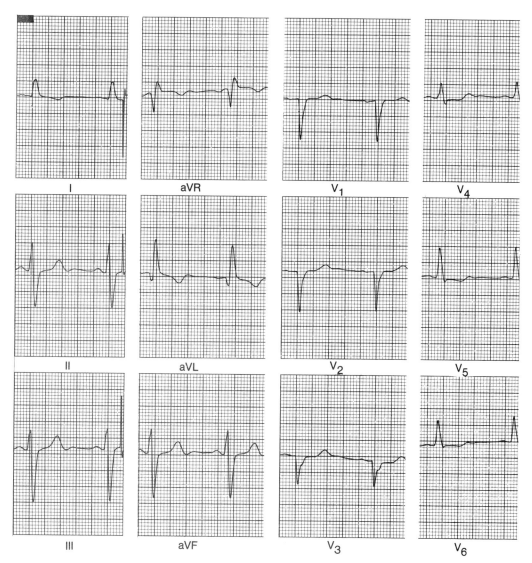

Fig 4-35.—Peri-infarction block.

REFERENCES

1. Rosenbaum MB, Elizari MV, Lazzari JO: *The Hemiblocks*. Tarpon Springs, Fla, Tampa Tracings, 1970, pp 18-39.

2. Goldman MJ: *Principles of Clinical Electrocardiography,* ed 10. Los Altos, Calif, Lange Medical Publications, 1979, p. 185.

3. Friedman HH: *Diagnostic Electrocardiography and Vectorcardiography,* ed 2. New York, McGraw-Hill Book Co, 1977, p 434.

4. Peter T: The electrocardiographic recognition of the Wenckebach phenomenon in sites other than the atrioventricular junction. *Heart Lung* 1976;5:747.

5. Marriott HJL: *Workshop in Electrocardiography*. Tarpon Springs, Fla, Tampa Tracings, 1972, p 389.

6. Schamroth L: *The Disorders of Cardiac Rhythm*. Oxford, England, Blackwell Scientific Publications, 1971, p 171.

7. Pelletier GB, Marriott HJL: Atrioventricular block: Incidence in acute myocardial infarction and determinants of its "degrees." *Heart Lung* 1977;6:327.

8. Uhley HN: Comparison of A-V block due to acute myocardial infarction and chronic conduction system disease. *Heart Lung* 1975;4:430.

9. Rosenbaum M: Intraventricular trifascicular block. *Heart Lung* 1972;1:216.

## Chapter 5

Aberrant Conduction

Aberrant conduction is a term applied to the abnormal intraventricular conduction of supraventricular impulses caused by a transient functional delay or block in one or more of the conducting fascicles. This functional block is due to differences in refractoriness existing in various portions of the ventricular conduction system and is usually related to the heart rate.[1]

Physiological Basis of Aberrant Conduction

The repolarization rate of the fascicles of the ventricular conduction system is not homogeneous. The RBB, the longest and thinnest of the fascicles, normally has a slightly longer refractory period than the left ventricular conduction system. For this reason, most aberrant QRS complexes exhibit an RBBB configuration.

The length of each refractory period varies directly with the length of the preceding cycle. The longer the R-R interval, the longer is the refractory period following the second beat. When ventricular depolarization occurs shortly after a preceding long R-R interval, it often exhibits aberrant conduction. This accounts for the frequent aberrantly conducted QRS complexes seen in atrial fibrillation, in which there is great variation in cycle length. The pattern of an aberrantly conducted beat occurring shortly after a preceding long cycle is called the Ashman phenomenon (Fig 5-1).[2]

Very premature supraventricular beats frequently arrive before the entire ventricular conduction system has had time to repolarize and are, therefore, conducted in an aberrant manner. Rapid supraventricular tachycardias may be conducted aberrantly for the same reason, but this phenomenon is not seen as frequently because, with short cycle lengths, the refractory period of the AV node tends to be longer than that of the ventricular conduction system, so very rapid atrial impulses are generally blocked in the junctional area, rather than causing aberrant ventricular conduction.

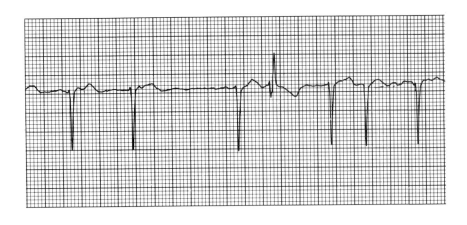

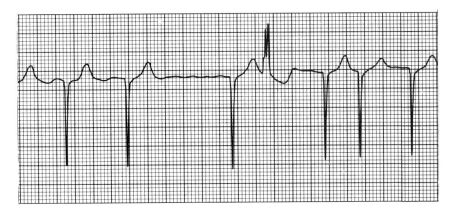

Fig 5-1.—Ashman phenomenon.

When one or more ventricular conducting fascicles are impaired by ischemia or pathology, their rate of repolarization may be slowed considerably, and aberrant ventricular conduction may be seen at relatively slow rates. The heart rate at which aberrant conduction occurs in such a patient is often referred to as his or her critical rate.

Aberrant conduction may, at least theoretically, result in a reentrant tachycardia, although this phenomenon is not often seen. The mechanism for this type of reentry is illustrated in Figure 5-2a.

A similar mechanism with concealed conduction into the previously blocked fascicle may result in persistence of the functional block,[3] as shown in Figure 5-2b. By this mechanism the functional block may be sustained, although the heart rate returns to normal.

This postulated mechanism may explain the persistent aberrant conduction seen in Figure 5-3. The first two beats show sinus tachycardia at a rate of 150 beats/min, with normal ventricular conduction. The next beat is clearly a PAC with a widened, abnormal QRS complex, indicating aberrant ventricular conduction.

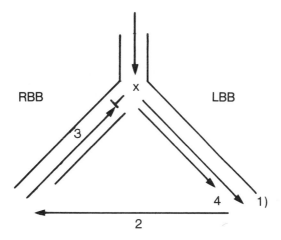

Fig 5-2a.—Diagram illustrating reentry due to aberrant conduction. Impulse arriving at x cannot be conducted through right bundle branch (RBB) due to temporary refractoriness but is conducted normally through left bundle branch (LBB)(1). It is then propagated to the right (2) and finding RBB now able to conduct, it returns in a retrograde manner to x (3). If LBB is capable of conducting at this time, reentrant beat (4) may occur, but this phenomenon is rare.

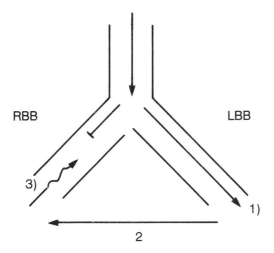

Fig 5-2b.—Diagram illustrating concealed conduction into previously blocked fascicle. Impulse cannot penetrate refractory right bundle branch (RBB) but is conducted normally through left bundle branch (LBB)(1). It then reaches right side of heart (2) and partly penetrates previously refractory RBB (3). This partial depolarization of RBB renders it again refractory, so it is unable to conduct next supraventricular impulse.

This is followed by sinus tachycardia, which shows persistent aberrant conduction, although the rate is the same as that of the earlier, normally conducted beats. A further PAC terminates the run of aberrant beats. Apparently the slight compensatory pause following the PAC allows the conduction system to repolarize completely, and the last two beats are once again normal.

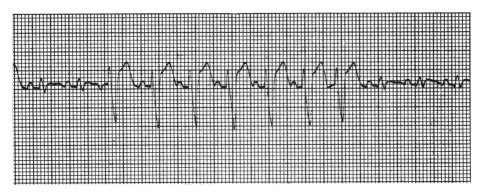

Fig 5-3.—Sinus tachycardia with premature atrial contraction followed by aberrant conduction.

A Word of Caution

When I took my first coronary care course, everything was very simple: wide, early beats were PVCs, and narrow, early beats were supraventricular. Since then it has been learned that wide, early, bizarre beats may be supraventricular in origin. Unfortunately, some people have become overenthusiastic and are inclined to call rhythms supraventricular and aberrant without the slightest justification. The safety of the patient demands that all premature, wide beats be considered ventricular in origin, unless it can be *proved* that they are supraventricular. Any other course is dangerous and exposes the patient to unnecessary risk.

Mistaken identification of aberrantly conducted supraventricular beats as PVCs may lead to cessation of necessary digitalis therapy. This can be avoided by careful analysis of the rhythm and good clinical judgment. It has also been shown that the administration of lidocaine may shorten the AV refractory period in some patients; thus, the ventricular response to a supraventricular tachycardia may be increased by erroneous administration of this drug. In most instances, however, lidocaine does not affect AV conduction.[4] On the other hand, untreated ventricular arrhythmias may significantly increase morbidity and mortality, and therefore, appropriate treatment is required.

Thus, bizarre QRS complexes should not be attributed to aberrant conduction, especially in tachycardias, unless there is convincing evidence to substantiate this conclusion.

Identification of Isolated Premature Beats

Numerous criteria have been advanced to help in distinguishing PVCs from aberrantly conducted supraventricular beats. These criteria include QRS configuration, presence of fixed coupling, degree of prematurity, presence of compensatory pause, and initial 0.02-second vector.[5] Studies utilizing His bundle electrograms have given further insight into the origin of abnormal premature QRS complexes.[6,7] The following ECG criteria are generally thought to be helpful in separating the sheep from the goats.

P Waves

Abnormal QRS complexes that are preceded by a premature P wave with a reasonable P-R interval are generally supraventricular with aberrant conduction.

The early, abnormal QRS complexes in Fig 5-4 are preceded by premature P′ waves and are clearly atrial in origin. Note that the earlier the P′ wave falls, the more aberrant the QRS appears.

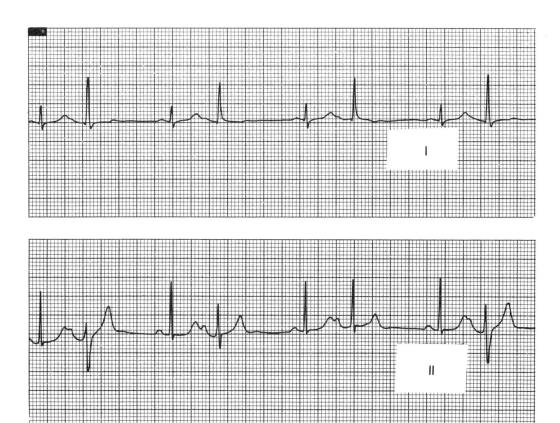

Fig 5-4.—Atrial bigeminy with various degrees of aberrant conduction.

The presence of a P wave preceding the QRS is not sufficient to guarantee the supraventricular origin of ventricular depolarization. The P-R interval must be long enough to permit AV conduction.

It might be assumed that the abnormal beats in Figure 5-5 are due to aberrant conduction of the preceding P′ wave. Close inspection shows, however, that the P′-R interval of the second abnormal QRS complex is only 0.08 second, whereas that of the first is 0.12 second. This interval is not long enough to favor the interpretation of supraventricular origin of the QRS in a patient who has a great many impulses blocked in the junction.

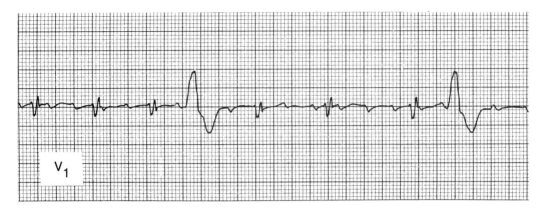

Fig 5-5.—Atrial tachycardia with variable conduction and premature ventricular contractions.

The tracing in Figure 5-6 is a more complex example, showing the importance of the P-R interval in deciding whether the QRS complex is aberrant. The tracing indicates that early PACs are conducted normally in this patient. Therefore, it is likely that beat D is a PVC or a fusion beat. This opinion is substantiated because D closely resembles beats A, B, and C in lead II.

QRS Configuration

Right Bundle Branch Block Pattern

Since aberrant conduction of premature supraventricular beats is usually due to refractoriness of the RBB, an RBBB pattern favors the diagnosis of aberrant conduction.[8] The classic RBBB pattern consists of an RSR' pattern in lead V_1 (Fig 5-7a). In Figure 5-7b, the beats that are different from the others are supraventricular in origin. They are preceded by premature P' waves with a reasonable P-R interval and show a classic RBBB configuration. In the tracing in Figure 5-8, some of the premature P' waves occur so early that they cannot be conducted to the ventricles, whereas the PACs that occur slightly later are conducted with an RBBB pattern. This is another typical example of aberrant conduction.

Left Bundle Branch Block Pattern

A configuration that resembles LBBB in lead V_1 but shows a noticeable initial R wave is generally a right ventricular PVC (Fig 5-9).

Left "Rabbit Ears"

The QRS complexes that are wide, notched, and positive in lead V_1, with the left point taller than the right, are PVCs. These are the famous "left rabbit ears" of Marriott et al[9,10] that generally indicate left ventricular ectopy.

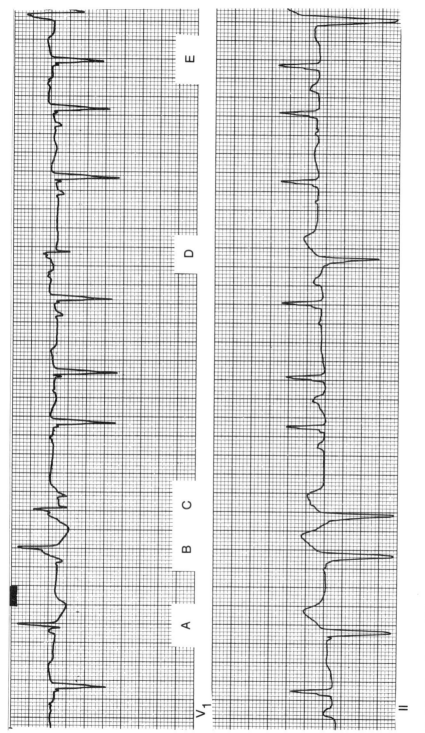

Fig 5-6.—Sinus rhythm with frequent premature atrial contractions and premature ventricular contractions (PVCs). Beats A, B, and C are clearly PVCs. QRS complex D is preceded by P wave, and may be aberrant. P wave of QRS complex E is equally premature; yet, E shows normal conduction.

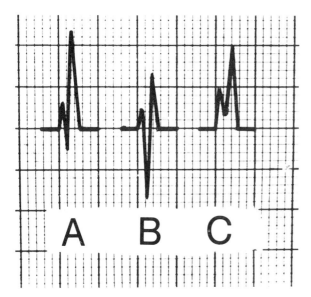

Fig 5-7a.—Diagram illustrating various RSR′ patterns in lead V_1. Beats A and B show classic right bundle branch block pattern. Beat C does not, since an S wave must, by definition, descend below the baseline. Pattern in C is just as likely to be a PVC originating from left ventricle. Reprinted by permission from Sweetwood HM, Boak JG: Aberrant conduction. *Heart Lung* 1977;6:675.

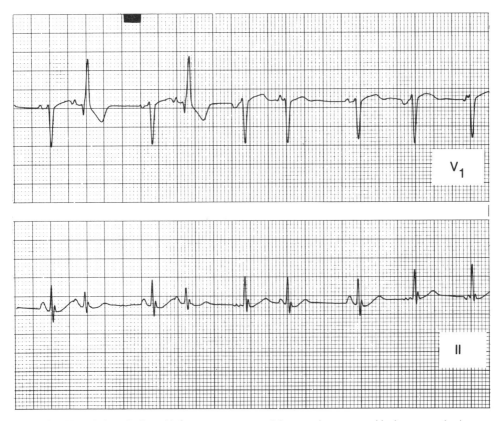

Fig 5-7b.—Normal sinus rhythm with frequent premature atrial contractions, some with aberrant conduction.

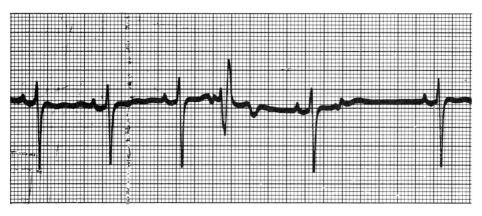

Fig 5-8.—Normal sinus rhythm with premature atrial contractions.

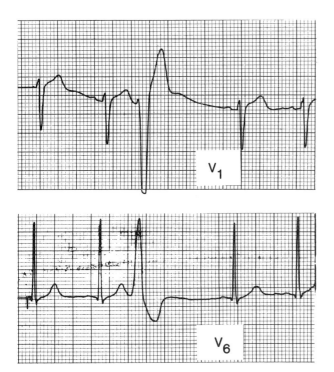

Fig 5-9.—Right ventricular premature ventricular contraction.

The configuration of the early QRS complexes in the tracing in Figure 5-10 indicates left ventricular ectopy. Do not be misled by the presence of the P waves that precede most of the abnormal complexes. The P-R interval preceding the abnormal beats is much shorter than this patient's normal P-R interval, and the P waves themselves are not premature. The abnormal beats are late diastolic PVCs.

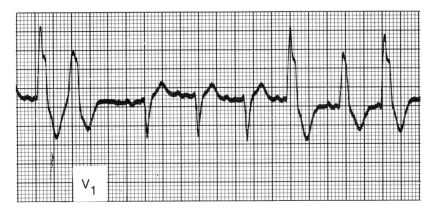

Fig 5-10.—Sinus tachycardia with frequent premature left ventricular contractions.

The Ashman Phenomenon

The tracing in Figure 5-11 illustrates the Ashman phenomenon. The early beats that follow a long R-R interval are conducted with an RBBB pattern, whereas the early beats that follow a short R-R interval are conducted normally. In this tracing (lead V_5) the RBBB pattern is indicated by the wide, deep S waves.

Initial Vector

Some investigators believe that when the initial 0.02-second deflection of the abnormal QRS is identical to that of the normal beats, the abnormal QRS is probably aberrantly conducted. This criterion does not always hold true. His bundle studies indicate that the most that can be said is that an initial 0.02-second vector opposite that of the normal beats usually suggests ventricular ectopy.[6]

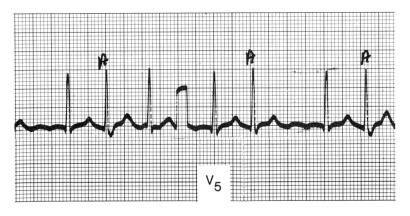

Fig 5-11.—Atrial flutter with variable atrioventricular conduction. A = aberrant.

The tracing in Figure 5-12 looks like a form of bigeminy; however, the P-P intervals are regular, and P-R intervals are identical. This patient conducts every second beat with complete LBBB. Unlike the fairly common RBBB type of aberrancy, LBBB generally implies that some form of heart disease is present. The initial deflection of the wide beats is the same as that of the normal beats. There is also one PVC (arrow), and you will note that its initial vector is opposite that of the normal beats.

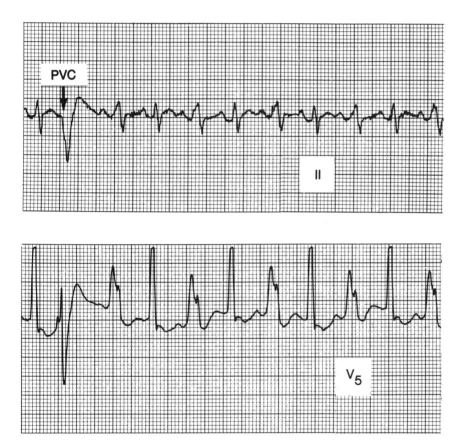

Fig 5-12.—Sinus tachycardia with alternating aberrant conduction and 1 premature ventricular contraction (arrow).

Figure 5-13 is another example of sinus rhythm in which every other beat shows LBBB. The initial vector, especially in the left ventricular leads (I, aVL, V_5, and V_6), is not the same in the wide beats as it is in the normal beats. This can be explained by the fact that the septal Q wave disappears in complete LBBB. There is one premature beat (arrow) that represents a PVC, yet its initial vector is the same as that of the normal beats, showing that the initial vector is not a very useful criterion.

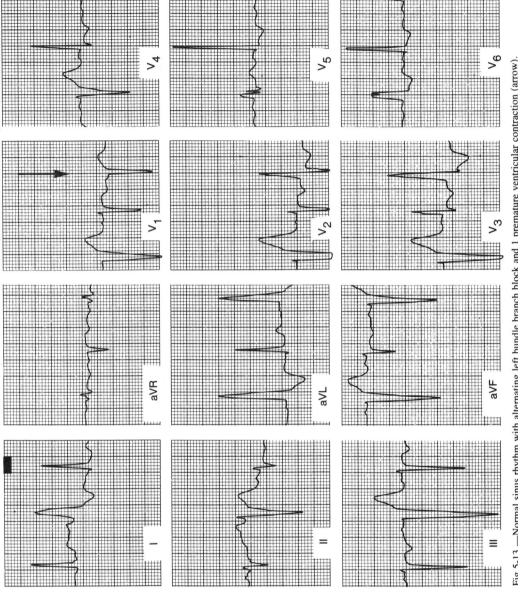

Fig 5-13.—Normal sinus rhythm with alternating left bundle branch block and 1 premature ventricular contraction (arrow).

Compensatory Pause

The presence or absence of a compensatory pause is not especially helpful in diagnosis. Most PVCs are followed by a fully compensatory pause, whereas this is generally not true for PACs. Interpolated PVCs (Fig 5-14) are occasionally seen, however, so this criterion is not especially helpful either.

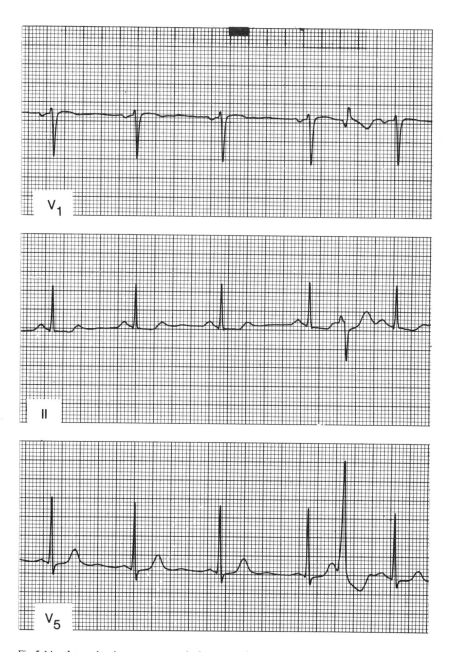

Fig 5-14.—Interpolated premature ventricular contraction.

Critical Rate

Impairment of a conducting fascicle by disease or ischemia may cause the appearance of aberrant conduction when a faster rate increases oxygen demand.

In this patient with known coronary insufficiency, LBBB is seen when the heart rate is 70 beats/min, whereas normal conduction returns when the sinus rate drops to 62 beats/min (Fig 5-15).

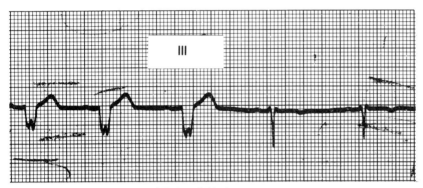

Fig 5-15.—Rate-dependent left bundle branch block.

Figure 5-16 shows the tracing in a patient with LBBB in whom the compensatory pause following a PVC allows the conduction system to recover so that the beat following the PVC shows more nearly normal conduction. This tracing again demonstrates the effect of heart rate on an impaired or ischemic conduction system.

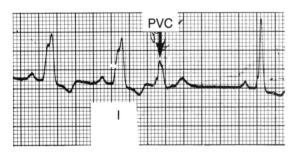

Fig 5-16.—Effect of heart rate on intraventricular conduction.

Paradoxical Aberrancy

It has been postulated that the relative refractory period of the ventricle is followed by a very brief period of "supernormal" conduction. This term is not meant to imply that normal conduction will become faster during this portion of the cycle. It means that in patients whose conduction is usually impaired, beats falling into this supernormal period are conducted in a more nearly normal manner.[3]

In the tracing in Figure 5-17, there is a pronounced intraventricular conduction defect of the LBBB type.

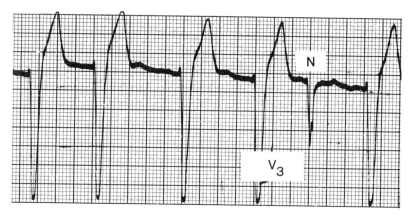

Fig 5-17.—Atrial fibrillation with left bundle branch block. Earliest beat (N) is apparently in supernormal period and is conducted in nearly normal manner.

Ectopy versus Aberrancy in Atrial Fibrillation

In the presence of atrial fibrillation, particular care must be taken to distinguish between ectopy and aberrant conduction. The following criteria may be helpful.

Coupling Intervals

Since the ventricular response to atrial fibrillation is characteristically very irregular, a constant coupling interval between normal and abnormal beats suggests ventricular ectopy.

In the tracing in Figure 5-18, each of the sequences is preceded by a long R-R interval, suggesting an Ashman phenomenon, but prolonged cycle length also favors the development of ventricular ectopy (rule of bigeminy). In the setting of atrial fibrillation, the presence of a compensatory pause is difficult to determine, but PVCs are usually followed by a fairly long pause, as is seen in beat 1 of this tracing. Beat 2, which is slightly different, is probably aberrant due to prematurity, and beats 1 and 3 show the characteristic left rabbit ear configuration seen with left ventricular origin.

Compare With Other Long-Short Sequences

The abnormal beats represented on the tracing in Figure 5-19 show a fixed coupling interval, indicating ventricular ectopic origin. In addition, there is one beat that is even more premature than the abnormal beats, and it is conducted normally. This supports the conclusion that the abnormal beats are ventricular in origin.

In Figure 5-20, the configuration of the abnormal beat suggests left ventricular ectopy. The last beat of the tracing follows very soon after a very long R-R interval; yet, it is conducted normally. This confirms the ectopic origin of the abnormal beat.

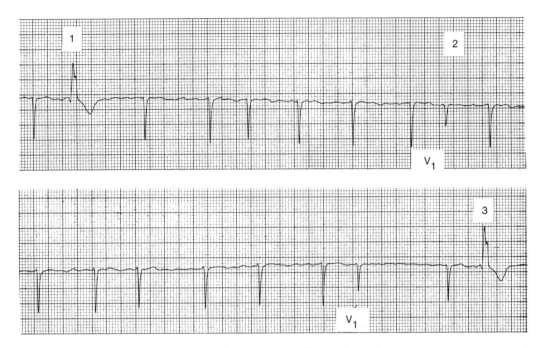

Fig 5-18.—Atrial fibrillation with premature ventricular contractions. Coupling interval between abnormal complexes (beats 1 and 3) and preceding normal QRS complex is constant.

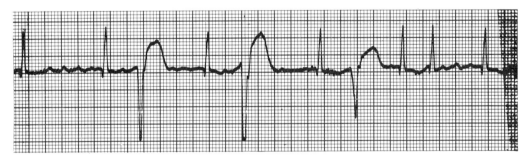

Fig 5-19.—Atrial fibrillation with premature ventricular contractions.

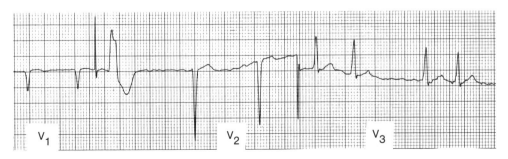

Fig 5-20.—Atrial fibrillation with 1 premature ventricular contraction. Continuous tracing of leads V_1 through V_3; straight lines are artifacts due to lead changes.

Identification of Tachycardias

If a patient who shows a tachycardia with wide, abnormal beats loses consciousness and palpable pulses, time should not be wasted trying to identify the rhythm. Electric cardioversion should be used to terminate this dangerous arrhythmia. If, on the other hand, the patient maintains consciousness, indicating that there is adequate cerebral perfusion, the following guidelines may be used in an attempt to discover the origin of the dysrhythmia.

There is a tendency to call an arrhythmia supraventricular and aberrant if the rate is relatively slow or if the patient does not immediately lose consciousness. Neither of these criteria are reliable. Although ventricular tachycardia usually occurs at a rate of 140 to 180 beats/min, slower rates may be encountered.

The following criteria are quite reliable, but any tachycardia with wide, abnormal QRS complexes must be considered to be ventricular in origin, unless there is evidence to prove otherwise.

Conducted P Waves

The P waves in the tracing in Figure 5-21 are obviously conducted; therefore, this tracing represents sinus tachycardia in a patient with a ventricular conduction defect.

Regularity of Rhythm

Ventricular tachycardia is usually fairly regular. The considerable R-R variations in Figure 5-22 indicate that the underlying rhythm must be atrial fibrillation. The width of the QRS complexes is due to an intraventricular conduction defect.

Features Favoring Diagnosis of Ventricular Tachycardia

Indeterminate Axis

An indeterminate axis, between $-90°$ and $+180°$, favors the interpretation of ventricular tachycardia (Figure 5-23).[11]

R on T Phenomenon

Tachycardias that start with the first abnormal QRS falling on the ''vulnerable'' portion of the preceding T wave are ventricular in origin.[11] Compare the first beat in Figure 5-24, which sets off a run of ventricular tachycardia, with the atrial premature beat in Figure 5-3, which starts a run of aberrant conduction.

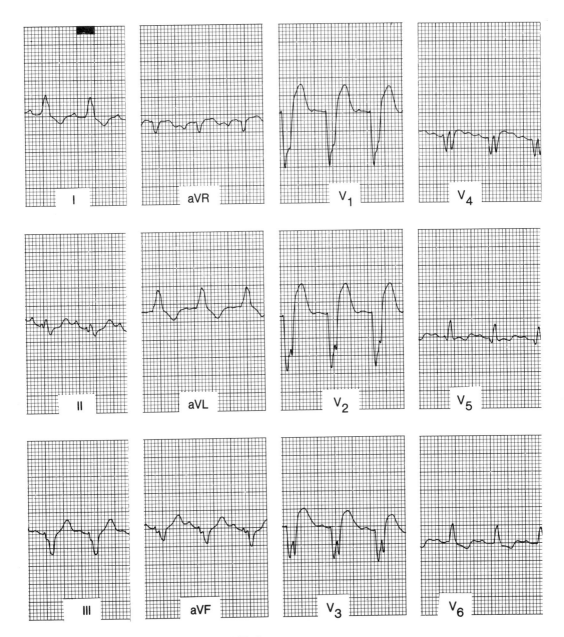

Fig 5-21.—Sinus tachycardia with bundle branch block.

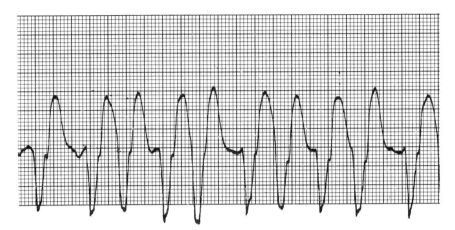

Fig 5-22.—Atrial fibrillation with bundle branch block.

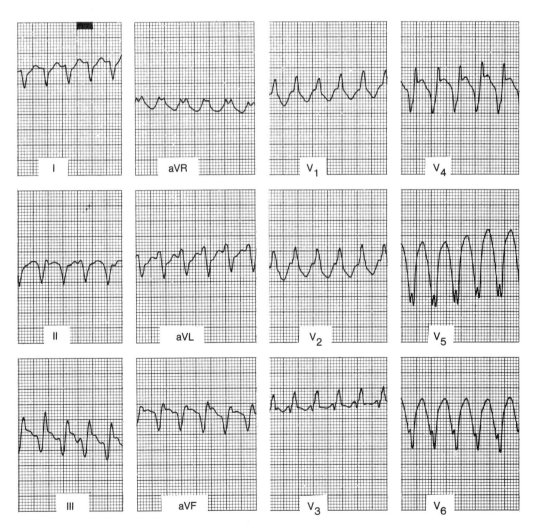

Fig 5-23.—Ventricular tachycardia.

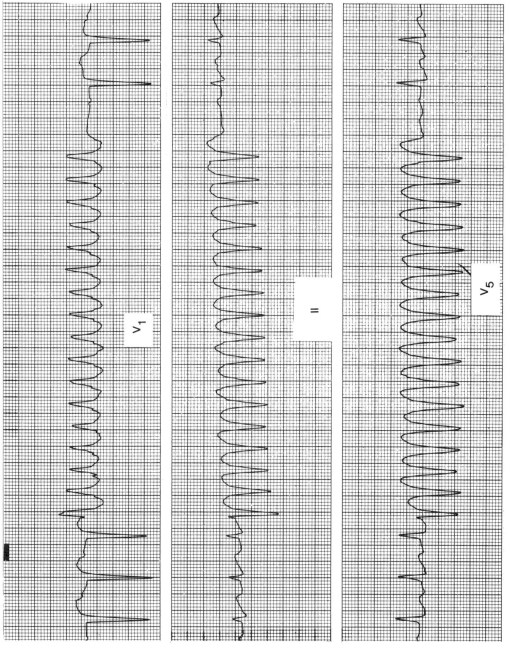

Fig 5-24.—Ventricular tachycardia.

Independent Atrial Rhythm

At times it is possible to demonstrate an independent atrial rhythm that is regular, slower than the ventricular rate, and unrelated to it (Fig 5-25). This occurs because the ectopic ventricular impulses are rarely conducted in a retrograde manner to the atria; thus, the atrial rhythm is not disturbed.

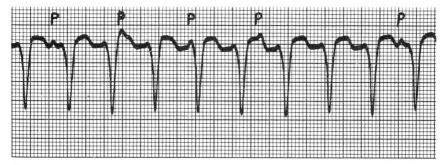

Fig 5-25.—Ventricular tachycardia showing independent atrial rhythm. P = P wave.

Figure 5-26 is another example of ventricular tachycardia at a rate of 200 beats/min, with an atrial rate of 100 beats/min. The independent atrial rhythm cannot always be found, but if it is present, the rhythm is almost certain to be ventricular tachycardia. It may be junctional tachycardia with a bundle branch block, but that is not nearly as likely, since in most instances of junctional rhythm there is retrograde conduction to the atria, as well as forward conduction to the ventricles.

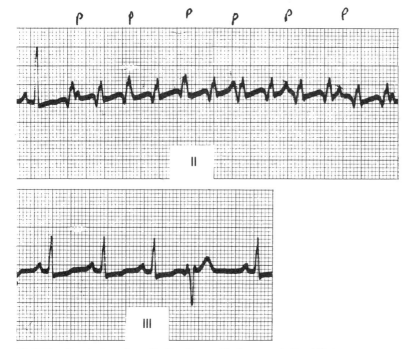

Fig 5-26.—Ventricular tachycardia. P = P wave. The bottom strip (Lead III shows return to normal sinus rhythm. Note that the P-P interval seen during sinus rhythm is the same as that seen during ventricular tachycardia.

Rosenbaum's "Normal" Pattern

Rosenbaum's normal pattern consists of LBBB configuration in the precordial leads, with right axis deviation in the frontal plane, a very unusual combination (Fig 5-27). In addition, the initial R wave in lead V_1 is often wider than is usual in LBBB.[12(p226)]

Fusion Beats and Capture Beats

Occasionally, a run of rapid, wide, bizarre beats is interrupted by a single normal beat. Such beats represent ventricular capture by a properly timed sinus impulse. At other times, a sinus impulse may arrive at the ventricles simultaneously with a ventricular ectopic impulse. In such cases, both impulses contribute to the depolarization of the ventricles, producing a QRS complex that looks more normal than the ventricular ectopic beats surrounding it. Such beats are referred to as fusions. The appearance of capture and fusion beats strongly supports the diagnosis of ventricular tachycardia.[3]

Concordance of Precordial Leads

It is rare to see a tracing in which the QRS complexes from leads V_1 to V_6 are either all positive or all negative. This finding is termed concordance and suggests that the rhythm is ventricular tachycardia.[11,12(p224)]

Ventricular tachycardia with concordance was called supraventricular and aberrant by several health professionals who studied the tracing in Figure 5-28, although none of them could give a convincing reason for the conclusion. Close inspection reveals at least four criteria for ventricular tachycardia. Aberrant conduction must be proved; hope alone is not enough.

Rapid, Regular Ventricular Rhythm in Atrial Fibrillation

A sudden regular ventricular response to atrial fibrillation indicates that there is a problem. If the ventricular complexes are wide, rapid, and bizarre, they may represent ventricular tachycardia. This is the case in Figure 5-29, as well as Figure 5-28. There is no reason to suspect aberrant conduction in the patient whose tracing is shown in Figure 5-29, since more rapid beats are conducted normally, even when they follow a slight pause.

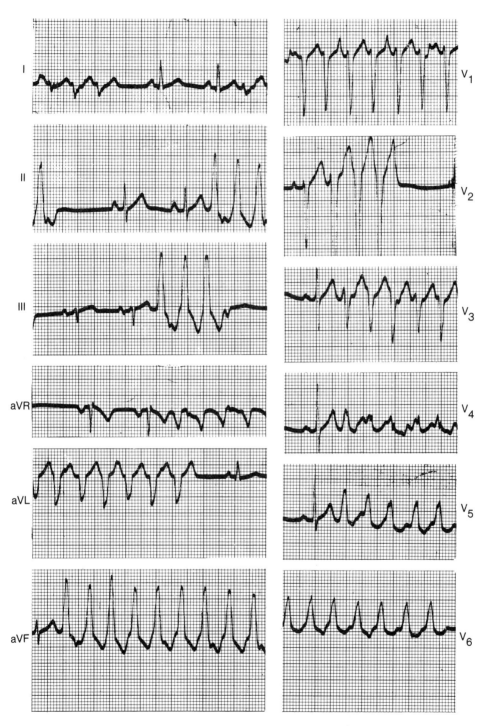

Fig 5-27.—Bursts of ventricular tachycardia showing Rosenbaum's normal pattern.

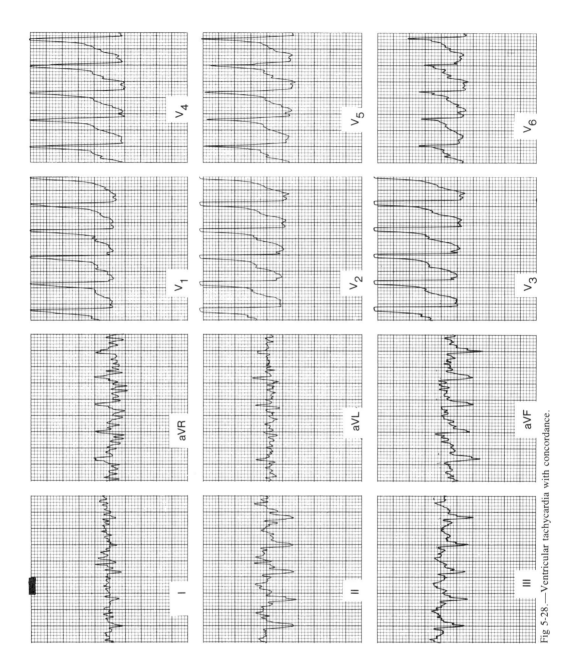

Fig 5-28.—Ventricular tachycardia with concordance.

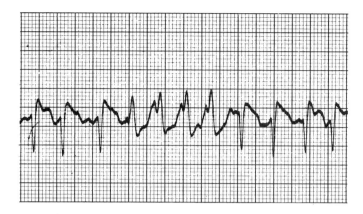

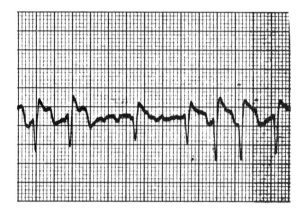

Fig 5-29.—Atrial fibrillation with bursts of ventricular tachycardia.

Examination of Previous Tracings

When a patient develops sudden tachycardia, there may not be time to examine previous tracings. The inspection of rhythm strips and 12-lead tracings obtained on preceding shifts should be part of the routine intershift report. For example, when there are several documented PVCs and the patient develops a tachycardia with QRS complexes resembling those PVCs, the diagnosis is ventricular tachycardia.

Previous Bundle Branch Block

The tracing shown in Figure 5-30a reveals that the patient has LBBB while he is in sinus rhythm. Another ECG (Fig 5-30b) was obtained from the same patient during a bout of rapid tachycardia. This is supraventricular tachycardia, since the configuration of the QRS complexes remains the same.

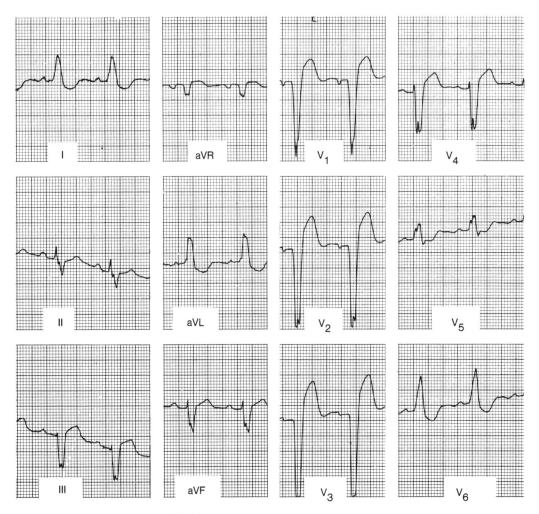

Fig 5-30a.—Normal sinus rhythm with left bundle branch block.

The tracing in Figure 5-31 shows tachycardia at a rate of 128 beats/min with wide, abnormal QRS complexes. No P waves can be identified. Since this is the usual undetermined "monitoring" lead, neither the QRS morphology nor some of the other factors cited are helpful. Fortunately, it was known that the patient had an intraventricular conduction defect, and this supraventricular tachycardia was treated with propranolol. Figure 5-31 (bottom) shows sinus rhythm, with the same abnormal QRS complexes.

Clinical Maneuvers

When all attempts to identify the rhythm by ECG criteria fail, some clinical maneuvers can be tried, provided that the patient is in a stable condition.

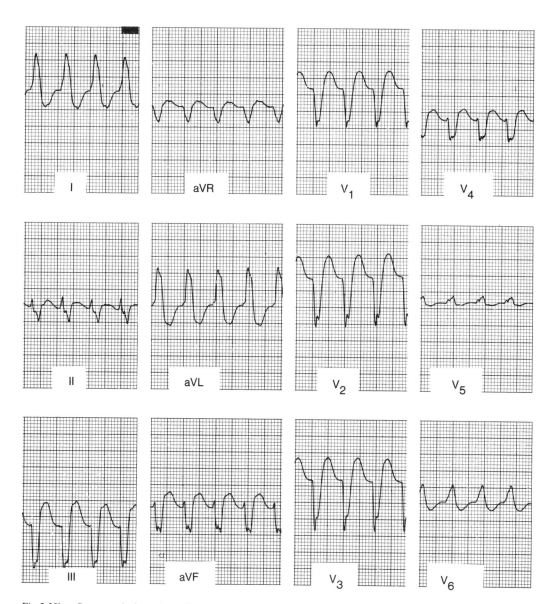

Fig 5-30b.—Supraventricular tachycardia with left bundle branch block.

Vagal Maneuvers

If the heart rate slows even temporarily as a result of a Valsalva maneuver or carotid sinus pressure, the arrhythmia is supraventricular in origin. The vagus nerve affects the discharge of the SA node and speed of transmission of impulses across the AV node, but it does not usually affect the rate of discharge of an ectopic ventricular focus.

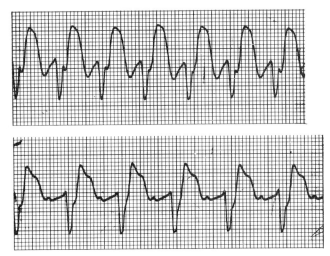

Fig 5-31.—Tracing for identification.

In this tachycardia the ventricular rate is cut in half by carotid sinus pressure (Fig 5-32). The QRS complexes remain wide during the slower rate, suggesting the presence of a bundle branch block. The irregularity of the baseline reveals the presence of atrial fibrillation. The regularity of the ventricular response in the presence of atrial fibrillation indicates that there is complete AV block and a junctional pacemaker. Since this arrhythmia is usually due to digitalis toxicity, there is a serious problem, but at least it is not ventricular tachycardia.

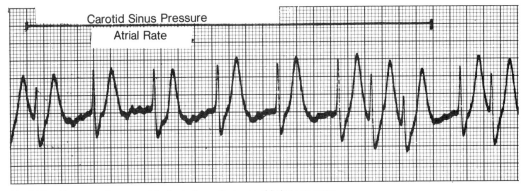

Fig 5-32.—Response of supraventricular tachycardia to carotid sinus pressure.

Clinical Examination

Since there is usually an independent atrial rhythm in ventricular tachycardia, the normal synchronization of sequential atrial and ventricular contraction is lost. Atrial contraction will occur at times when the atrioventricular valves are closed during ventricular systole. This loss of synchronous action may cause variations in the intensity of the first heart sound, as well as the occasional appearance of "cannon a waves" in the jugular veins.[4]

"Narrow" Premature Ventricular Contractions

Premature ventricular contractions are generally characterized by their wide, bizarre QRS configuration. There are, however, situations in which PVCs arising in the proximal portions of the intraventricular conduction system may not meet the usual criteria. For example, an impulse arising from the RBB may be conducted normally to the right ventricle and in a retrograde manner to the left with only a slight delay, producing a pattern of incomplete LBBB. Similarly, an impulse produced by a focus in the anterior fascicle of the LBB may be conducted with a modified RBBB with an LPH pattern.[3]

This is merely mentioned as a curiosity, since a single monitoring lead is insufficient to diagnose such patterns. There would have to be a 12-lead ECG with one of these beats occuring in each lead, if the diagnosis is to be certain.

Judging by the absence of a P wave and its position in the cycle, the premature beat in Figure 5-33 must be a PVC. Yet, it is much narrower than the patient's normal beats. The tracing shows RBBB during sinus rhythm. This leaves two possible explanations for the narrow beat: it may be a junctional premature beat that occurs in the supernormal period of conduction, and is, therefore, conducted normally, or it is a PVC, arising in the conduction system of the left ventricle, that is not conducted to the right side of the heart, since that is still refractory.

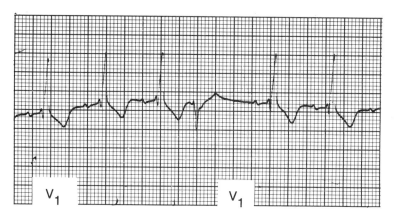

Fig 5-33.—Unidentified premature beat.

Figure 5-34 shows simultaneous tracings (leads V_1, II, and V_5) of an arrhythmia and a conduction defect of the LBBB type. The underlying rhythm is atrial tachycardia with 2:1 conduction and there are frequent PVCs. The QRS complexes are numbered. Beats 3, 6, and 9 appear to be narrower and more normal than the patient's general pattern, at least in some leads. The possibility of supernormal conduction can be discounted, since the QRS complexes in question are too far away from the preceding T waves. It is possible that these beats represent fusion beats between supraventricular impulses and PVCs originating from the distal portion of the LBB. If this were the case, the left ventricle, or at least a portion of it, would be depolarized by the PVC, while the remainder of the ventricular musculature would be depolarized by the supraventricular impulse.

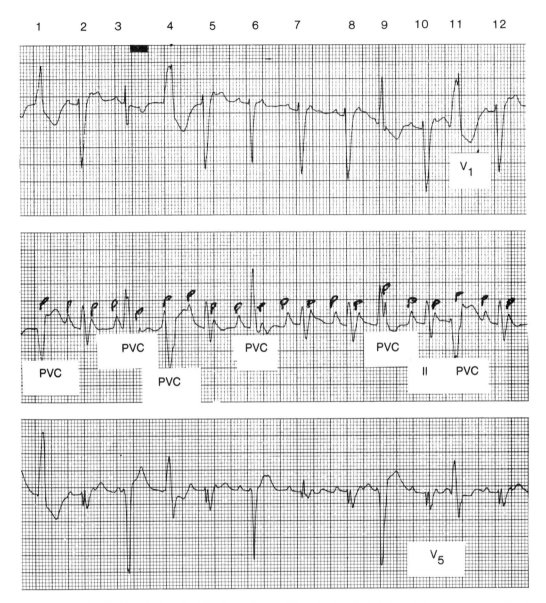

Fig 5-34.—Tracing for identification of atrial tachycardia with 2:1 conduction. Beats 1, 4, and 11 are premature ventricular contractions. Beats 2, 5, 7, 8, 10, and 12 are conducted in the patient's normal pattern of atypical LBBB. Beats 3, 6, and 9 do not conform to the patient's general pattern. P = P wave.

This would account for the shorter duration of depolarization in a patient with LBBB. The slight differences in the configurations of beats 3, 6, and 9 might be attributed to their varying relation to the preceding P wave, which would alter the time of arrival and the effect of the supraventricular component of depolarization.

This interpretation is purely speculative and is presented in an attempt to explain the concept of narrow PVCs. Theories explaining narrow PVCs have little practical applicability, but you should at least be acquainted with them.

REFERENCES

1. McKibbin J, Schamroth L: Phasic aberrant ventricular conduction manifesting as right bundle branch block with left anterior hemiblock. *Heart Lung* 1975;4:441.

2. Gouaux JL, Ashman R: Auricular fibrillation with aberration simulating ventricular paroxysmal tachycardia. *Am Heart J* 1947;34:366.

3. Schamroth L: *The Disorders of Cardiac Rhythm.* Oxford, England, Blackwell Scientific Publications, 1971.

4. Helfant RH: *Bellet's Essentials of Cardiac Arrhythmias,* ed 2. Philadelphia, WB Saunders Co, 1979.

5. Sandler IA, Marriott HJL: The differential morphology of anomalous ventricular complexes of RBBB type in lead V_1. *Circulation* 1965;31:551.

6. Kennedy HL, Underhill SJ: Electrocardiographic recognition of ventricular ectopic beats in lead V_1—a preliminary report. *Heart Lung* 1975;4:921.

7. Aranda JM, Befeler B, Castellanos A, et al: His bundle recordings: Their contribution to the understanding of human electrophysiology. *Heart Lung* 1976;5:907.

8. Sweetwood HM, Boak JG: Aberrant conduction. *Heart Lung* 1977;6:673.

9. Marriott HJL, Fogg E: Constant monitoring for cardiac dysrhythmias and blocks. *Mod Concepts Cardiovasc Dis* 1970;39:103.

10. Gozensky C, Thorne D: Rabbit ears: An aid to distinguishing ventricular ectopy from aberration. *Heart Lung* 1974;3:634.

11. Vera Z: His bundle electrography for evaluation of criteria in differentiating ventricular ectopy from aberrancy in atrial fibrillation. *Circulation* 1972;46(suppl II):90.

12. Marriott HJL: *Workshop in Electrocardiography.* Tarpon Springs, Fla, Tampa Tracings, 1972.

## Chapter 6

Preexcitation

Preexcitation is the premature depolarization of ventricular myocardium by a supraventricular impulse. Numerous theories have been advanced to account for this phenomenon. The most widely accepted view is that this activation occurs via anomalous conducting pathways.[1]

Since the conduction time of the anomalous pathways is usually shorter than that of the AV node, impulses from the atria may traverse these fibers and initiate depolarization of a portion of ventricular myocardium before excitation proceeding through the AV nodal system has arrived at the ventricles—hence, the term preexcitation.

Based on ECG characteristics, preexcitation can be divided into three groups: Wolff-Parkinson-White (WPW) syndrome, Lown-Ganong-Levine syndrome, and conduction over Mahaim fibers.

Wolff-Parkinson-White Syndrome

The most frequently seen form of preexcitation is WPW syndrome, first described as a clinical entity by Wolff, Parkinson, and White in 1930.[2] Some authors use this term to include the entire spectrum of preexcitation.

The incidence of the syndrome is about 1/1,000 population. It occurs approximately twice as frequently in males as in females and is seen in all age groups, with the majority of cases found in young adults. It is possible that heredity plays a role in the etiology of this disorder, and 30% to 50% of pediatric patients with preexcitation have associated congenital heart disease, notably Ebstein's anomaly.[3]

Anatomical Considerations

In the normal heart the annulus fibrosus provides effective electrical insulation between the atria and the ventricles. Impulses arising in the sinus node or atria must, therefore, pass through the AV node and the bundle of His to reach the ventricles. Relatively slow conduction through the AV node causes a delay in ventricular excitation that facilitates the synchronized, sequential depolarization of atria and ventricles. Pathological, surgical, and electrophysiological studies of patients with WPW syndrome have revealed one or more fibrous "bridges" between the atrial and ventricular myocardium. These accessory pathways, first described by Kent,[4] are generally located on the periphery of the heart.

Electrocardiogram

ECG characteristics (Fig 6-1)

- short P-R interval
- delta wave
- abnormally wide QRS complex
- abnormal T wave, usually

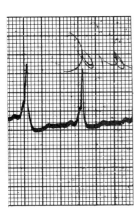

Fig 6-1.—ECG complex showing characteristics of Wolff-Parkinson-White preexcitation.

P-R Interval

Since impulses travel very rapidly across the accessory pathway, the P-R interval is shortened in WPW syndrome and usually measures less than 0.12 second. Longer P-R intervals may occasionally be seen in patients who have an abnormally long P-R interval during normal conduction.

Delta Wave

An impulse reaching ventricular myocardium via an accessory pathway causes depolarization by fiber-to-fiber propagation. This slow spread of excitation is reflected in the thickening and slurring of the initial portion of the QRS complex, called the delta wave.

QRS Complex

In most cases of WPW conduction, only a portion of the ventricles is depolarized via the bypass fibers, while the remainder of the ventricular myocardium is depolarized by impulse propagation through the normal conduction system (Fig 6-2). Thus, the QRS complex generally represents a fusion between normal and anomalous excitation.

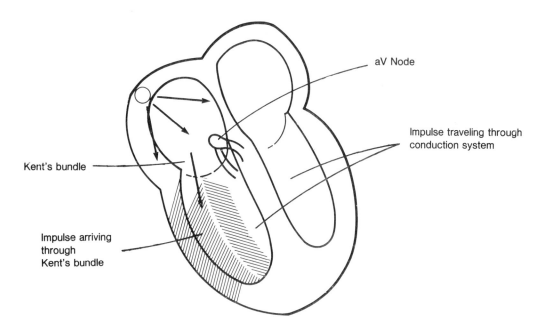

aV Node

Impulse traveling through conduction system

Kent's bundle

Impulse arriving through Kent's bundle

Fig 6-2.—Diagrammatic representation of ventricular depolarization in WPW preexcitation. SA = sinoatrial node, AV = atrioventricular node, RBB = right bundle branch, and LBB = left bundle branch. Depolarization of shaded area produces delta wave, while excitation of unshaded area is reflected in remainder of QRS complex.

The addition of the delta wave prolongs the QRS complex, usually to about 0.11 to 0.12 second. The width of the QRS complex is dependent on the proportion of ventricular myocardium depolarized via the anomalous pathway. This, in turn, depends on the speed with which the stimulus traverses the bypass fibers. Therefore, the delta wave generally becomes more pronounced and the QRS complex widens as the P-R interval grows shorter. When the entire ventricular myocardium is depolarized via Kent's bundle, the resulting QRS may measure up to 0.20 second. The relationship between the length of the P-R interval and the width of the QRS complex is shown in Figure 6-3.

In some patients, conduction may vary from normal to different degrees of preexcitation (Fig 6-4). Such changes may be due to administration of drugs, vagal influences, exercise, or tachycardia, or they may occur spontaneously for no apparent reason.

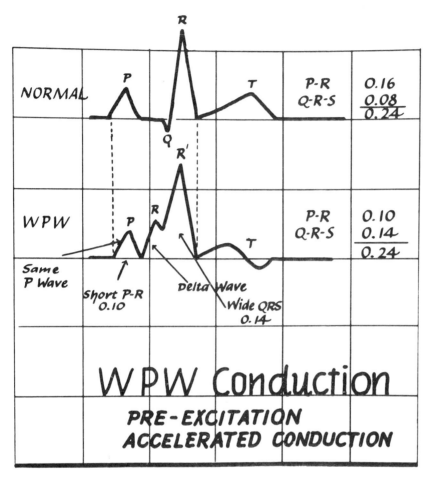

Fig 6-3.—Diagrammatic illustration of relationship between length of P-R interval and width of QRS complex in Wolff-Parkinson-White preexcitation. T = T wave. Reprinted by permission from Sweetwood HM: *The Patient in the Coronary Care Unit*. Copyright 1976 by Springer Publishing Co, Inc, New York, p 398.

T Wave

Repolarization during WPW conduction is frequently abnormal, and S-T segment depression and flattening or inversion of the T wave are often seen. Figure 6-4 shows an example of S-T segment depression and T wave inversion in leads II, III, and aVF during WPW conduction; this is not seen in the patient's normally conducted beats.

Classification

Efforts have been made to classify types of WPW syndrome according to QRS configuration and to determine the anatomical location of the bypass fibers by ECG findings. For example, Boineau et al[5] described five different locations with specific ECG patterns, whereas Sherf and Neufeld[3] listed four. The most frequently used and generally accepted classification divides WPW preexcitation into type

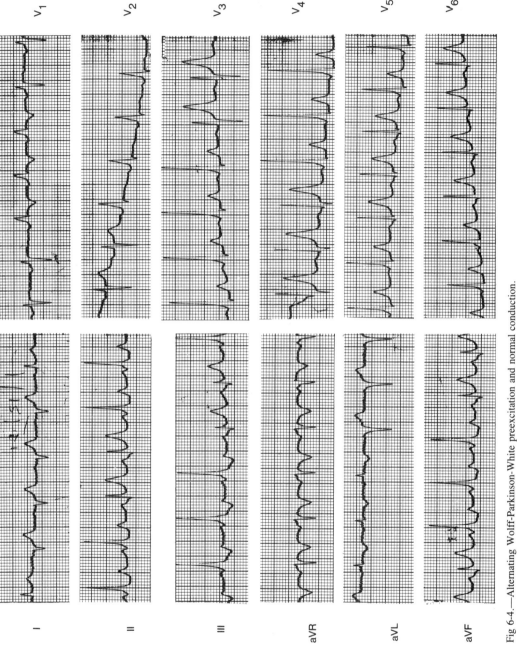

Fig 6-4.—Alternating Wolff-Parkinson-White preexcitation and normal conduction.

A, with a positive QRS complex in lead V_1 (Fig 6-5), and type B, characterized by a negative ventricular complex in lead V_1 (Fig 6-6). The bypass fibers in type B usually connect the anterior or lateral aspects of the right atrium and ventricle; in type A they bridge the posterior aspects of the right or left atrium and ventricle.

Tachycardias

WPW conduction per se is not detrimental; problems arise only when the individual develops a tachyarrhythmia. Unfortunately, persons with WPW syn-

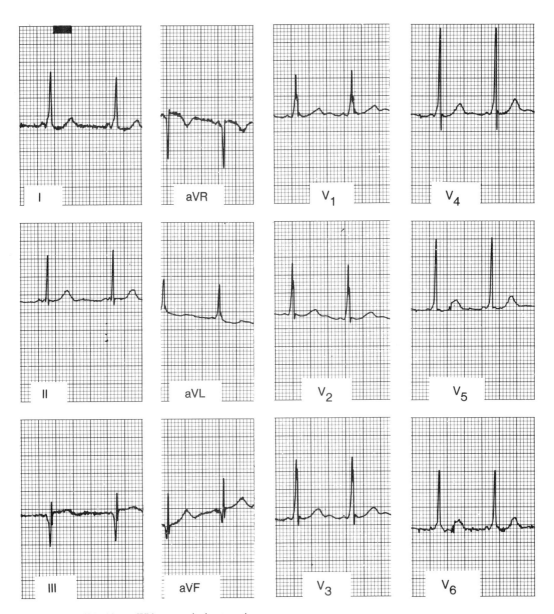

Fig 6-5.—Wolff-Parkinson-White preexcitation type A.

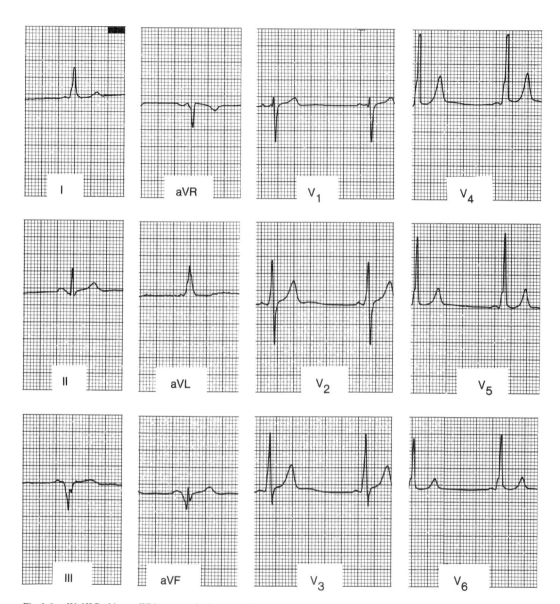

Fig 6-6.—Wolff-Parkinson-White preexcitation type B.

drome are prone to this complication. Between 40% and 80% of patients studied have rhythm disturbances either documented by ECG or suggested by a history of palpitations, dizziness, and similar complaints.

Atrial Tachycardia

About 70% of tachycardia occurring in this patient group has been identified as paroxysmal atrial tachycardia (PAT). A widely accepted theory explaining the initiation of PAT is illustrated in Figure 6-7.

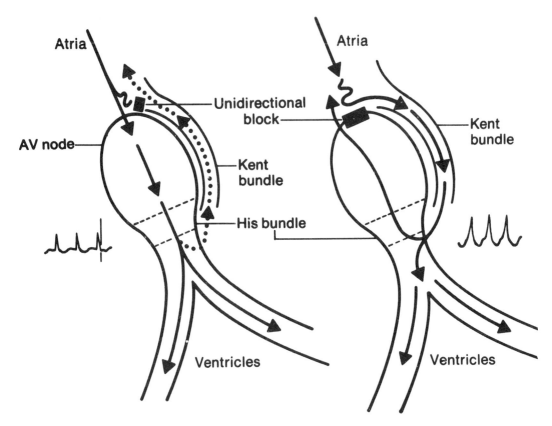

Fig 6-7.—Diagrammatic representation of initiation of paroxysmal atrial tachycardia in Wolff-Parkinson-White preexcitation. The pathogenesis of supraventricular tachycardia in the WPW syndrome. In the form shown at the left, the impulse reaches the ventricles by the normal pathway down the AV node and His bundle, and a normal QRS complex results; the impulse then reenters the atria via the Kent bundle (in this case the Kent bundle offers unidirectional block to impulses proceeding in antegrade fashion). In the form at the right, the impulse is blocked in the normal pathway and enters the ventricles via the Kent bundle. The ventricles are preexcited. Note the wide QRS complexes with delta waves (from Singh[6]).

A premature atrial impulse is conducted through the AV node but is unable to penetrate the accessory bundle. As activation of the ventricles proceeds, the wave front reaches the anomalous pathway and is able to conduct in a retrograde manner to the atrium. If the AV node is fully repolarized at this time, a circus movement is set up. Very rapid reentry tachycardias are produced in this way.

The precipitating premature impulse may be atrial or ventricular in origin, and ventricular depolarization may occur via the normal or the anomalous pathway. If antegrade conduction occurs through the AV pathway, the QRS complex may be normal and may give no indication that the patient has WPW syndrome.

Impulses originating from a ventricular focus may penetrate in a retrograde manner to the atrium through the AV node or through bypass fibers and may reenter the ventricle through the alternate route, thereby setting up a circus movement.

In Figure 6-8, the QRS complexes look completely normal and the characteristics of WPW conduction become apparent only when sinus rhythm is restored by carotid sinus pressure. In this patient, antegrade conduction obviously occurred

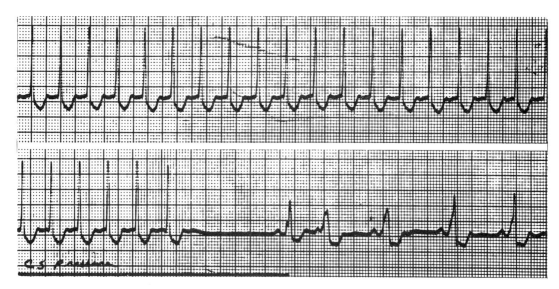

Fig 6-8.—Paroxysmal atrial tachycardia in patient with Wolff-Parkinson-White preexcitation terminated by carotid sinus pressure (courtesy Anthony Damato, MD).

through the normal AV conduction system, whereas reentry to the atria took place in a retrograde manner via the anomalous pathway.

It is also possible for reentry to occur through the AV nodal pathway, with antegrade conduction through Kent's bundle, although this type of circus movement is seen less frequently. During tachycardia (Fig 6-9b) the QRS complexes look similar to those seen during normal sinus rhythm with WPW conduction (Fig 6-9a), suggesting that forward propagation occurs through the anomalous pathway.

Lead V_6 of this tracing (Fig 6-9b) shows how reentry tachycardias start. The first two beats are of sinus origin. The T wave following the second QRS complex looks slightly different and probably contains a P' wave caused by retrograde conduction to the atrium. This sets up a circus movement, with antegrade conduction through Kent's bundle and retrograde conduction through the AV node.

Thus, current evidence indicates that sustained reentry is dependent on the synchronization of alternating refractoriness of the two pathways and on their respective conduction time. The circus movement is interrupted when the refractoriness and/or conduction time of either pathway is changed either spontaneously or through therapeutic intervention.

Refractoriness of the AV node is increased by vagal maneuvers and administration of digitalis, propranolol, or verapamil, whereas refractoriness and/or conduction time of the accessory pathway are prolonged by administration of procainamide, quinidine, or lidocaine.

In very rapid atrial tachycardia, the QRS complexes may become wide and bizarre due to rate-related aberrancy, even if antegrade conduction occurs across the normal AV pathway. The P waves may merge with the T waves, and the fast regular rhythm with abnormal QRS complexes and absent P waves is easily mistaken for ventricular tachycardia.

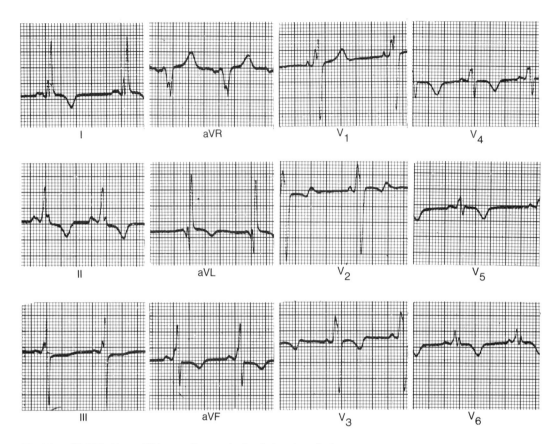

Fig 6-9a.—Wolff-Parkinson-White type B preexcitation during sinus rhythm.

Case Report. A 24-year-old man was admitted to the emergency department in obvious, severe distress, complaining of chest pain, palpitations, and shortness of breath of sudden, recent onset. He was unable to give a clear history due to his state of near collapse.

The first tracing obtained (Fig 6-10a) showed a tachycardia rate of 240 beats/min with relatively wide QRS complexes and no identifiable P waves. The age of the patient and the extremely fast heart rate suggested the possibility of supraventricular tachycardia with aberrant conduction. The possibility of WPW syndrome was also considered but could not be substantiated due to the absence of delta waves, the patient's inability to give a history, and the clinical necessity for rapid intervention, which precluded a search for previous tracings.

Since vagal maneuvers (Valsalva maneuver and carotid sinus pressure) did not affect the rhythm, a 50-mg bolus of lidocaine was administered intravenously. The immediate results are shown in Figure 6-10b.

The tachycardia ceased within seconds of lidocaine administration. The beat following the first longer R-R interval (arrow) shows a short P-R interval, suggesting the possibility of WPW preexcitation. The slight abnormalities of rhythm seen before resumption of normal sinus rhythm, ie, apparent PVC and sinus pause, are not unusual after sudden interruption of very rapid tachycardias.

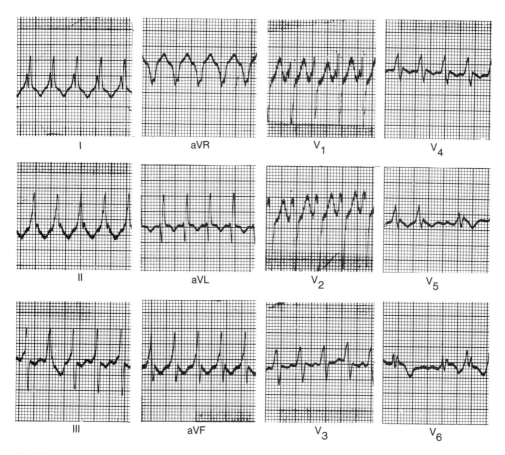

Fig 6-9b.—Tracing of same patient as in Fig 6-9a, during tachycardia.

A 12-lead tracing obtained shortly after termination of the tachycardia (Fig 6-10c) was completely normal; however, a search of our records revealed an ECG (Fig 6-10d) obtained 4 years earlier that showed WPW syndrome type B.

The wide, bizarre ventricular complexes of the tachycardia do not resemble the QRS complexes seen during WPW conduction, either in configuration or axis. It was concluded that the tachycardia represented atrial reentry with antegrade propagation through the AV pathway and aberrant conduction through the ventricles, due to the extremely rapid rate. Alternative, less likely, interpretations include the possibilities that the patient has more than one anomalous pathway and that this episode was ventricular tachycardia. Both of these phenomena have been reported in patients with WPW syndrome.

Administration of lidocaine is normally not effective in supraventricular tachycardias, but it can be useful in tachycardias produced by reentry across an anomalous pathway, by slowing conduction.

If the response to lidocaine had not been so immediate in this patient, the next step in treatment would have been synchronized electric countershock. This is probably the safest, most effective means of terminating rapid tachyarrhythmias of unknown origin that cause severe cardiovascular symptoms.

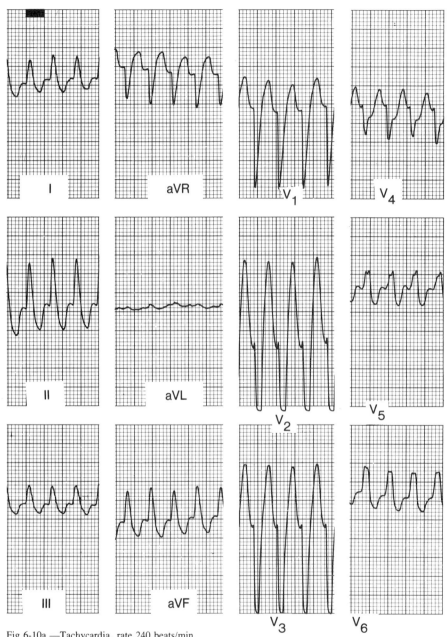

Fig 6-10a.—Tachycardia, rate 240 beats/min.

Atrial Flutter

This arrhythmia is relatively rare in patients with WPW syndrome, but when it occurs, it can cause serious hemodynamic consequences. In the adult, atrial flutter is rarely conducted on a 1:1 basis across the normal AV pathway, so the resulting ventricular rate is generally 150 beats/min or less. Conduction time across the accessory pathway is frequently very short, and 1:1 conduction of rates of 300 beats/min has been reported.[3]

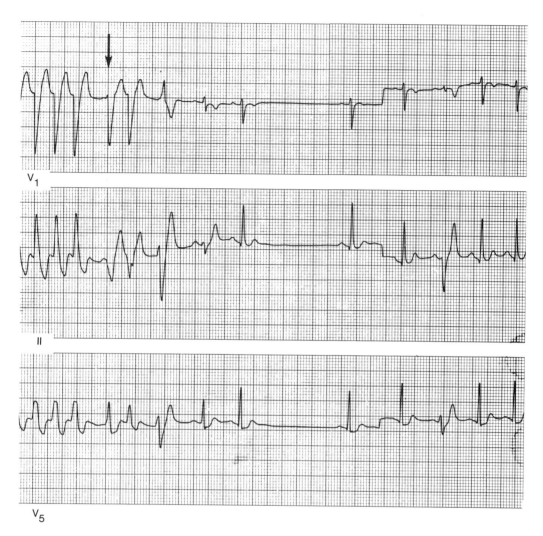

Fig 6-10b.—Interruption of rapid tachycardia by bolus of lidocaine 50 mg (arrow).

Atrial Fibrillation

Up to 20% of patients with WPW preexcitation have one or more attacks of atrial fibrillation.[3] This may occur as a consequence of concomitant heart disease or may be triggered by the reentry of a premature impulse during the relative refractory period of the atria.

Because the AV node usually permits only a fraction of atrial fibrillatory impulses to reach the ventricles, the ventricular response to atrial fibrillation rarely exceeds 180 beats/min in the adult. The bypass fibers in the patient with WPW syndrome, however, readily conduct a much greater number of impulses directly into the ventricular myocardium. The resulting ventricular response may be in excess of 300 beats/min.[7]

This is not only detrimental from a hemodynamic point of view, but it may result in ventricular fibrillation, as rapid, irregular impulses reach myocardial

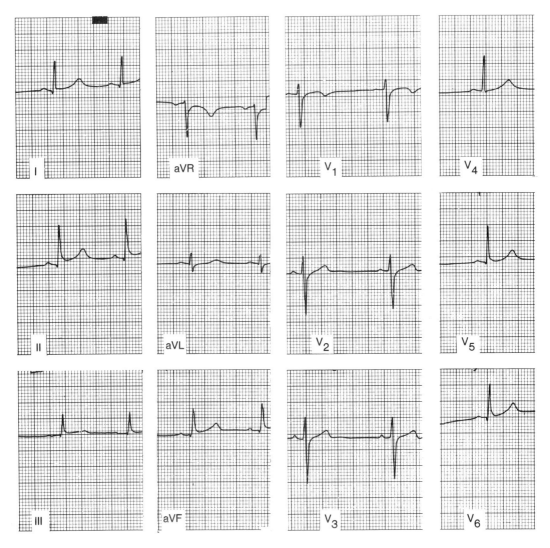

Fig 6-10c.—Normal ECG.

fibers in various stages of repolarization. A number of cases of ventricular fibrillation have been reported in otherwise healthy young persons with WPW preexcitation.[8]

When atrial fibrillation is conducted across the accessory pathway, the ECG shows wide, bizarre QRS complexes occurring at a very fast rate and with slight irregularity. Except for this irregularity, the rhythm might readily be mistaken for an unusually rapid ventricular tachycardia or ventricular flutter. Such an error would probably not harm the patient, since the means generally used to terminate ventricular tachycardia—lidocaine, procainamide, and especially synchronized countershock—would most likely terminate the arrhythmia. On the other hand, digitalis, the drug normally used to slow the ventricular response to atrial fibrillation, may actually increase conduction to the ventricles in this situation and may lead to ventricular fibrillation.[8]

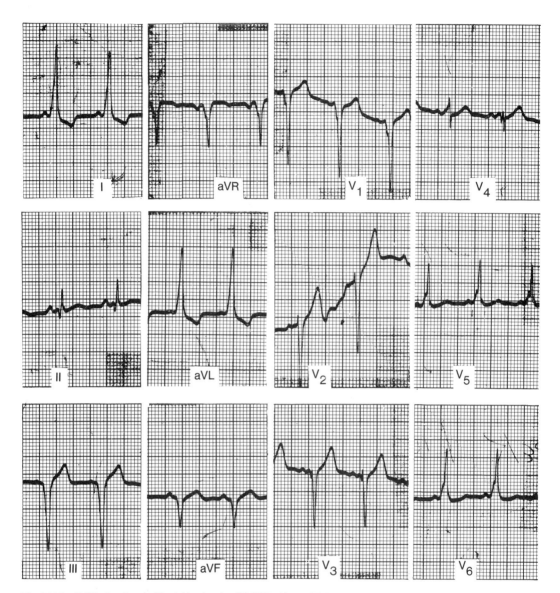

Fig 6-10d.—ECG of patient in Fig 6-10a showing Wolff-Parkinson-White type B preexcitation.

Heart Block

Various types of heart block have been reported in WPW syndrome.[9] Delay or block may occur in either pathway or in both. When block occurs in the AV nodal system, conduction through the bypass fibers may maintain cardiac rhythm. When conduction fails in the bypass fibers, the ECG is normal if AV conduction is present.

In some instances, it is possible that a block in the bypass fibers may account for the intermittency of WPW conduction. For example, WPW preexcitation seen in a bigeminal pattern may be due to 2:1 block in the anomalous pathway (Fig 6-11).

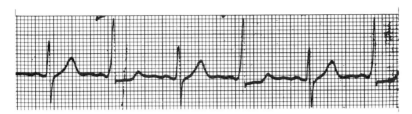

Fig 6-11.—Alternating Wolff-Parkinson-White preexcitation and normal conduction.

Congenital versus Acquired Syndrome

Occasionally, WPW syndrome has been diagnosed in individuals of advanced age, following the onset of cardiac disease. This has given rise to speculation concerning the possibility of acquired WPW syndrome. Since actual anatomical structures can be identified, however, it seems likely that these were present from birth. Some authors describe muscular bridges between the atrium and the ventricle in the normal fetal and newborn heart; these generally disappear by age 6 months.[10] It is possible that the persistence of one or more of these bridges beyond that age is the anatomical basis of WPW syndrome. The late appearance of this syndrome in an individual may be explained by several factors.

1. About 50% of persons with WPW syndrome have no symptoms and ECGs are not usually obtained in young, healthy people. Paul Dudley White[11] has quoted a colleague reporting an incidence of 1:100 in naval cadets. One must assume that these young men were in good health, since they were inducted into the navy.
2. Babies and young children are either unable to complain of symptoms or unable to describe their discomfort with any degree of accuracy.

Case Report. A four-year-old boy complained that his chest hurt. His mother, a member of our hospital staff, checked his pulse and found it to be above 180 beats/min. The subsequent thorough cardiological examination showed the boy to be in excellent health, except for the ECG shown in Figure 6-12. The youngster was placed on small doses of propranolol, and the mother was taught several vagal maneuvers as a precaution. The child has been well for several years, with no further instances of tachycardia reported. The case is described to stress the importance of following up on the frequently vague complaints of young children.

3. WPW preexcitation is intermittent in many patients, as has been shown in a number of tracings in this chapter. Even several normal ECGs do not rule out the presence of this anomaly in a patient.
4. Schamroth[12] suggests a possible explanation for intermittency or late appearance of WPW syndrome as follows. The diameter of the bypass tract is very small in comparison to the portion of myocardium in which it terminates, and the small amount of electricity passing through may not be sufficient to effect ventricular depolarization, due to mismatch impedance. If AV nodal conduction is slowed or inhibited due to disease or other factors, a greater share of the activation front will be transmitted across the accessory

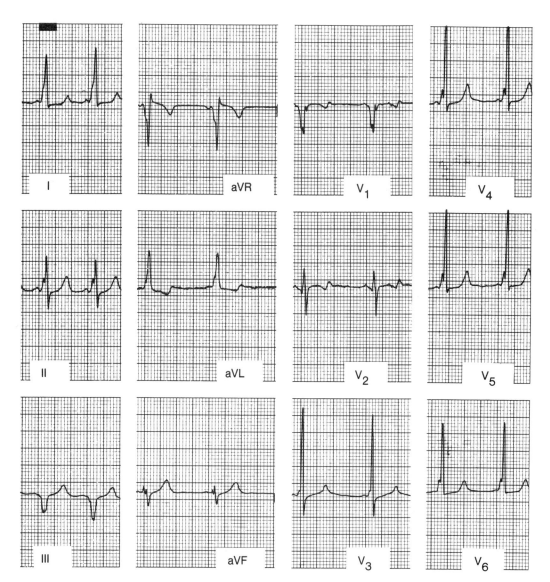

Fig 6-12.—Wolff-Parkinson-White type B preexcitation.

pathway and may be sufficient to depolarize all of, or a portion of, the ventricular myocardium. This view is supported by the results of one series of autopsies[3] in which fibrosis, inflammation, and other pathological changes were found in or near the AV nodal system in about 50% of persons with WPW syndrome.

Case Report. A 32-year-old man was brought to the emergency department with a stab wound of the chest. He had cardiac arrest almost immediately on arrival. The chest was opened, and a large amount of blood was removed from the pericardium. Mechanical ventilation, open-chest cardiac massage, defibrillation, and transfusion of large amounts of plasma and blood restored the patient sufficiently to permit transportation to the operating room. A laceration of the ascending aorta in the area immediately above the valve was closed, and the patient made a good initial recovery. About 10 days after the injury, congestive heart failure developed and was treated with digitalis and diuretics. It was at this point that the ECG first showed signs of WPW preexcitation (Fig 6-13).

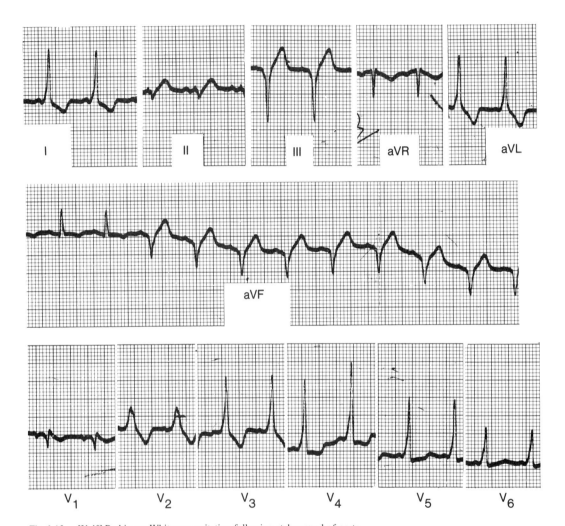

Fig 6-13.—Wolff-Parkinson-White preexcitation following stab wound of aorta.

While this was seen only intermittently in the first tracing, subsequent tracings showed WPW preexcitation throughout. No tachycardia occurred, and the patient was discharged and told to take 0.1 mg of digitoxin per day. Four years later, when he was entirely well and not taking any medications, the ECG was completely normal, with no sign of WPW syndrome or complaint of tachycardia. The incident occurred in 1966, and the patient has since been lost to cardiological followup, but his family physican reports no further problems.

Since this young man never had an ECG prior to his injury, it is impossible to determine whether the abnormality had always been present or whether it surfaced only transiently due to his injury and/or attendant treatment.

Concealed Wolff-Parkinson-White Syndrome

Kent's bundle may be present without ever giving rise to the characteristic WPW conduction; yet, it may still provide evidence of its existence by causing paroxysmal supraventricular tachycardia. The mismatch impedance previously cited may prevent antegrade conduction across the bypass fibers, but this same principle does not necessarily apply to retrograde conduction into the atrium. In such cases, the characteristic delta wave is never seen, and the QRS complexes generally look normal. This possibility should be considered in patients who have frequent, unexplained PAT. The diagnosis is made on the basis of intracardiac stimulation and recording techniques and His bundle ECGs that reveal the origin and conduction of electrical impulses within the heart.

The most common sign of reentry across Kent's bundle is the appearance of the P′ wave behind the QRS complex during tachycardia.[13] Other less characteristic signs include a negative P wave in lead I or LBBB type of aberration during tachycardia. While these findings are suggestive, it must be emphasized that they are not diagnostic or retrograde conduction across an accessory pathway.

In the tracing in Figure 6-14, the QRS complexes are completely normal, and no delta waves are seen during sinus rhythm or tachycardia. The P wave is inverted and appears immediately behind the QRS complex during the tachycardia. Electrophysiological studies proved that impulses reached the atria immediately following ventricular depolarization, without passing through the AV node.

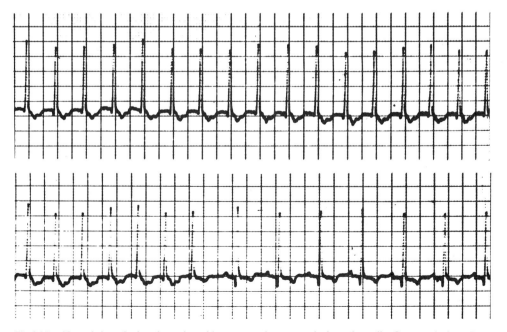

Fig 6-14.—Normal sinus rhythm alternating with paroxysmal supraventricular tachycardia. Courtesy Anthony Damato, MD.

Misleading ECG Findings

The QRS configuration in WPW preexcitation may mimic a number of other abnormalities, notably myocardial infarction.

The impressive Q waves in leads II, III, and aVF in Figure 6-15 might lead to the erroneous diagnosis of IWMI, unless the short P-R interval and the delta wave are recognized. This is not an unusual finding, and it is also seen in Figures 6-6 and 6-10.

Stress tests frequently produce false-positive results in patients with WPW syndrome. Many of these patients have depressed S-T segments in a number of

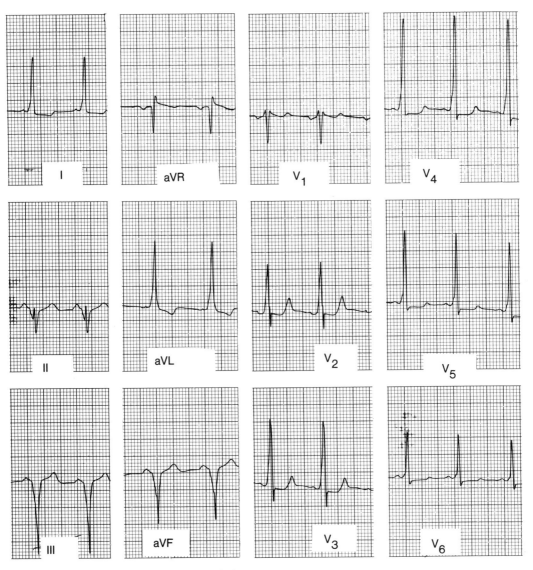

Fig 6-15.—Wolff-Parkinson-White type B preexcitation.

leads at rest, and this abnormality is further enhanced by exercise. For this reason, S-T segment depression or T wave abnormalities in these patients are not considered a sign of coronary artery disease, unless they occur in beats showing normal conduction.

On the other hand, conduction normalizes during exercise in many patients with WPW preexcitation, as shown in Figures 6-16a and 6-16b.

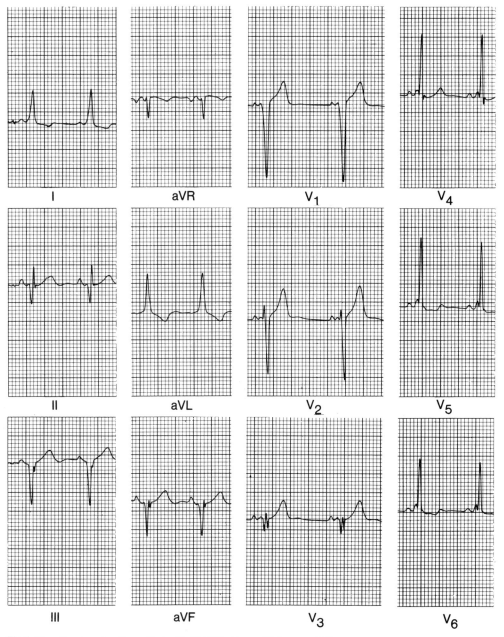

Fig 6-16a.—Tracing of resting patient with Wolff-Parkinson-White preexcitation.

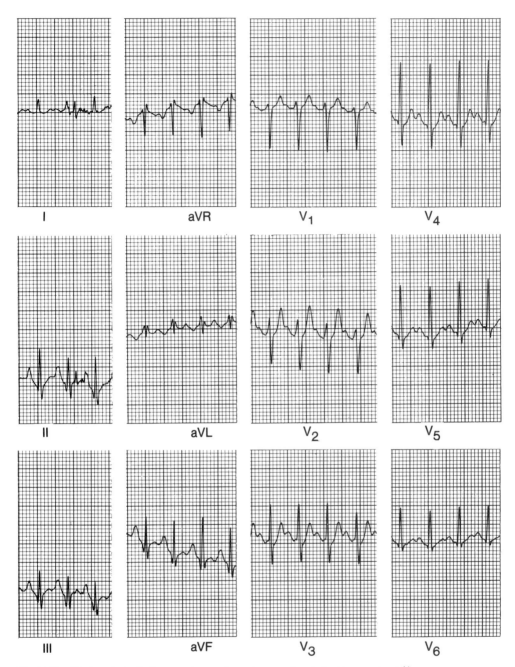

I   aVR   V₁   V₄

II   aVL   V₂   V₅

III   aVF   V₃   V₆

Fig 6-16b.—Tracing obtained after ten minutes of exercise according to the Bruce protocol.[14]

Treatment and Prognosis

Both treatment and prognosis depend on the presence of concomitant heart disease and the occurrence of tachyarrhythmias. Asymptomatic, healthy individuals require no treatment and should be encouraged to pursue a normal lifestyle. Their life expectancy is the same as that of other healthy persons of their age group.

Infants with tachycardias require prompt treatment, since their extremely rapid ventricular rates quickly cause severe heart failure, cardiovascular collapse, and death. Tachycardia in infants is usually of the reentry type, and it can safely be treated with digitalis.

Paroxysmal atrial tachycardia in the adult can often be terminated by simple vagal maneuvers or synchronized electric countershock. Intravenous propranolol, procainamide, verapamil, or lidocaine have all proved effective. Digitalis should be used only if there is certainty that the tachycardia is of the reentry type. The drug of choice for preventing tachycardia is usually propranolol. Oral quinidine, too, is effective in many patients.

Atrial flutter or fibrillation with rapid conduction through bypass fibers is most safely terminated by electric cardioversion. Intravenous administration of procainamide may terminate the arrhythmia, and lidocaine has been recommended as the drug of choice by some authors.[8] The use of digitalis is definitely contraindicated in this situation, since it may enhance conduction through the anomalous pathway and precipitate ventricular fibrillation.

Patients with severe tachycardias, especially flutter-fibrillation, require careful study, management, and education, since sudden deaths have been reported in this group, and the mortality of young patients in this group is considerably greater than is common for the age group.[1] Electrophysiological studies may be required to determine the mechanism of the arrhythmia and the most effective drug treatment for the individual patient.

Surgical intervention and the use of externally controlled pacemakers[3,8] are beyond the scope of this discussion. Interested readers will find details in the references cited.

Lown-Ganong-Levine Syndrome

Lown-Ganong-Levine (LGL) syndrome[15] is a relatively rare form of preexcitation.

Anatomical Considerations

Conduction in LGL is thought to occur across bypass fibers (first described by James[16]) that connect the atrium to the lower portion of the AV node or the bundle of His.

Electrocardiogram

ECG characteristics

- abnormally short P-R interval, followed by normal QRS complex

The P-R interval is short because the anomalous fibers bypass the AV node. Conduction occurs through the normal pathways from the bundle of His to the ventricles, so the QRS complex is normal.

Short P-R intervals may be due to an ectopic atrial pacemaker. To allow the diagnosis of LGL, the P wave must be normal, as distinguished from the abnormal P waves of ectopic atrial or junctional rhythms. Documentation or good historical evidence of tachycardia is also required to confirm the diagnosis.

Treatment and Prognosis

Treatment and prognosis are similar to that of WPW syndrome. Rare, mild tachycardia often requires no treatment, and the prognosis is excellent.

The tracing in Figure 6-17, which was obtained in a young technician at our hospital, shows a short P-R interval as an isolated abnormality. The patient reports occasional bouts of tachycardia, but these are of such short duration that we have never been able to document them. She continues in excellent health without medication.

Severe, frequent tachycardias require treatment as previously described.

Case Report. The tracing in Figure 6-18a was obtained in a girl less than 1 year of age. It shows an irregular sinus rhythm (sinus arrhythmia is very common in this age group) with very short P-R intervals of 0.08 second.

The tracing obtained during tachycardia (Fig 6-18b) shows a ventricular rate of precisely 300 beats/min, suggesting atrial flutter with 1:1 conduction.

Digitalis was used to control the tachycardia during infancy, and propranolol prophylaxis was begun when the girl became older. She has been readmitted several times with bouts of tachycardia, due to the mother's occasional failure to comply with the medical regimen.

The prognosis in these cases hinges on the ability to prevent and treat the tachycardia.

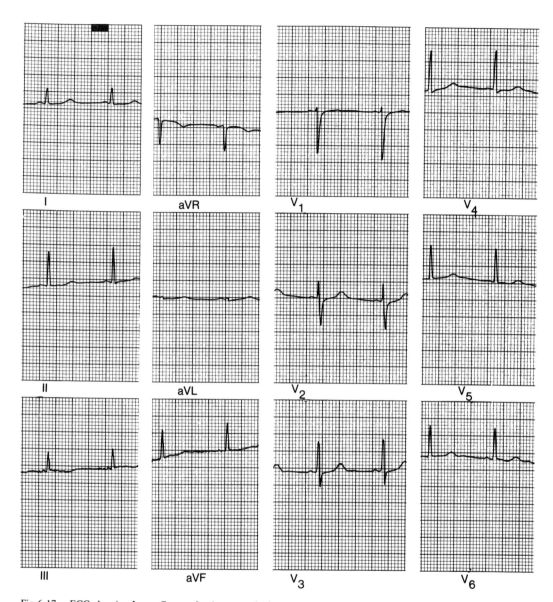

Fig 6-17.—ECG showing Lown-Ganong-Levine preexcitation.

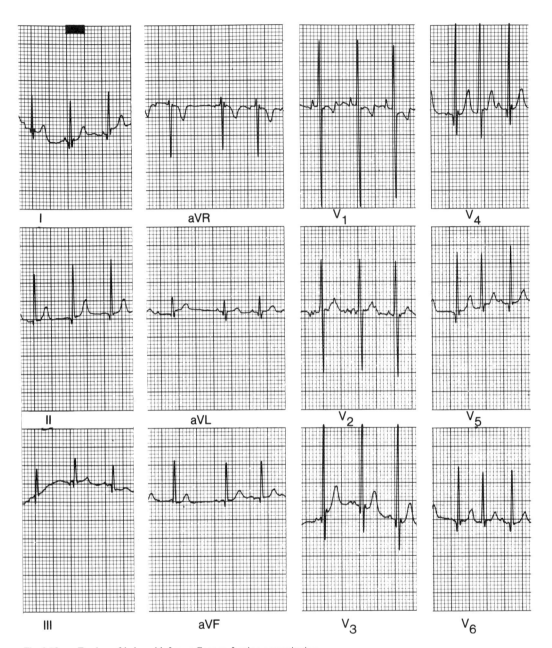

Fig 6-18a.—Tracing of baby with Lown-Ganong-Levine preexcitation.

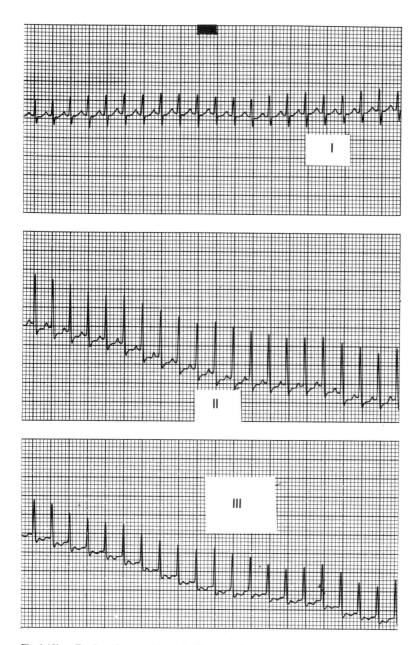

Fig 6-18b.—Tracing of same child as in Figure 6-18a during tachycardia.

Conduction through Mahaim Fibers

Conduction through Mahaim fibers is rare, and its clinical significance, if any, is rarely discussed.

Cause

- paraspecific fibers of Mahaim[17] emerge from lower nodal area, bundle of His, or bundle branches and terminate in ventricular myocardium

Electrocardiogram

ECG characteristics

- normal P-R interval, since bypass fibers begin below AV node
- QRS widened by addition of distinct delta wave caused by fiber-to-fiber impulse propagation through portion of ventricular myocardium

Case Report. A 37-year-old man underwent a stress test because of a complaint of chest pain related to exercise. The resting ECG (Fig 6-19a) shows a normal P-R interval of 0.18 second. There is distinct slurring of the ascending portion of the R wave in leads II, V_5, and V_6. The first three beats of the tracing, leads I, II, and III, show progressive widening of the QRS complex and a pronounced shift of the frontal plane QRS vector from $+60°$ to $+10°$. Such beat-to-beat variations, reflecting changes in the proportion of myocardium depolarized via bypass fibers, is not uncommon in preexcitation. If there is alternating widening and narrowing, it is referred to as a "concertina" effect.

After eight minutes of exercise, with a heart rate of 160 beats/min, the QRS width is normal and the delta wave has disappeared (Fig 6-19b). Three minutes into the recovery period, when the rate drops to 105 beats/min, the wide QRS and delta waves are again seen.

Clinical Significance

This particular form of preexcitation appears to have little clinical significance. The location of the bypass fibers below the AV node precludes both the reentrant PAT and the atrial fibrillation with rapid ventricular response that may cause serious consequences in other forms of preexcitation.

Combined Forms of Preexcitation

If a patient has several types of bypass fibers, combinations of several forms of preexcitation may be seen. For example, cases have been described in which the short P-R interval is due to conduction across James fibers, while the ventricle is depolarized in part via Mahaim fibers, producing a delta wave. In another instance,[18] electrophysiological studies showed that an apparent case of conduction through Mahaim fibers was due to abnormally slow impulse propagation through Kent's bundle. Such variations cannot be detected on the surface ECG but must be diagnosed through sophisticated electrophysiological examination.

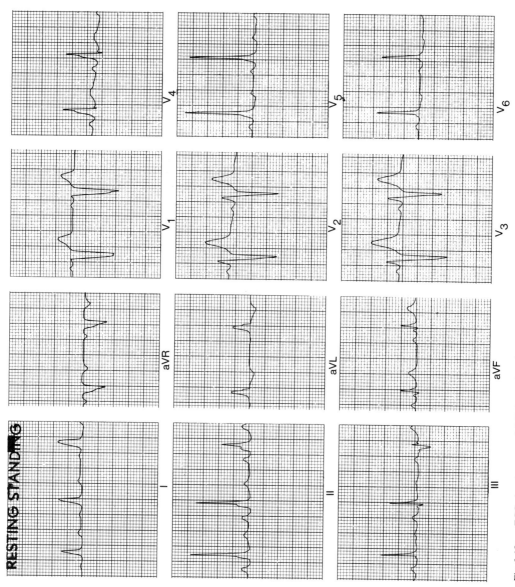

Fig 6-19a.—ECG showing normal P-R interval and delta wave.

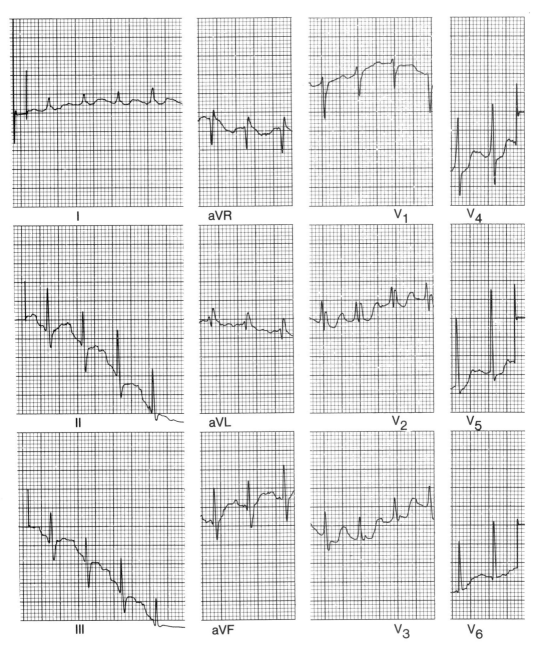

I   aVR   V₁   V₄

II   aVL   V₂   V₅

III   aVF   V₃   V₆

Fig 6-19b.—Tracing of same patient as in Fig 6-19a after 8 minutes of exercise.

Comment

The treatment and prognosis of preexcitation have been discussed in greater detail than is customary in a textbook of electrocardiography because many nurses are not as familiar with this syndrome as they are with the other abnormalities described. The fatal outcome in two young patients in the author's personal experience serves as a reminder that preexcitation is not always a benign electrocardiographic curiosity and that the role of the nurse in patient and family education is essential.

REFERENCES

1. Castellanos A, Agha AS, Castillo CA, et al: Ventricular activation in the presence of Wolff-Parkinson-White syndrome, in Dreifus LS, Watanabe Y (eds): *Cardiac Arrhythmias*. New York, Grune & Stratton, Inc, 1973, p 457.

2. Wolff L, Parkinson J, White PD: Bundle branch block with short P-R interval in healthy young people prone to paroxysmal tachycardia. *Am Heart J* 1930;5:685.

3. Sherf L, Neufeld H: *The Pre-excitation Syndromes: Facts and Theories*. New York, Yorke Medical Books, 1978.

4. Kent AFS: Researches on the structure and function of the mammalian heart. *J Physiol* 1893;14:233.

5. Boineau JP, Moore EN, Spear JF, et al: Basis of clinical ECG variation in right and left ventricular pre-excitation, in Dreifus LS, Watanabe Y (eds): *Cardiac Arrhythmias*. New York, Grune & Stratton, Inc, 1973, p 421.

6. Singh BN: The genesis of arrhythmias, in *Cornell Postgraduate Course in Cardiac Arrhythmias*. New York, Medcom, Inc, 1979, p 20. Reprinted by permission.

7. Gallagher JJ, Gilbert M, Svenson RH, et al: The Wolff-Parkinson-White syndrome. *Circulation* 1975;51:767.

8. Papa LA, Saia JA, Chung EK: Ventricular fibrillation in Wolff-Parkinson-White syndrome, type A. *Heart Lung* 1978;7:1015.

9. Dreifus LS, Watanabe Y: AV conduction block associated with Wolff-Parkinson-White syndrome, in Dreifus LS, Watanabe Y (eds): *Cardiac Arrhythmias*. New York, Grune & Stratton, Inc., 1973, p 467.

10. Wolff G, Han J, Curran J: Wolff-Parkinson-White syndrome in the neonate. *Am J Cardiol* 1978;41:559.

11. White PD: Wolff-Parkinson-White syndrome, in Sandoe E, Jensen EF, Olesen KH (eds): *Cardiac Arrhythmias*. Södertälje, Sweden, AB Astra, 1970, p 368.

12. Schamroth L: *The Disorders of Cardiac Rhythm*. Oxford, England, Blackwell Scientific Publications, 1971, p. 233.

13. Farshidi A, Josephson ME, Horowitz LN: Electrophysiologic characteristics of concealed bypass tracts: Clinical and electrocardiographic correlates. *Am J Cardiol* 1978;41:1052.

14. Bruce RA, Irving JB: Exercise electrocardiography, in Hurst JW (ed): *The Heart*. New York, McGraw-Hill Book Co, 1978, p 336.

15. Lown B, Ganong WF, Levine SA: The syndrome of short P-R interval, normal QRS complex and paroxysmal rapid heart action. *Circulation* 1952;5:693.

16. James TN: Morphology of the human atrioventricular node, with remarks pertinent to its electrophysiology. *Am Heart J* 1961;62:756.

17. Mahaim A: Kent fibers and the paraspecific conduction through the upper connection of the bundle of His-Tawara. *Am Heart J* 1947;33:651.

18. Rosen KM, Arostegui FL, Pouget JM: Pre-excitation with normal P-R intervals. *Chest* 1972;62:581.

## Chapter 7

Coronary Artery Disease

The ECG changes caused by coronary artery disease (CAD) are often referred to as ischemia, injury, and infarction. These terms correspond to, but are not synonymous with, pathological changes caused by clinical disease.

Electrophysiological Considerations

Injured or ischemic cells have a decreased resting potential, for example, -70 mV instead of -90 mV, due to loss of intracellular potassium. This slows the depolarization of the affected cells, and the resultant delay in intraventricular conduction may be reflected in widening or slurring of the QRS complex. In severely injured cells the resting potential may decrease to -60 mV or less; such cells can no longer be depolarized, and they become electrically "dead." These cells may recover, however, and resume electrical activity; thus, electrical necrosis is not identical with pathological cellular death. Cells that have been destroyed by lack of blood supply will remain unable to participate in electrical activity, even after healing and scar formation have taken place.

In the normal heart, repolarization currents move from epicardium toward endocardium. The presence of ischemia interferes with this orderly process of repolarization, and changes in the S-T segments and T waves are seen in the leads reflecting the electrical activity of the affected portion of the myocardium.

Localization of the Problem

The left ventricle may be visualized as a cone composed of the intraventricular septum and the anterior, lateral, and posterior walls. The aspects of this cone are reflected on the ECG as shown in Figure 7-1 and in Table 7-1.

193

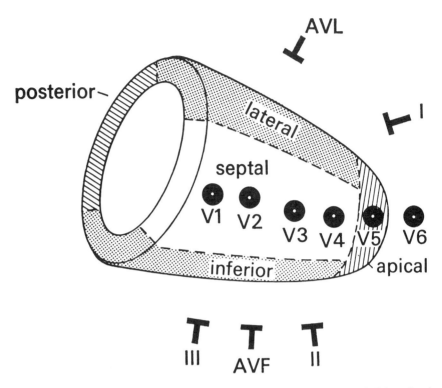

Fig 7-1.—Diagrammatic representation of various surfaces of left ventricular anatomical "cone" and their relationship to frontal and horizontal plane leads (from Schamroth[1(p17)]).

Table 7-1.—Relationship of Left Ventricular Anatomical Cone Surfaces to ECG Leads

Surface	Lead
Anteroseptal area	V_1 to V_3 or V_4
Anterior wall	V_2 to V_5 or V_6
Lateral wall	I and aVL*
Inferior (diaphragmatic)	II, III, and aVF
Posterior	V_7 to V_9
Apical	V_5 and V_6

*May include V_5 and V_6

Since all surfaces terminate at the apex, leads V_4, I, or II may be affected by disease processes involving the apex.

Myocardial ischemia and injury may be subendocardial, subepicardial, or transmural. The relative location of the problem within the muscular wall is indicated by the nature of the changes occurring in the S-T segment and T wave, as shown in Figure 7-2.

In most cases of chronic angina, the problem is subendocardial, whereas acute events such as a Prinzmetal's angina episode or a myocardial infarction are generally subepicardial or transmural.

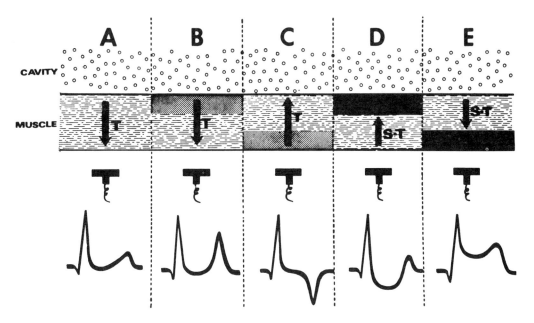

Fig 7-2.—Diagrammatic illustration of: A, the normal endocardial to epicardial T wave vector; B, the T wave vector of subendocardial ischemia; C, the T wave vector of subepicardial ischemia; D, the S-T segment vector of subendocardial injury; and E, the S-T vector of subepicardial injury (from Schamroth[1(p7)]).

Myocardial Ischemia

Ischemia usually interferes with repolarization first[1(p17)] and causes changes in the S-T segment and the T or U wave. Less frequently, the QRS complex and cardiac rhythm are also affected; however, these latter changes are not diagnostic. The ECG signs of coronary insufficiency may be permanent, or they may occur transiently during chest pain, exercise, or emotional stress.

Some controversy exists concerning the criteria used to establish the diagnosis of myocardial ischemia or injury. The most commonly used criteria and terminology are used here.

Changes in Repolarization

The normal *S-T segment* measures less than 0.12 second. It leaves the baseline shortly after its junction with the terminal portion of the QRS complex (the J point) and merges smoothly and imperceptibly with the upstroke of the T wave (Fig 7-3).

The most commonly described change with myocardial ischemia is S-T segment depression of 1 mm or more below the baseline, persisting for 0.08 second or more beyond the J point,[2] with the depressed portion horizontal, sloping downward, or showing a sagging, concave upward appearance.

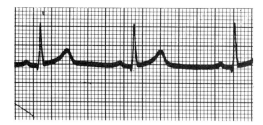

Fig 7-3.—Normal QRS-T configuration.

The rhythm strips shown in Figure 7-4 were obtained in a patient with severe coronary insufficiency. Lead I, recorded during supraventricular tachycardia, shows a depressed S-T segment with upward concavity, whereas lead V_5 of the same tracing, with the patient in sinus rhythm, shows pronounced horizontal S-T depression.

Another characteristic change occasionally described[1(p8)] shows an S-T segment that remains horizontal for 0.12 second or more and forms a distinct, sharp angle with the upstroke of the T wave. This configuration is shown in leads I, II, and aVF of Figure 7-5.

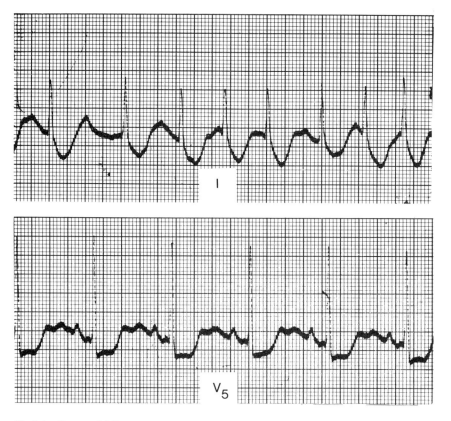

Fig 7-4.—Depressed S-T segment.

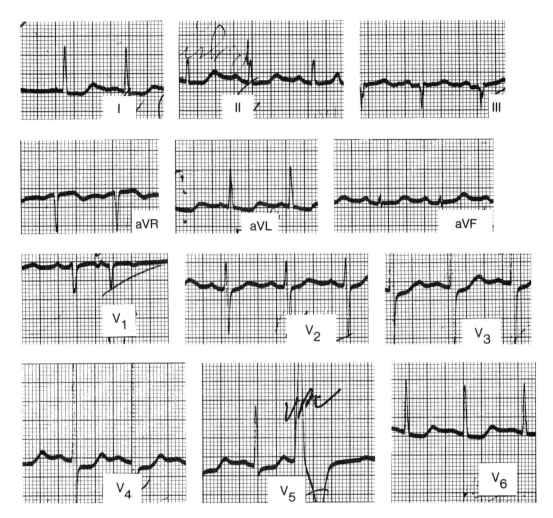

Fig 7-5.—ECG showing prolonged, flat S-T segments in several leads.

The normal *T wave* is asymmetrical, with a slow upward slope, a relatively blunt apex, and a fairly rapid descent of the distal limb (Fig 7-3). The main vector of the T wave is similar to that of the QRS complex in most leads, so that positive QRS complexes are followed by positive T waves.

The most frequent change seen as a result of ischemia is inversion of the T wave, as shown in Figure 7-6. The T wave may sometimes become more symmetrical and taller, with a narrow base and pointed apex. Inversion of the T wave of the first QRS following a premature ventricular complex, *postectopic T wave inversion* is considered to be characteristic of CAD (Fig 7-7).

Occasionally, *U waves* are seen as small deflections following the T wave. They normally measure no more than 1 mm in height and have the same vector as the QRS complex and the T wave. Inverted U waves may be caused by several pathological conditions, but U wave inversion following exercise is considered characteristic of CAD.[2(p301)]

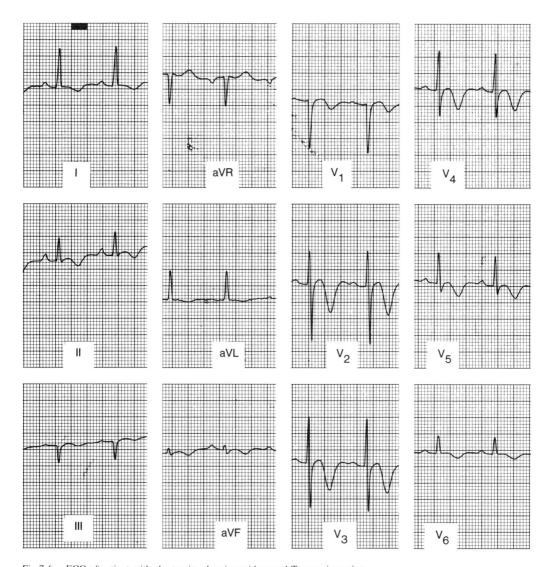

Fig 7-6.—ECG of patient with chest pain, showing widespread T wave inversion.

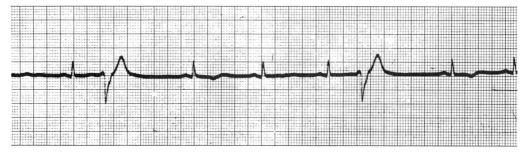

Fig 7-7.—Postectopic T wave inversion.

The tracing in Figure 7-8 shows a number of characteristics of myocardial ischemia: the S-T segment hugs the baseline for more than 0.12 second (V_3 to V_6); the T waves are tall, symmetrical, and pointed (V_3, V_4); and the initial portion of the U wave is inverted (V_2 through V_4).

The *Q-T interval* is directly proportionate to the preceding R-R interval, growing shorter with increasing heart rates. Normal Q-T intervals are shown in Table 7-2. When the T wave is inverted due to ischemia, the Q-T interval is frequently prolonged (Figs 7-5 and 7-6). Q-T prolongation per se is not a specific sign of myocardial ischemia, since it may be caused by a number of other factors.

In most cases of myocardial ischemia, several of these changes are present, as shown in Figures 7-5, 7-6, and 7-8. Improvement or worsening of the patient's condition may be reflected by changes seen in tracings obtained at different times.

Table 7-2.—Q-T Interval: Normal Range for Various Heart Rates and Cycle Lengths

Heart rate, min	Cycle length (R-R interval), s	Men and children, s	Women, s
40	1.50	0.45 - 0.49	0.46 - 0.50
43	1.40	0.44 - 0.48	0.45 - 0.49
46	1.30	0.43 - 0.47	0.44 - 0.48
48	1.25	0.42 - 0.46	0.43 - 0.47
50	1.20	0.41 - 0.45	0.43 - 0.46
52	1.15	0.41 - 0.45	0.42 - 0.46
55	1.10	0.40 - 0.44	0.41 - 0.45
57	1.05	0.39 - 0.43	0.40 - 0.44
60	1.00	0.39 - 0.42	0.40 - 0.43
63	0.95	0.38 - 0.41	0.39 - 0.42
67	0.90	0.37 - 0.40	0.38 - 0.41
71	0.85	0.36 - 0.38	0.37 - 0.41
75	0.80	0.35 - 0.38	0.36 - 0.39
80	0.75	0.34 - 0.37	0.35 - 0.38
86	0.70	0.33 - 0.36	0.34 - 0.37
93	0.65	0.32 - 0.35	0.33 - 0.36
100	0.60	0.31 - 0.34	0.32 - 0.35
109	0.55	0.30 - 0.33	0.31 - 0.33
120	0.50	0.28 - 0.31	0.29 - 0.32
133	0.45	0.27 - 0.29	0.28 - 0.30
150	0.40	0.25 - 0.28	0.26 - 0.28
172	0.35	0.23 - 0.26	0.24 - 0.26

Table 7-2 is adapted from Friedman.[2(p601)] Used by permission of the American Heart Association.

The tracing in Figure 7-9 is from a patient with CAD; the S-T segment following a prolonged R-R interval is depressed but horizontal, whereas the complexes with a shorter R-R interval show down-sloping of the S-T segment and frank inversion of the T wave. This probably reflects worsening of ischemia, as an increase in myocardial work increases the demand for oxygen.

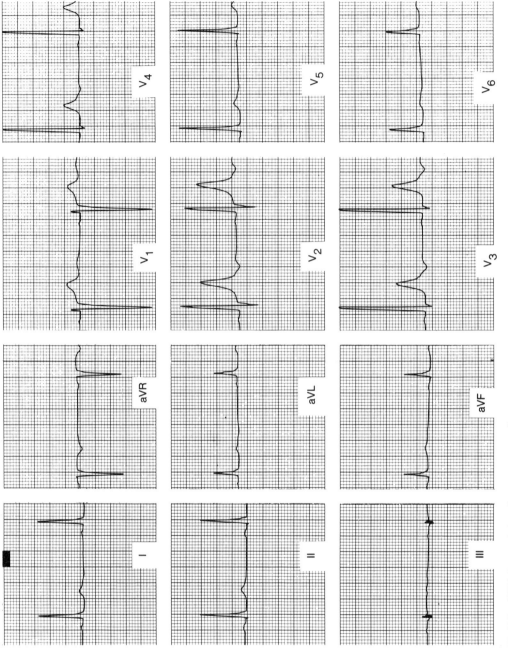

Fig 7-8.—ECG characteristics of coronary artery disease.

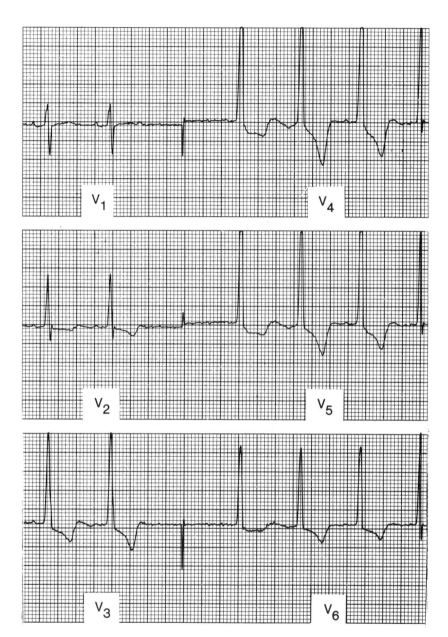

Fig 7-9.—Depressed S-T segment and T wave inversion related to heart rate.

Occasionally, T wave inversion may be a *normal variant*.[3] An example of this phenomenon is shown in a series of ECGs in Figures 7-10a through c obtained from a healthy 34-year-old woman.

The tracing in Figure 7-10a was obtained with the woman in a standing position. The tracing obtained in a supine position (Fig 7-10b) shows ''improvement'' of the T wave inversion, and an ECG obtained following ten minutes of exercise (Fig 7-10c) is nearly normal. This sequence clearly illustrates the importance of evaluating all ECG changes in light of the total clinical picture.

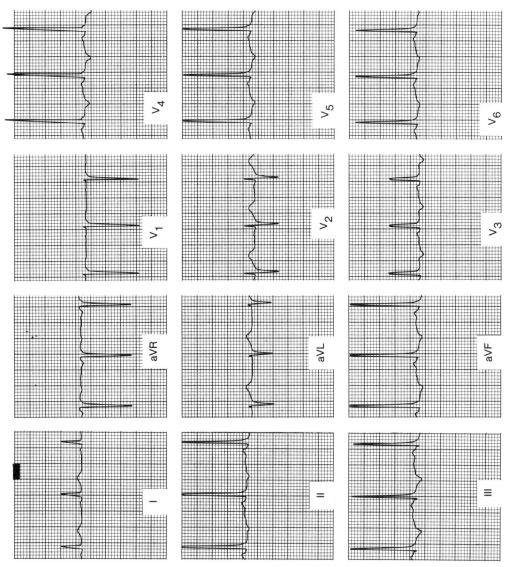

Fig 7-10a.—ECG of healthy young woman in standing position, showing T wave inversion.

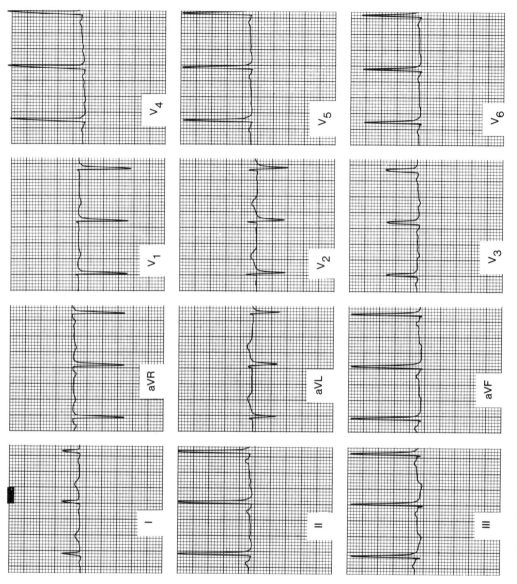

Fig 7-10b.—ECG of patient in Fig 7-10a, in supine position.

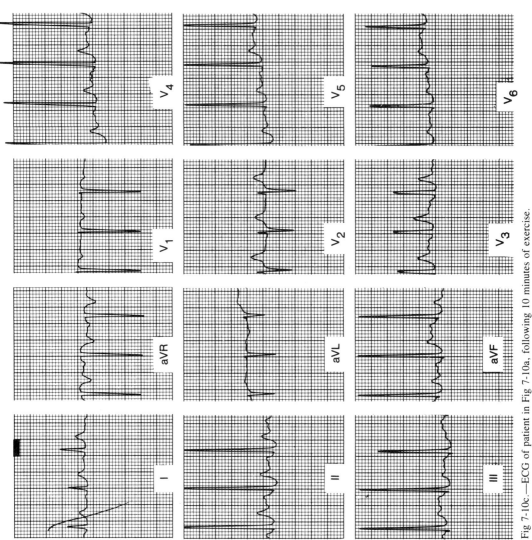

Fig 7-10c.—ECG of patient in Fig 7-10a, following 10 minutes of exercise.

Clinical Comment

All abnormalities of repolarization must be viewed in light of several factors

- administration of cardiac drugs, diuretics, and antihypertensive agents
- presence of LBBB or left ventricular hypertrophy
- electrolyte disturbances

Changes in QRS Complex

Both RBBB and LBBB as well as LAH may be due to coronary insufficiency.[1(p140)] Although such conduction defects are not a specific sign of ischemia, the sudden appearance of LBBB, in particular, should be viewed with great suspicion, since it is usually a sign of advanced coronary and/or hypertensive heart disease. Forty-eight percent of the 51 patients in the Framingham study[4] who suddenly developed LBBB also showed clinical signs of CAD or congestive heart failure for the first time.

Cardiac Arrhythmias

Myocardial ischemia may cause all types of arrhythmias, such as AV conduction defects and ventricular ectopy. Acute, severe ischemia may precipitate ventricular tachycardia and fibrillation, causing sudden death in patients who do not exhibit pathological evidence of myocardial infarction.

Exercise Stress Tests

Many patients with significant CAD have a normal ECG during asymptomatic periods, making accurate diagnosis difficult. Exercise causes an increase in myocardial oxygen demand and usually precipitates myocardial ischemia in patients with coronary insufficiency. The exercise stress test is designed to obtain evidence of this event under controlled conditions.

The test consists of performance of increasing, standardized work loads on a specially equipped treadmill or bicycle.[5] The ECG and physiological factors such as blood pressure and, at times, oxygen consumption are monitored throughout the test, and 12-lead tracings are obtained before and at specific intervals during and after the test. The patient is also encouraged to verbalize any symptoms. The test may be terminated by the cardiologist because of unfavorable physiological or ECG changes or by the patient because of symptoms or fatigue.

The factors considered in establishing the diagnosis of CAD are ECG changes, unfavorable physiological response, and subjective symptoms.

ECG Changes

There is considerable controversy concerning the degree of change required to make a definite diagnosis of CAD.[6] Test results may be interpreted with great specificity, that is, the criteria for a positive test can be so strict that there will be very few false-positive results. By this method a number of individuals with definite CAD will have normal results. On the other hand, the sensitivity of the test can be increased by using minimal criteria. This will ensure that all persons with CAD are identified, but this method produces many false-positive results. For example, Masters et al[7] considered an S-T depression greater than 0.5 mm in any lead as a positive sign, but this degree of depression occurs in up to 25% of normal individuals.[1(p160)] It is essential to use criteria and methods that identify individuals with CAD, while avoiding a false-positive diagnosis that may turn a healthy individual into a "cardiac cripple." The following criteria are used in many institutions. To avoid errors in diagnosis, they must be interpreted in the light of the patient's total clinical picture.

Horizontal S-T depression of 1 mm or more that continues for 0.08 second or more is characteristic of CAD and constitutes a positive stress test.

The series of tracings in Figures 7-11a through c shows the typical exercise response of a patient with CAD. The resting tracing (Fig 7-11a) shows only minor, nonspecific abnormalities. After three minutes of exercise (Fig 7-11b), there was beginning S-T segment depression in leads II, III, and aVF and in the left precordial leads. After six minutes of exercise, the S-T depression was marked, and the test was terminated.

J point depression occurs with increasing heart rates in many normal individuals. It is a sign of CAD only if the S-T segment remains more than 2 mm below the baseline for more than 0.08 second.[6] Figure 7-12 shows some J point depression in a healthy young woman after nine minutes of exercise with a heart rate of 190 beats/min.

The S-T segment slopes steeply upward from the J point and merges with the T wave in a smooth curve. An imaginary parabola drawn from the down stroke of the P wave continues smoothly to the upstroke of the T wave. This is not the case if the depression is due to ischemia. The difference is clearly illustrated in Figure 7-13.

Figure 7-14a is the tracing of a 29-year-old marathon runner, showing sinus arrhythmia and pronounced sinus bradycardia at rest. After 17½ minutes of exercise (a feat that is not often achieved), the heart rate is about 165 beats/min (Fig 7-14b), and there is a normal, physiological S-T depression.

S-T segment elevation of 1 mm or more during or immediately following exercise is a sign of subepicardial ischemia or injury.

T wave inversion occurring during exercise is usually a sign of CAD, especially if the T wave is symmetrical, pointed, and deeper than 2 mm.

An increase in the height of the T wave and a more symmetrical configuration may reflect subendocardial ischemia. This change is often accompanied by S-T depression. If it occurs as an isolated finding, it must be interpreted with caution, since the height of the T wave may increase with exercise in healthy individuals.

A U wave inversion during or following exercise is a positive sign.

Intraventricular conduction defects may develop but are not a specific sign.

An increase in the height of the R wave has also been described as an indication of CAD.[8]

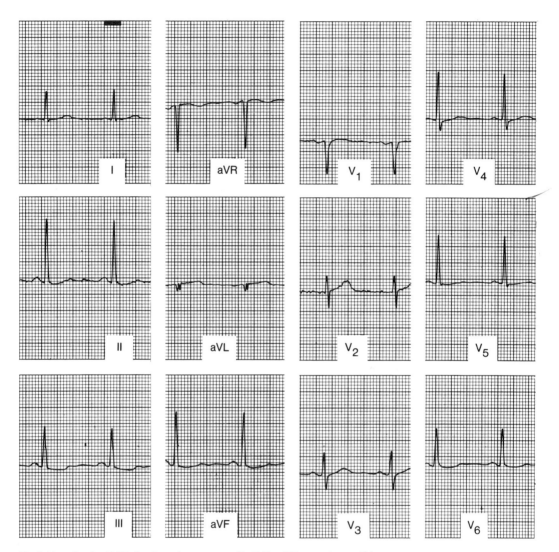

Fig 7-11a.—Resting ECG showing minor, nonspecific S-T and T wave abnormalities.

S-T segment and T wave changes during exercise must be interpreted with caution in patients with such clinical problems as left ventricular hypertrophy and preexcitation.

Cardiac Arrhythmias

Supraventricular arrhythmias are seen in normal subjects as frequently as in patients with cardiovascular disease.[9]

Ventricular arrhythmias occur in healthy persons, as well as in patients with valvular, organic, and ischemic heart disease. The incidence of ventricular arrhythmias increases with increasing sinus rates; at rates above 170 beats/min,

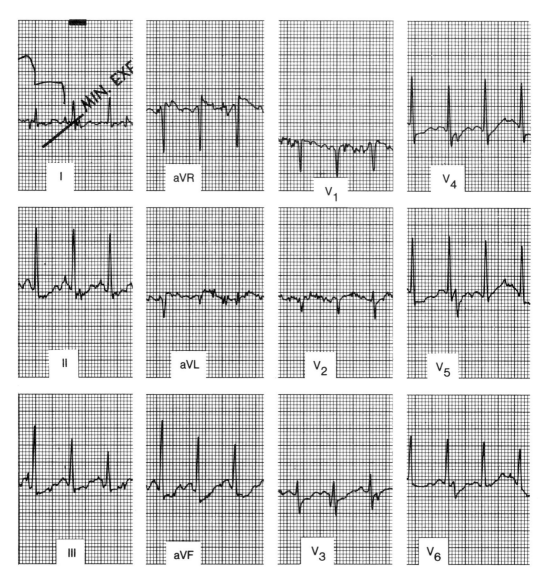

Fig 7-11b.—Tracing of patient in Fig 7-11a after 3 minutes of exercise.

ventricular ectopic activity has been seen in 44% of healthy individuals tested.[9] Two major differences between normal subjects and those with CAD have been reported. At sinus rates below 130 beats/min, ventricular arrhythmias occurred in only 6% of healthy persons but in 27% of patients with CAD. The latter group tends to exhibit more complex arrhythmias, such as multifocal or coupled PVCs and ventricular tachycardia.[9] We have also noted that these ventricular arrhythmias may occur immediately following, rather than during, exercise.

The appearance of PVCs as the sole abnormality during exercise does not permit the diagnosis of CAD. A patient who has multifocal and coupled ventricular

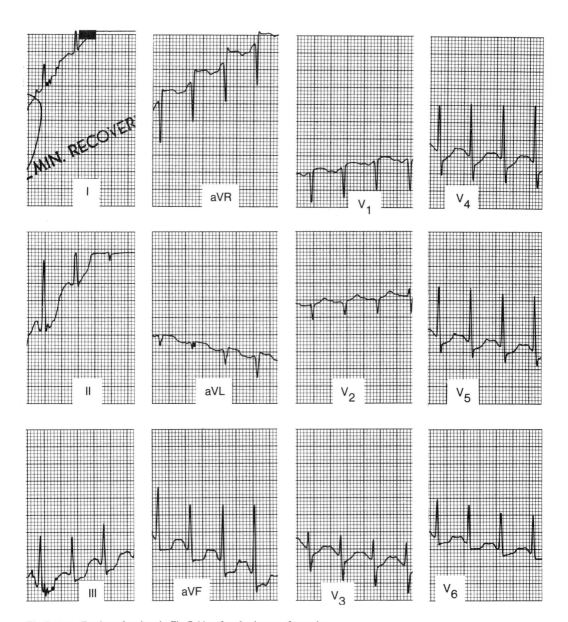

Fig 7-11c.—Tracing of patient in Fig 7-11a after 6 minutes of exercise.

extrasystoles and ventricular tachycardia should be examined further, even if the test appears to be otherwise negative. If there are additional positive signs, careful management is required, since a high incidence of sudden death has been reported in patients with CAD and complex ventricular arrhythmias.

AV conduction defects and bradycardia may occur during exercise (Fig 4-31b). These are not necessarily indicative of ischemic heart disease and must be evaluated in light of the total clinical findings.

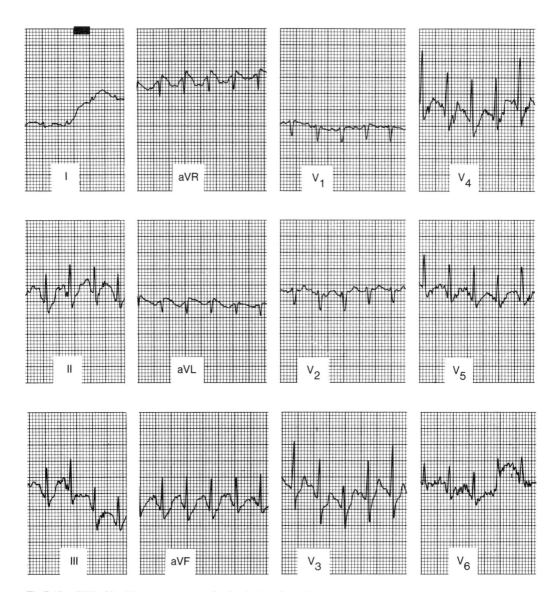

Fig 7-12.—ECG of healthy young woman after 9 minutes of exercise.

Physiological and Symptomatic Findings

Frequent signs of CAD are a decrease of systolic blood pressure or the development of characteristic *anginal discomfort,* that is, pain and/or pressure in the substernal area. These signs are used to substantiate ECG findings. But even in the absence of positive ECG signs, they require further investigation. In doubtful cases, a thallium stress test should be performed to confirm the diagnosis.[10,11]

A

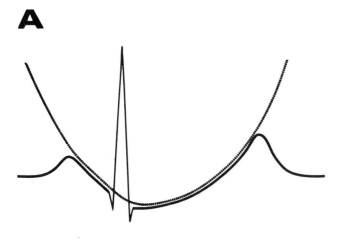

B

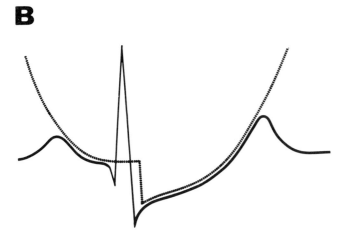

Fig 7-13.—Diagrams illustrating: A, the normal unbroken parabola of physiological junctional S-T segment depression; and B, the broken parabola of abnormal junctional S-T segment depression (from Schamroth[1(p160)]).

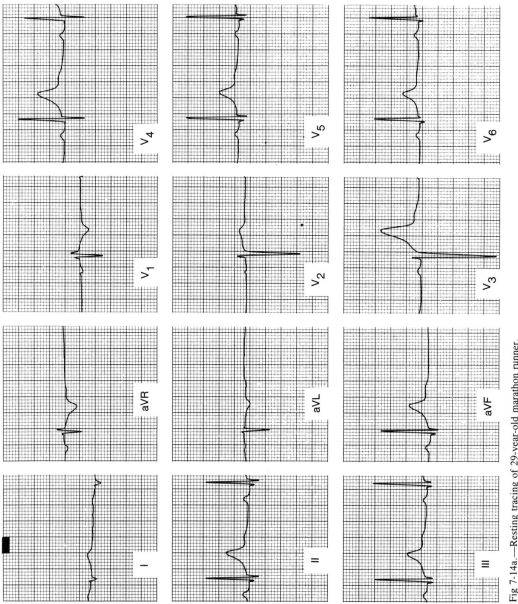

Fig 7-14a.—Resting tracing of 29-year-old marathon runner.

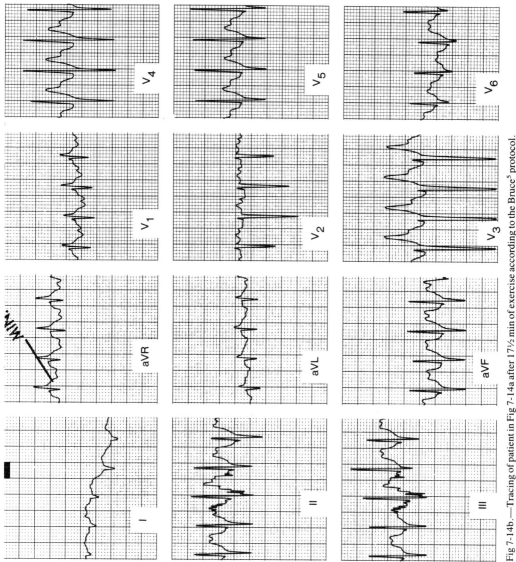

Fig 7-14b.—Tracing of patient in Fig 7-14a after 17½ min of exercise according to the Bruce[5] protocol.

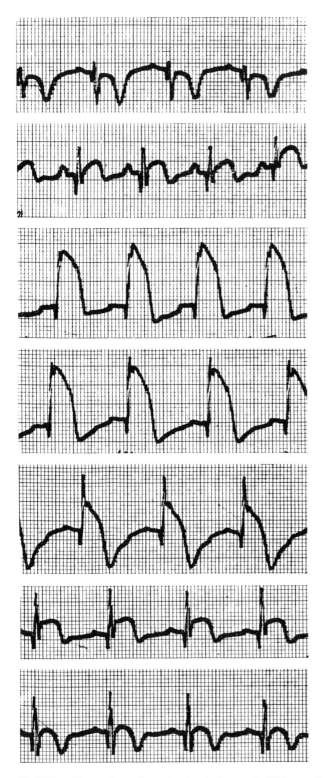

Fig 7-15a.—Consecutive tracings of patient during attack of Prinzmetal's angina.

Prinzmetal's Angina

A variant form of angina was first described by Prinzmetal et al in 1959.[12] It differs from the common form of myocardial ischemia in ECG appearance, precipitating factors, and pathology.

ECG characteristics

Prinzmetal's angina is characterized by sudden, pronounced, transient elevation of the S-T segment. The elevation occurs directly above the area of myocardium affected by insufficient blood flow and is usually accompanied by chest pain. This usually lasts for a short time, and then the ECG returns to normal.

The rhythm strips in Figures 7-15a and b were obtained during an attack of Prinzmetal's angina that lasted about 20 minutes.

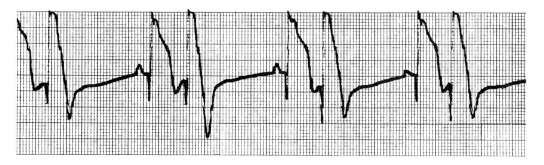

Fig 7-15b.—Ventricular bigeminy in patient in Fig 7-15a, during attack of angina.

Cardiac Arrhythmias

Attacks of Prinzmetal's angina are accompanied by cardiac dysrhythmias in as many as 40% of patients.[13] All types of arrhythmias may be seen, with ventricular ectopic activity predominating.[14] We have seen several instances of ventricular tachycardia beginning almost simultaneously with the sudden onset of S-T elevation. This may easily degenerate into ventricular fibrillation and result in sudden death if the patient is not hospitalized.

Precipitating Factors

Whereas the common form of angina is usually precipitated by physical stress, Prinzmetal's angina frequently occurs during sleep. We have observed several patients who were sleeping soundly when sudden S-T elevation was noted on the monitor. The patients awakened within seconds or minutes and complained of severe pain. Occasionally, it is possible to provoke this type of attack by exercise stress testing.[15]

The patient whose tracings are shown in Figures 7-16a and b was referred for a stress test because of severe nocturnal chest pain. The resting tracing (Fig 7-16a) shows minimal S-T depression in a number of leads, together with some flattening of the S-T segment in leads V_5 and V_6. While these changes may raise the suspicion of possible myocardial ischemia, especially in view of the history, they are not sufficient to allow the diagnosis of CAD.

After six minutes of exercise, the patient complained of increasing substernal pressure, and the tracing obtained at that time (Fig 7-16b) shows significant elevation of the S-T segment in leads V_2 through V_4. After an additional 1½ minutes of exercise, the heart rate and blood pressure began to fall, the substernal pressure increased, and the S-T elevation increased, leading to termination of the test.

The ECG signs and physical symptoms persisted during the first three minutes of recovery. At this time, nitroglycerin (0.4 mg) was administered sublingually, and the S-T segment returned almost immediately to preexercise level.

Pathology and Diagnosis

Angina pectoris is generally due to a fixed lesion in one or more coronary vessels, whereas Prinzmetal's angina is caused by spasm in a coronary artery segment. Until recently, this posed considerable diagnostic problems, since patients with Prinzmetal's angina frequently have normal resting and exercise ECGs, and it may not be possible to document the presence of spasm by coronary angiography or thallium stress testing. It is most important, however, that the problem be identified so that appropriate treatment can be started, since this variant form of angina may cause myocardial infarction and sudden death.[16]

To establish the diagnosis of Prinzmetal's angina, several methods have been used to provoke spasm under controlled circumstances. They include exercise stress testing,[14,15] Valsalva maneuvers,[14] cold pressure tests,[17] and injection of ergonovine maleate.[18,19]

The ergonovine test may be performed with continuous ECG monitoring in the coronary care unit (CCU) during cardiac catheterization, or with thallium scintigraphy. The evidence of the spasm becomes apparent as S-T elevation.

As soon as the spasm is documented, nitroglycerin is administered, usually intravenously, to prevent myocardial infarction and dysrhythmias. The effect of nitroglycerin injection is immediate, and all signs of spasm, including pain, disappear within seconds in most instances. This test is not without danger, however, and should only be performed under strictly controlled conditions, with emergency equipment and sufficient skilled help readily available. It should probably not be undertaken if the patient is known to also have fixed, severe coronary obstructions.[18,19]

Clinical Comment

The identification of coronary artery spasm is essential to the appropriate treatment of the patient. The β-blockers such as propranolol, which are so effective in the treatment of the usual form of angina, may actually cause a

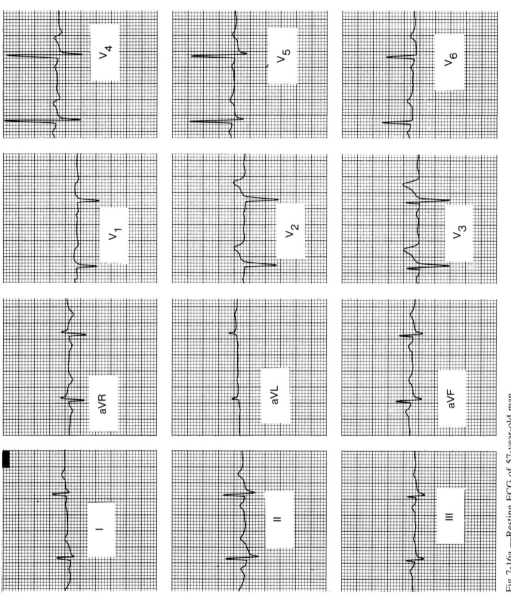

Fig 7-16a.—Resting ECG of 57-year-old man.

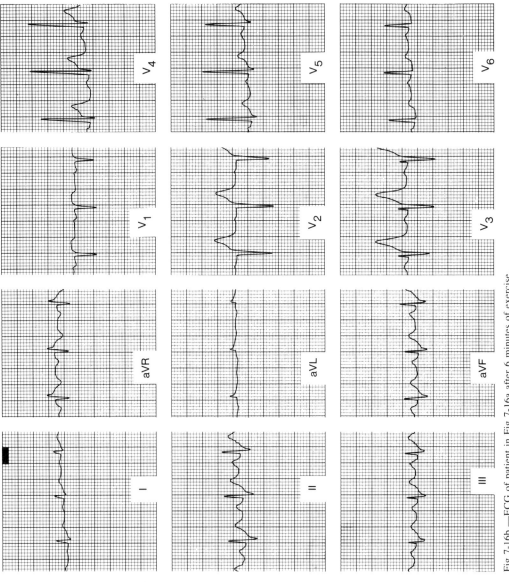

Fig 7-16b.—ECG of patient in Fig 7-16a after 6 minutes of exercise.

worsening in the condition of the patient with Prinzmetal's angina.[20] Instead, a relatively new group of medications, calcium antagonists (slow channel blockers), are increasingly used to prevent and treat coronary artery spasm. These include verapamil, nifedipine, and diltiazem.[14,20]

"Mixed" Lesions

Coronary spasm and fixed lesions may coexist in the same patient. Coronary angiography revealed that most of our patients with Prinzmetal's angina also had fixed obstructive lesions (Figs 7-15 through 7-17). It is also likely that an element of spasm is involved in many instances of myocardial infarction.[17]

The tracing in Figure 7-17a was obtained in a 54-year-old-man who was referred for evaluation of repeated episodes of substernal pressure and pain radiating to the jaw, which occurred both during activity and rest. At the time of the test, the patient was treated with nitroglycerin (Nitrobid ointment) and propranolol. The sinus bradycardia shown on the resting tracing is probably due to propranolol. The resting tracing was considered to be within broad normal limits.

After 1½ minutes of exercise, the patient complained of chest pain, and there were elevations of the S-T segments in leads II, III, and aVF and in leads V_1 through V_4. The test was terminated after two minutes of exercise, and oxygen and sublingual nitroglycerin were administered immediately.

Numerous PVCs began to appear, and a tracing obtained after ½ minute of recovery (Fig 7-17b) shows three consecutive PVCs. There were persistent S-T elevations in leads III and aVF, together with reciprocal changes in leads I and aVL. The S-T elevation in lead V_1 can still be seen in the tracing in Figure 7-17c, which was obtained one minute into the recovery period. The pain disappeared rapidly, and the tracing returned to normal within minutes.

Because the S-T elevation occurred during the stress test, it was decided that the patient probably had Prinzmetal's angina. This diagnosis was confirmed by the sequence of tracings in Figures 7-18a and b, which occurred spontaneously two days later while the patient was resting quietly in bed in the CCU.

The patient had undergone coronary angiography on the previous day and fixed lesions had been identified in the right coronary artery, as well as in the anterior descending branch of the left coronary artery.

An ergonovine test was performed at this time, to clearly demonstrate the presence of spasm in addition to the obstructive lesions. The results of this test are documented in the tracings shown in Figures 7-19a through c, which were obtained over a span of five minutes.

Immediately after injection of 0.1 mg of ergonovine, the S-T segments began to rise, and two minutes after injection, reached considerable height in leads II, III, aVF, and V_1 (Fig 7-19b).

Ventricular tachycardia then developed. Intravenous injection of nitroglycerin (1.6 mg) resulted in instantaneous resumption of normal sinus rhythm, rapid reduction of the pain, and improvement in the electrocardiogram. Within five minutes of the initial injection of ergonovine, the ECG had returned to normal.

The test recorded here not only demonstrates the presence of coronary artery spasm but is an effective illustration of the potential deadliness of acute myocardial ischemia.

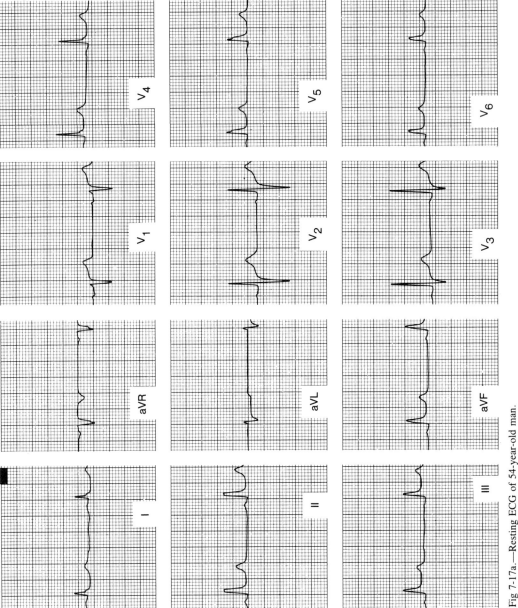

Fig 7-17a.—Resting ECG of 54-year-old man.

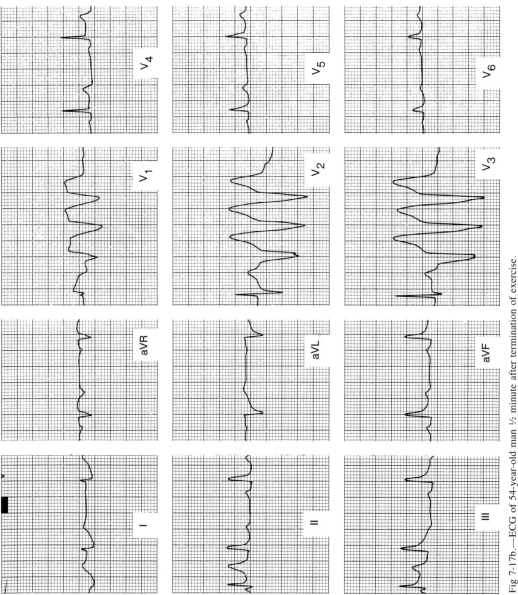

Fig 7-17b.—ECG of 54-year-old man ½ minute after termination of exercise.

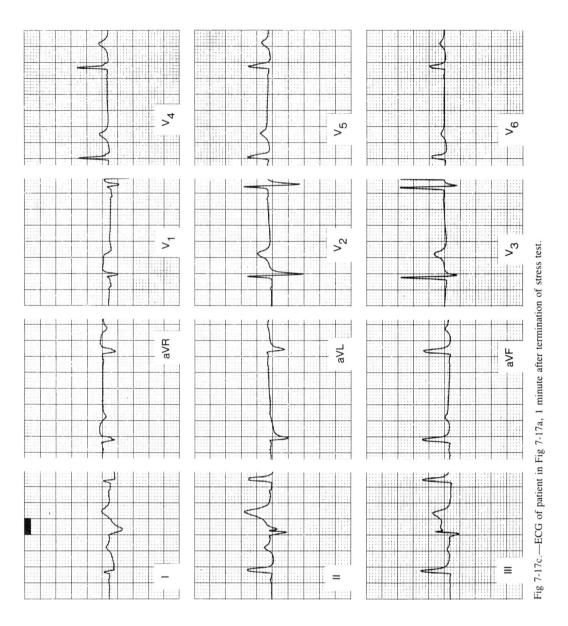

Fig 7-17c.—ECG of patient in Fig 7-17a, 1 minute after termination of stress test.

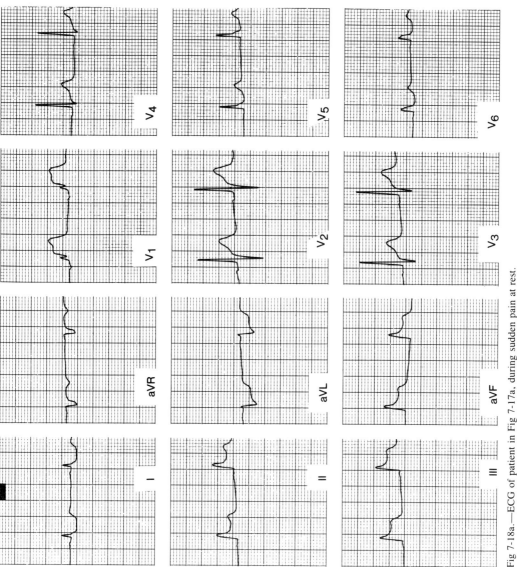

Fig 7-18a.—ECG of patient in Fig 7-17a, during sudden pain at rest.

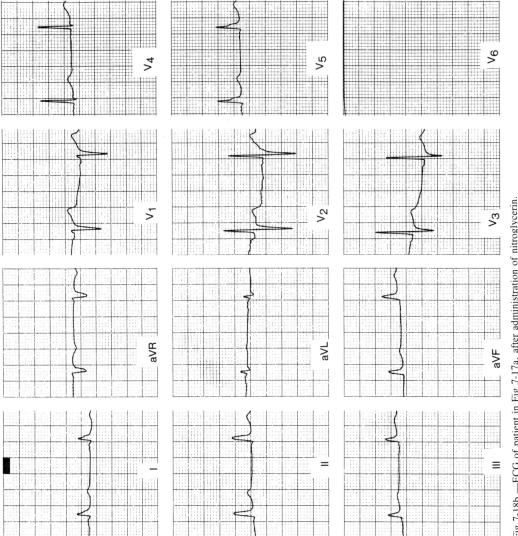

Fig 7-18b.—ECG of patient in Fig 7-17a, after administration of nitroglycerin.

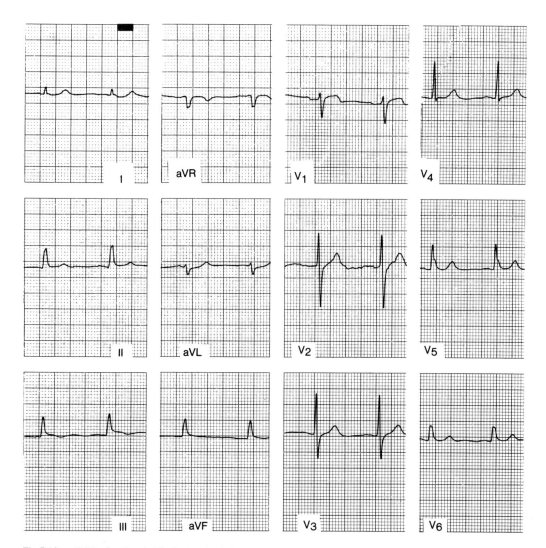

Fig 7-19a.—ECG of patient in Fig 7-18a after injection of ergonovine.

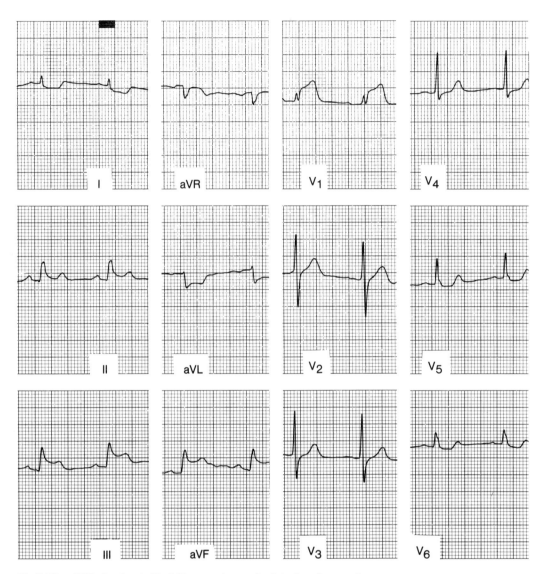

Fig 7-19b.—ECG of patient in Fig 7-18a two minutes after injection of ergonovine.

Subsequently, the patient began to receive nifedipine (20 mg four times a day) and did well. One week later the exercise stress test was repeated to evaluate the results of therapy. The results are shown in Figures 7-20a and b.

The test was terminated after four minutes because of chest pain. The tracing taken at this time (Fig 7-20b) shows slight S-T depression and T wave inversion in leads II, III, and aVF and in the left precordial leads. These changes are usually seen with angina in the presence of fixed obstruction. The administration of nifedipine obviously prevented the recurrence of the spasm previously document-ed, and the S-T and T wave changes on the last tracing are due to this patient's obstructive lesions, discovered during coronary angiography.

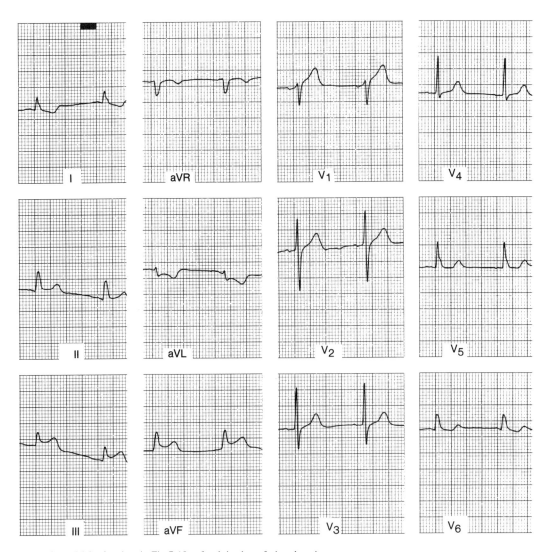

Fig 7-19c.—ECG of patient in Fig 7-18a after injection of nitroglycerin.

Clinical Comment

Today, follow-up studies of the patient with chest pain are much more vigorous and aggressive than they had been in the past. It is no longer acceptable to use a normal resting ECG as confirmation of the absence of CAD. Stress testing, thallium tests, and coronary angiography are used increasingly to determine the presence, location, and nature of obstruction of coronary blood flow. The results facilitate the institution of appropriate medical and/or surgical therapy, which will alleviate pain, and hopefully, prevent myocardial infarction.

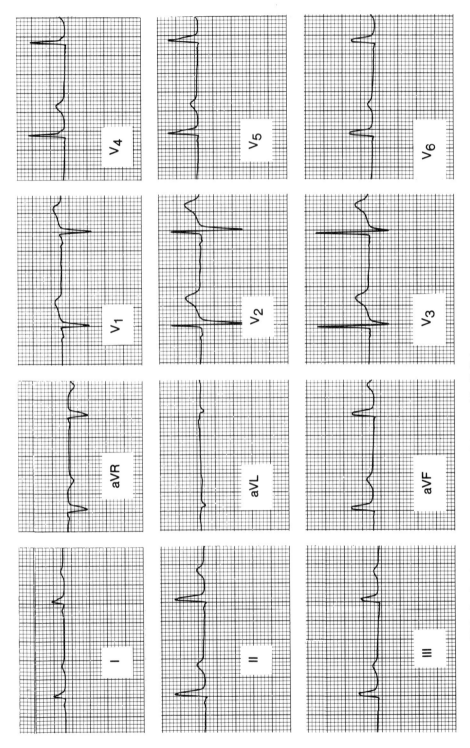

Fig 7-20a.—Resting ECG of patient in Fig 7-18a after 1 week of therapy with nifedipine.

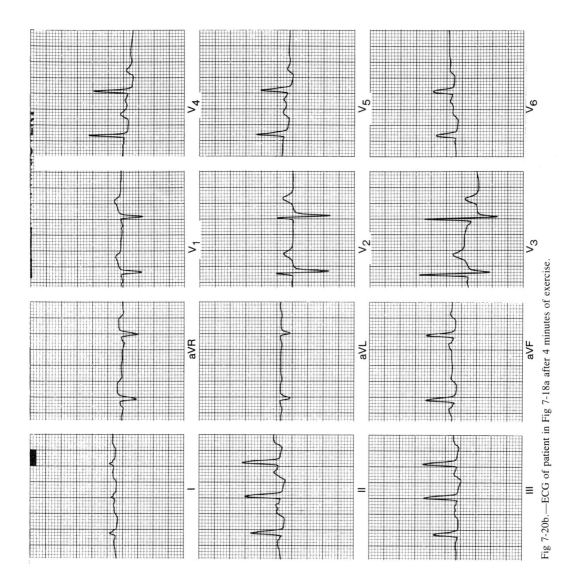

Fig 7-20b.—ECG of patient in Fig 7-18a after 4 minutes of exercise.

REFERENCES

1. Schamroth L: *The Electrocardiology of Coronary Artery Disease*. Oxford, England, Blackwell Scientific Publications, 1975. Reprinted by permission.

2. Friedman HH: *Diagnostic Electrocardiography and Vector Cardiography*, ed 2. New York, McGraw-Hill Book Co, 1977.

3. St Mary E, Virgin H, Castillo C, et al: The "variant normal" electrocardiogram of the professional football player. *Phys Sports Med* 1978;6:85.

4. Schneider JF, Thomas HE, Kreger BE, et al: Newly acquired left bundle branch block: The Framingham study. *Ann Intern Med* 1979;5:303.

5. Bruce RA, Irving JB: Special electrocardiographic examination of the heart, in Hurst JW (ed): *The Heart*. New York, McGraw-Hill Book Co, 1978, pp 336-348.

6. Zohman LR, Kattus AA: Exercise testing in the diagnosis of coronary heart disease: A perspective. *Am J Cardiol* 1977;40:243.

7. Master AM, Friedman R, Dack S: The electrocardiogram after standard exercise as functional test of the heart. *Am Heart J* 1942;24:777.

8. Berman JL, Wynne J, Cohn PF: Multiple lead QRS changes with exercise testing, diagnostic value and hemodynamic implications. *Circulation* 1980;61:53.

9. Favis JV, Morris SN: Detection, prevalence and significance of arrhythmias during exercise. *Heart Lung* 1981;10:644.

10. Botvinick EH, Taradash MR, Shames DM, et al: Thallium-201 myocardial perfusion scintigraphy for the clinical clarification of normal, abnormal and equivocal electrocardiographic stress tests. *Am J Cardiol* 1978;41:43.

11. Leppo J, Yipintsoi T, Blankstein R, et al: Thallium-201 myocardial scintigraphy in patients with triple-vessel disease and ischemic exercise stress tests. *Circulation* 1979;59:715.

12. Prinzmetal M, Ekmekci A, Kennaner R, et al: Angina pectoris I: A variant form of angina pectoris. *Am J Med* 1959;27:375.

13. Cain RS, Ferguson RM, Tillisch JH: Variant angina: A nursing approach. *Heart Lung* 1979;8:1122.

14. Kennedy GT: Variant angina: Clinical spectrum, pathophysiology, and management. *Heart Lung* 1981;10:1073.

15. Fuller CM, Raizner AE, Chahine RA, et al: Exercise-induced coronary arterial spasm: Angiographic demonstration, documentation of ischemia by myocardial scintigraphy and results of pharmacologic intervention. *Am J Cardiol* 1980;46:500.

16. Severi S, Davies G, Maseri A, et al: Long-term prognosis of "variant" angina with medical treatment. *Am J Cardiol* 1980;46:228.

17. Helfant RH: Coronary spasm. *Am J Cardiol* 1979;44:839.

18. Heupler FA: Provocative testing for coronary arterial spasm: Risk, method and rationale. *Am J Cardiol* 1980;46:335.

19. Fester A: Provocative testing for coronary arterial spasm with ergonovine malleate. *Am J Cardiol* 1980;46:338.

20. Freeman WR, Peter T, Mandel WJ: Verapamil therapy in variant angina pectoris refractory to nitrates. *Am Heart J* 1981;102:358.

## Chapter 8

Myocardial Infarction

The word infarction implies death of tissue. In clinical medicine the term myocardial infarction (MI) is used to describe a process that begins with myocardial injury and progresses to death of tissue and subsequent scar formation. This terminology is paralleled in electrocardiography with the terms "hyperacute infarction" and "acute infarction" to describe the initial signs of the process that are often seen before actual death of tissue has taken place. Subsequent changes are described as "evolution of infarction" until the pattern stabilizes into one of "old infarction."

Electrophysiological Considerations

In the left ventricular cone described in Chapter 7, depolarization currents move from the endocardium toward the epicardium so that the vector of depolarization of the free wall of the left ventricle is directly opposite that of the free wall of the right ventricle. An electrode placed in the appropriate position on the left lateral thorax will record electricity moving toward it through the left ventricular wall. If this area is unable to conduct electricity due to severe injury or tissue necrosis, the same electrode will now reflect current moving through the septum and the wall of the right ventricle, which is located opposite the affected area.

Since this current is moving away from the electrode, the resulting ventricular complex will be negative. This principle holds true for all segments of the left ventricle and explains the appearance of *pathological Q waves* in MI. This principle is illustrated in Figure 8-1.

Repolarization, too, occurs in opposing directions in opposite areas of the heart, and gross abnormalities of the S-T segment and T wave over one area will be reflected as a mirror image in leads showing the corresponding opposite section. Such abnormalities are called *reciprocal changes* and are shown in Figure 8-2, as well as in many of the ECGs in this chapter.

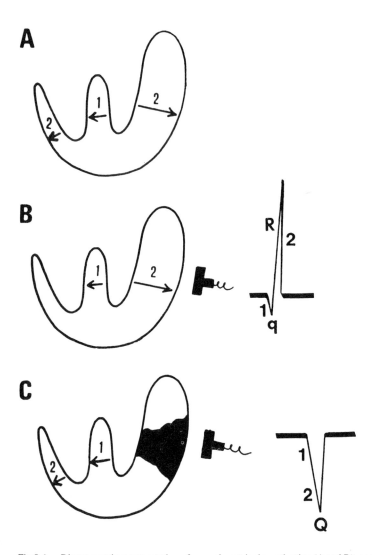

Fig 8-1.—Diagrammatic representation of normal ventricular activation (A and B), as reflected by qR complex in a lead oriented to left ventricle and ventricular activation associated with transmural necrosis, as reflected by QS complex in a lead oriented to left ventricle (C) (from Schamroth[1(p9)]).

Pathological and ECG Changes

Hyperacute Phase

In the hyperacute phase of MI there is usually severe, characteristic chest pain, as curtailment of blood flow and oxygen supply produce severe ischemia and injury in the affected portion of the ventricular myocardium. During this phase, there is increased ventricular automaticity, as well as considerable disparity in the

Effects of Cardiac Infarction, Injury, and Ischemia

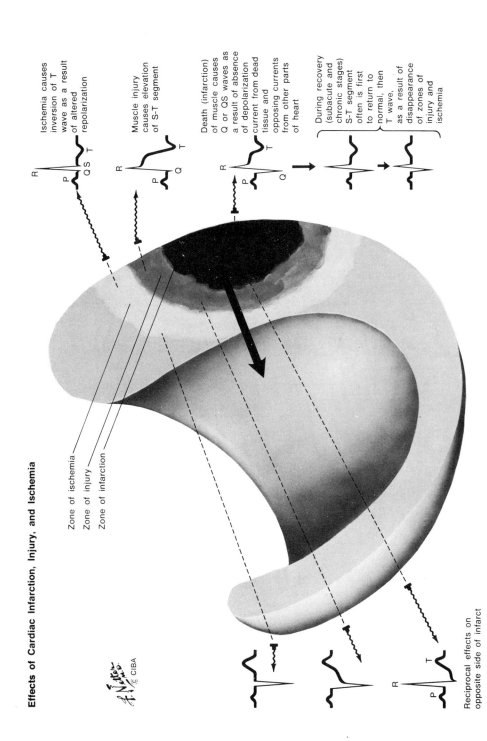

Zone of ischemia
Zone of injury
Zone of infarction

Ischemia causes inversion of T wave as a result of altered repolarization

Muscle injury causes elevation of S-T segment

Death (infarction) of muscle causes Q or QS waves as a result of absence of depolarization current from dead tissue and opposing currents from other parts of heart

During recovery (subacute and chronic stages) S-T segment often is first to return to normal, then T wave, as a result of disappearance of zones of injury and ischemia

Reciprocal effects on opposite side of infarct

Fig 8-2.—Effects of cardiac infarction, injury, and ischemia. Copyright 1969, 1978, CIBA Pharmaceutical Co, Division of CIBA-GEIGY Corp. Reprinted with permission from *The CIBA Collection of Medical Illustrations. The Heart,* vol 5, p 62; illustrated by Frank H. Netter, MD. All rights reserved.

speed of both depolarization and repolarization between healthy and ischemic myocardium. This may cause severe ventricular arrhythmias and/or conduction defects that pose a serious threat to life and may result in sudden death before a patient can reach a hospital.

There is usually some delay between the onset of pain and the patient's arrival at the hospital, so the ECG evidence of hyperacute infarction is not recorded in many cases.

Generally, the first definite ECG sign is *pronounced elevation of the S-T segment*. The S-T segment may extend upward in a nearly straight line from the R wave (Fig 8-4), may slope upward in a convex manner (Fig 8-5), or may be elevated and concave (Fig 8-6). Reciprocal changes are frequently seen in the opposing leads. ECG changes seen in the hyperacute phase are shown in Figures 8-3 through 8-6.

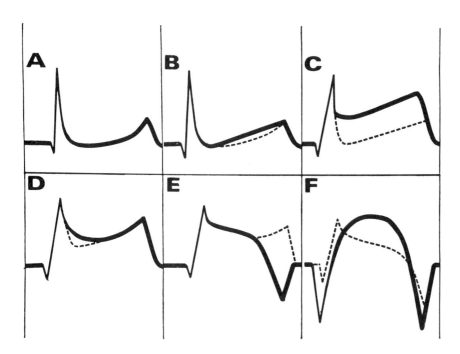

Fig 8-3.—Diagrams illustrating evolution of infarction pattern from normal (A), through various stages of hyperacute phase (B, C, and D), to fully evolved phase (F) (from Schamroth[1(p41)]).

The *T wave* may become abnormally tall, reflecting subepicardial ischemia. This prominent T wave may be the first ECG sign of the disease process, especially in anterior wall myocardial infarction (AWMI).[1(p29)] Tall T waves cannot be considered diagnostic, however, because they may be seen in healthy individuals or as a sign of electrolyte disturbance (chap 12). Nevertheless, very prominent T waves in a patient with chest pain should arouse suspicion of MI.

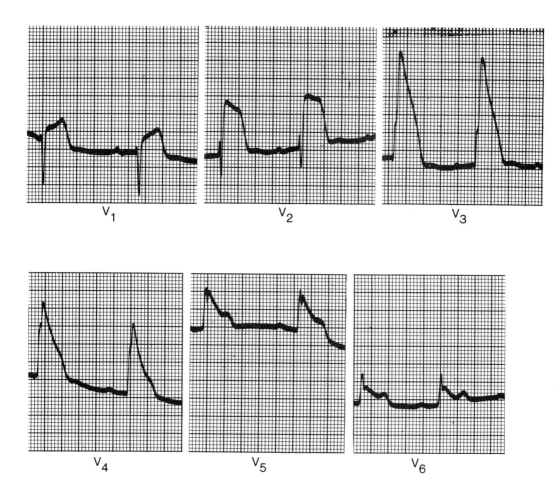

Fig 8-4.—Leads V_1 through V_6, showing hyperacute phase of anterior wall myocardial infarction.

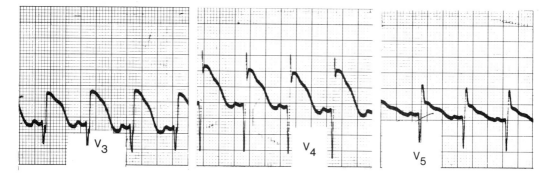

Fig 8-5.—Leads V_3 through V_5, showing hyperacute anterior wall myocardial infarction.

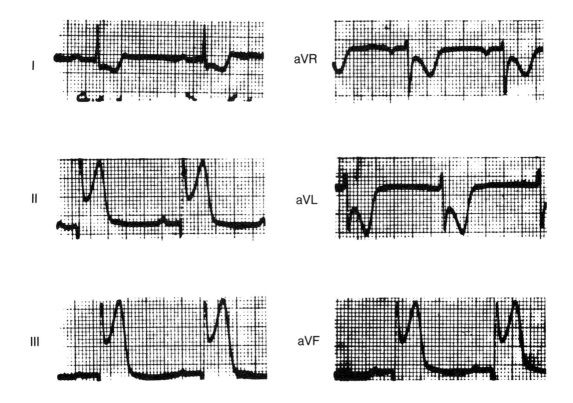

Fig 8-6.—Frontal plane leads showing hyperacute phase of inferior wall infarction, with pronounced reciprocal changes in leads I and aVL.

Figure 8-7a shows a 12-lead ECG obtained in a 51-year-old man with chest pain. It does not appear to be very abnormal; close inspection, however, reveals a 1 to 2 mm elevation of the S-T segments in leads V_2 through V_4. The reciprocal S-T segments, especially in lead aVF, while not actually depressed, tend to hug the baseline for more than 3 mm, and the T waves in V_2 through V_4 are pronounced. Although these findings are not precisely diagnostic, they should arouse suspicion. A patient should always be treated on the basis of clinical findings, even if the ECG is completely normal.

The wisdom of this course is proven by the ECG of the same patient taken the next day (Fig 8-7b).

Widening of the QRS complex, occasionally seen during the hyperacute phase, is often referred to as "acute injury block." This form of intraventricular conduction defect does not have the characteristics of either RBBB or LBBB. It consists of widening of the QRS complex, which may sometimes be accompanied by an initial increase in the height of the R wave. It is often difficult to discern the increase in the width of the QRS complex, due to the distortion of the S-T segment. This is true, for example, in Figure 8-8, but careful measurement shows a QRS of at least 0.11 second in several leads.

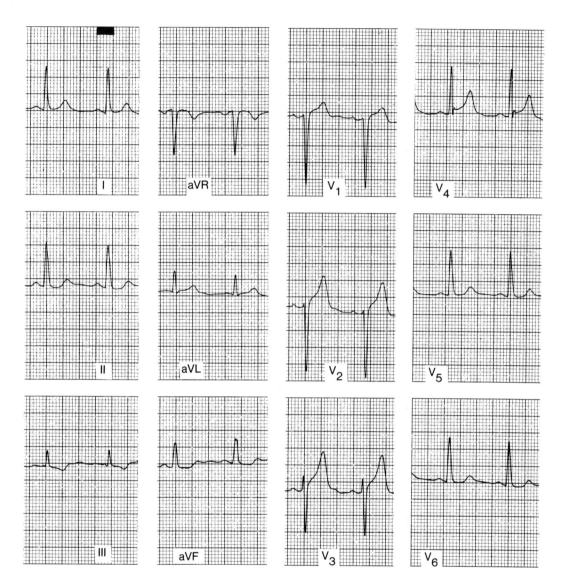

Fig 8-7a.—12-lead ECG of patient with chest pain at admission.

Acute Phase

The phase of MI that is usually seen when the patient arrives at the hospital is the acute phase. Pain persists and arrhythmias are common, as myocardial injury continues.

The pathological findings in the fully evolved stage are generally as shown in Figure 8-2. There is a central area in which cells are so severely damaged that they can no longer participate in electrical activity. This is surrounded by an area of injury, around which there is an ischemic zone.

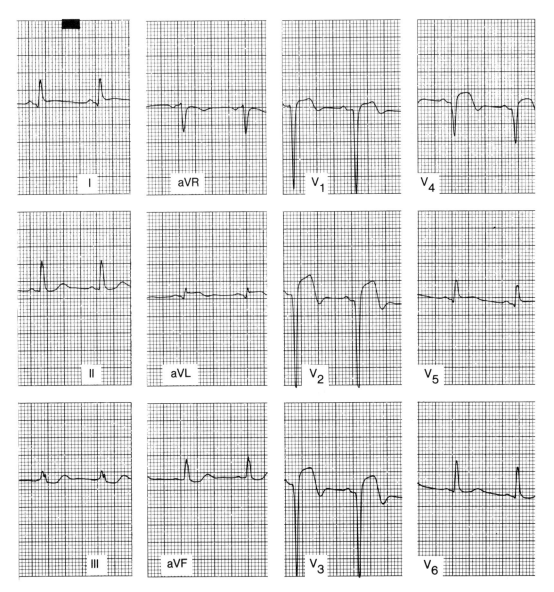

Fig 8-7b.—ECG tracing in patient in Fig 8-7a, showing evidence of acute anteroseptal myocardial infarction, with extension to lateral wall.

The S-T segment is elevated and coved upward, reflecting the injured zone. Reciprocal S-T depression in the opposing leads is frequently seen and substantiates the existence of an acute problem.

The T wave is symmetrical and inverted, the so-called "coronary" or Pardee T wave,[2(p239)] and it reflects the ischemic area.

Pathological Q waves appear in the leads over the affected area, where the myocardium is too severely injured to conduct electricity or where necrosis has set in.

These ECG findings of acute MI are well illustrated in Figure 8-7b.

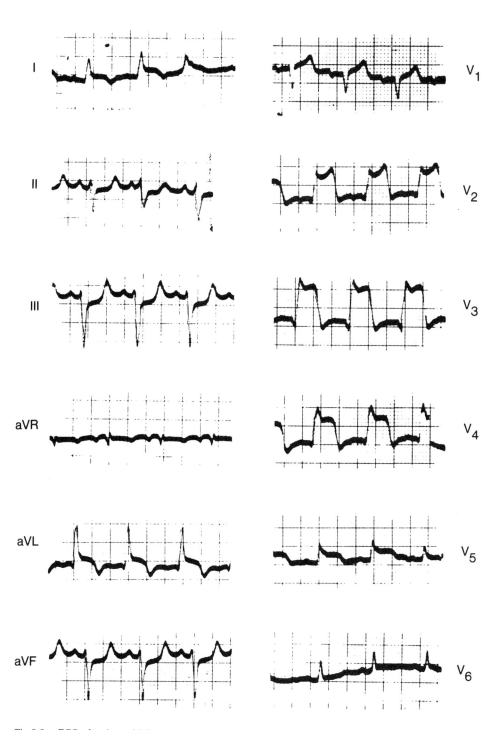

Fig 8-8.—ECG of patient with hyperacute anterior and lateral wall myocardial infarction.

Evolution of Myocardial Infarction

During the days and weeks that follow the initial insult, the patient's condition usually stabilizes, pain disappears, and arrhythmias are seen less frequently.

Several changes occur in the affected cells. The most favorable change is total recovery. Although this is rare, it is possible,[3] and clinical efforts are under way in many institutions to assist in recovery of injured cells.[4,5] If this effort is successful, the Q waves indicating electrical necrosis will disappear completely.

More frequently, actual pathological necrosis will occur in the areas most severely affected, and the Q waves will become a permanent feature of the patient's ECG.

The usual patterns of evolution are illustrated in Figure 8-9.

Under favorable circumstances, most of the cells located in the injury zone will recover, so Q waves may not appear in all of the leads that initially showed S-T segment elevation. Therapeutic interventions are intended to facilitate this "limitation of infarction."[6] The process of improvement in injured areas is illustrated in lead V_6 of Figure 8-9a through e.

The S-T segment gradually returns to the baseline, as the area of injury either heals or becomes necrotic. This change generally lasts less than 2 weeks[2(p239)] and often takes place within one to two days after infarction. Reciprocal changes usually disappear within one to two days as well.

The T wave initially remains inverted but gradually returns to its normal, upright position within several months to 1 year.

The Q wave may initially become deeper as more of the affected cells become necrotic, and the R wave may disappear completely. If necrosis involves the entire thickness of the ventricular wall (transmural infarct), Q waves will probably always remain prominent in the leads over the affected area. More frequently, Q waves become smaller, and an R wave follows the Q wave, indicating the presence of some viable, conducting muscle fibers in the damaged area. This R wave is generally smaller than that seen in preinfarction tracings of the same patient, as a result of loss of muscle mass.

These developments frequently occur in IWMI (Figs 8-10a through d and 8-11). The series of tracings (in Figures 8-10a through d) illustrates the evolution of IWMI. Leads V_5 and V_6, which indicated involvement of the apical area in the ischemic process, have returned to normal, and small R waves have returned in leads II and aVF, indicating survival of viable myocardium.

Old Myocardial Infarction

In uncomplicated cases, the necrotic area forms a scar, and the remaining portion of the myocardium returns to normal. If the affected area is not too large and if perfusion of other coronary vessels is adequate, the patient should be free from pain and arrhythmias and able to enjoy a normal, active life.

The only ECG evidence remaining at the end of 6 months to 1 year should be Q waves or QR complexes in the affected areas. This initial Q wave may be so small, especially after IWMI, that the ECG looks almost normal.

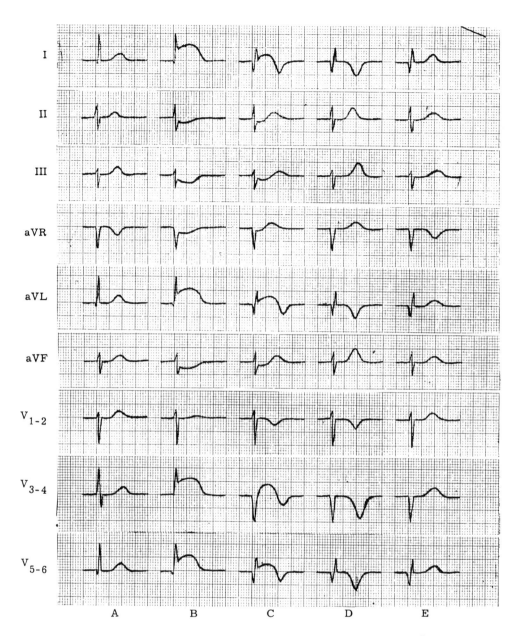

Fig 8-9.—Diagrammatic illustration of serial changes in anterolateral infarction (from Goldman[7]).

A. Normal tracing.

B. Very Early Pattern (Hours After Infarction): ST segment elevation in I, aVL, and V_{3-6}; reciprocal ST depression in II, III, and aVF.

C. Later Pattern (Many Hours to a Few Days): Q waves have appeared in I, aVL, and V_{5-6}. QS complexes are present in V_{3-4}. This indicates that the major transmural infarction is underlying the area recorded by V_{3-4}; ST segment changes persist, but are of lesser degree, and the T waves are beginning to invert in those leads in which the ST segments are elevated.

D. Late Established Pattern (Many Days to Weeks): The Q waves and QS complexes persist; the ST segments are iso-electric; the T waves are symmetrical, and deeply inverted in leads which had ST elevation and tall in leads which had ST depression. This pattern may persist for the remainder of the patient's life.

E. Very Late Pattern: This may occur many months to years after the infarct. The abnormal Q waves and QS complexes persist. The T waves have gradually returned to normal.

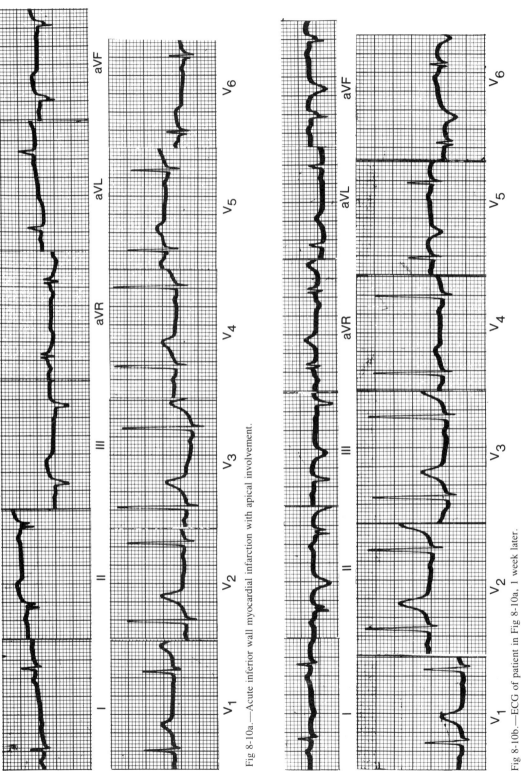

Fig 8-10a.—Acute inferior wall myocardial infarction with apical involvement.

Fig 8-10b.—ECG of patient in Fig 8-10a, 1 week later.

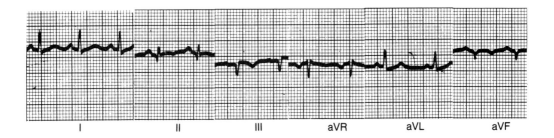

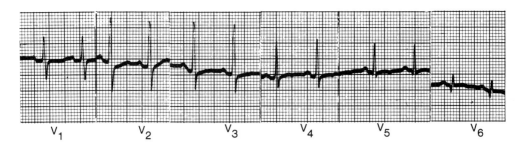

Fig 8-10c.—ECG of patient in Fig 8-10a, 2 months after infarction.

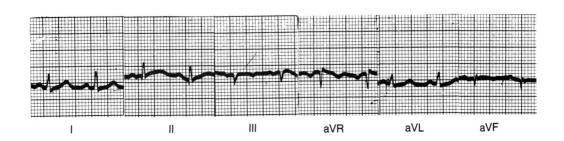

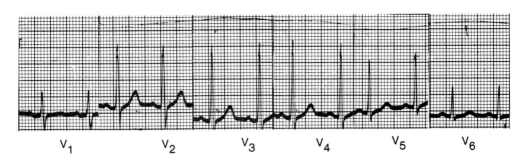

Fig 8-10d.—ECG of patient in Fig 8-10a, 3 months after infarction.

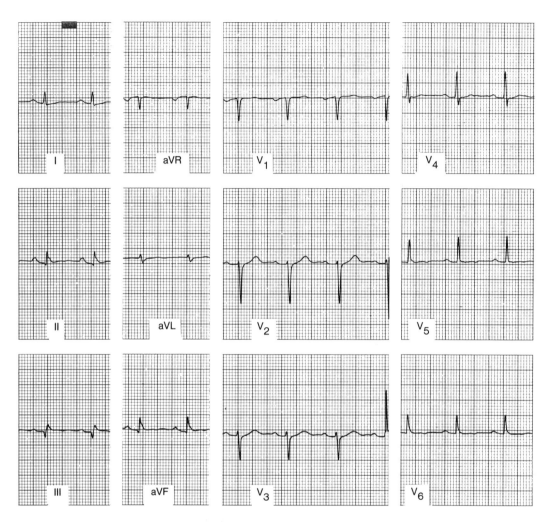

Fig 8-11.—ECG obtained 6 months after inferior wall infarction with lateral and apical involvement.

Localization of Myocardial Infarction

The site of infarction is identified by the leads in which the characteristic ECG changes are seen (chap 7). Leads II, III, and aVF reflect the inferior or diaphragmatic portion of the left ventricle (Figs 8-6, 8-10, and 8-11). Anteroseptal and anterior wall damage is seen in the precordial leads (Figs 8-4, 8-5, and 8-7). Lateral wall infarcts are identified by changes in leads I and aVL. These rarely appear as an isolated finding but are usually accompanied by involvement of the apical, anterior, or inferior area (Fig 8-12).

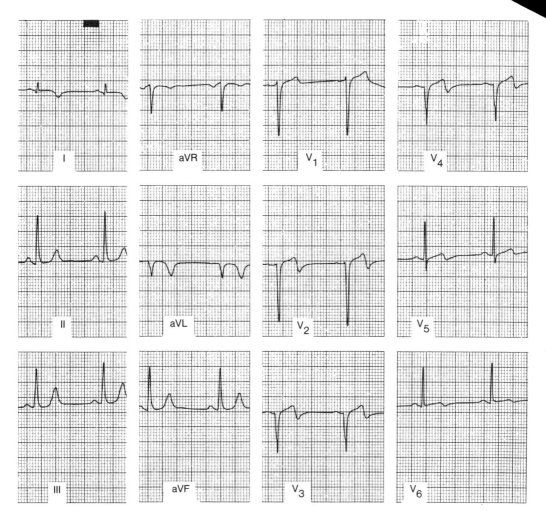

Fig 8-12.—Anterolateral infarction.

True Posterior Wall Infarction

The true posterior wall of the heart is not reflected directly in the leads normally obtained in a 12-lead ECG. The position of this aspect of the left ventricle is shown in Figure 8-13.

The initial diagnosis of true posterior wall infarction is based on the reciprocal changes produced in the standard leads. These changes, usually best seen in leads V_1 through V_3, consist of a depressed S-T segment, an upright T wave, and increased height of the R wave,[8] as shown in Figure 8-14a.

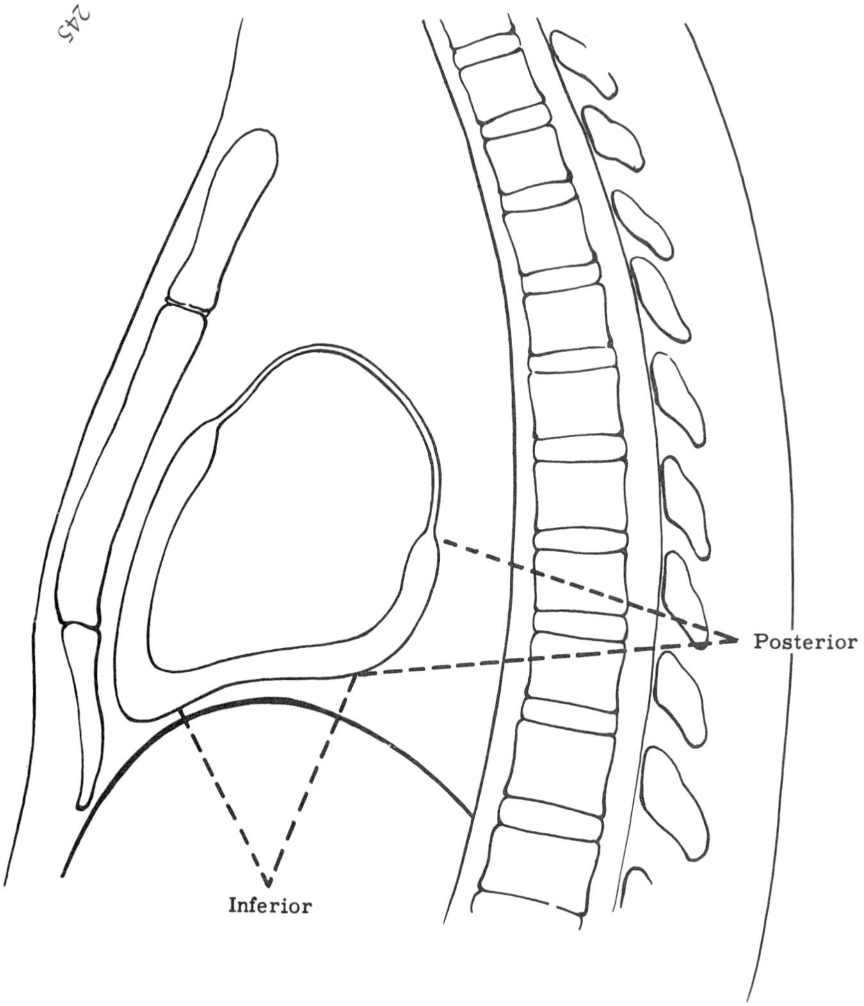

Fig 8-13.—Inferior and posterior locations (from Goldman[7(p176)]).

The characteristic findings described represent the mirror image of the S-T elevation, inverted T wave, and pathological Q wave seen in the leads directly over the affected area, leads V_7 through V_9 (Fig 8-14b).

Posterior wall infarction is frequently seen in combination with infarction of the inferior and/or apical portions of the heart, as shown in Figures 8-15a through c.

The current of injury seen in the earlier tracing (Fig 8-15a) has subsided considerably. The S-T segments in leads V_1 through V_3 have returned to the baseline as well, but there is a fairly tall R wave in lead V_1 that was not present in

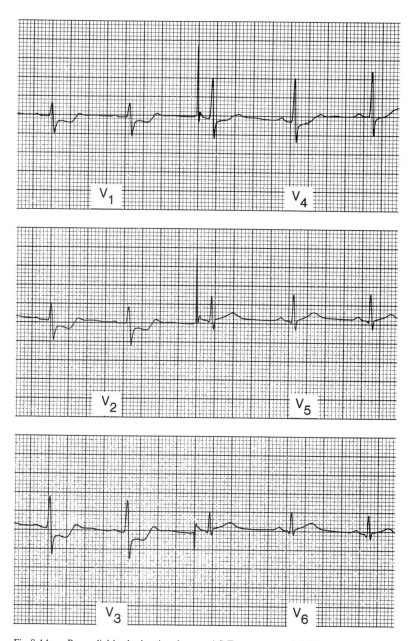

Fig 8-14a.—Precordial leads showing depressed S-T segment, upright T wave, and tall R waves in leads V_1 through V_4.

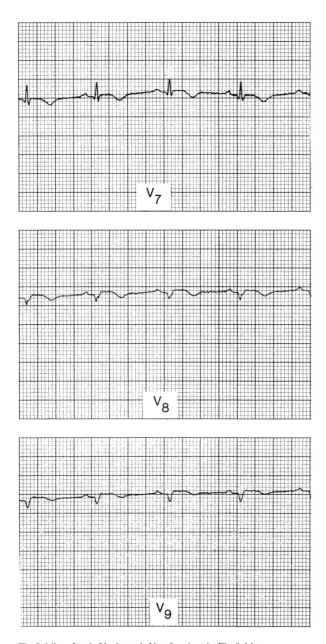

Fig 8-14b.—Leads V$_7$ through V$_9$ of patient in Fig 8-14a.

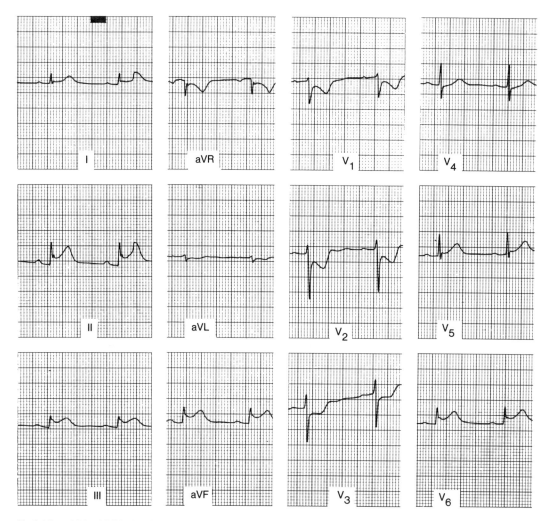

Fig 8-15a.—12-lead ECG showing acute inferior and apical injury, as well as pronounced S-T depression in right precordial leads.

the previous tracing. This indicates that the S-T depressions seen in V_1 through V_3 were not simply reciprocal changes due to injury in the inferior portion of the heart but probably reflected an active process taking place in the posterior portion of the left ventricle. The tracing shown in Figure 8-15c confirms this suspicion.

In light of this information, it is obvious that the patient whose ECG is shown in Figure 8-10a had a true posterior wall infarction, as well as damage in the inferior apical portion of the heart.

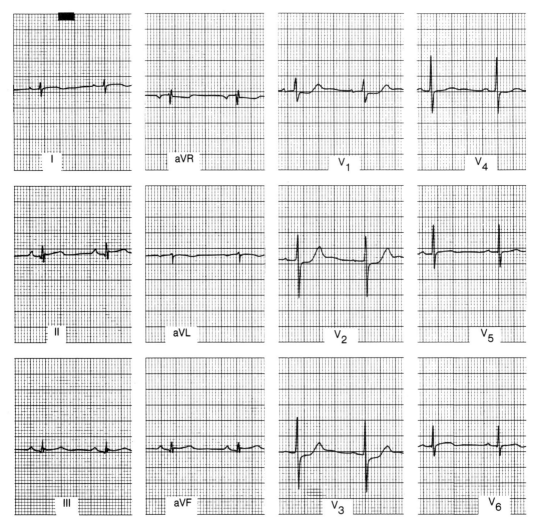

Fig 8-15b.—12-lead ECG obtained from patient in Fig 8-15a, 24 hours later.

Right Ventricular Infarction

Infarction of the right ventricle has recently gained renewed interest and discussion.[9] It is most usually associated with IWMI. The diagnosis of this complication is based primarily on clinical and hemodynamic findings and diagnostic studies such as enzyme assays and echocardiography.[10] Leads V_{3R} and V_{4R} may show the characteristic Q waves and ST segment changes of myocardial infarction. This type of infarction is frequently associated with some form of heart block.

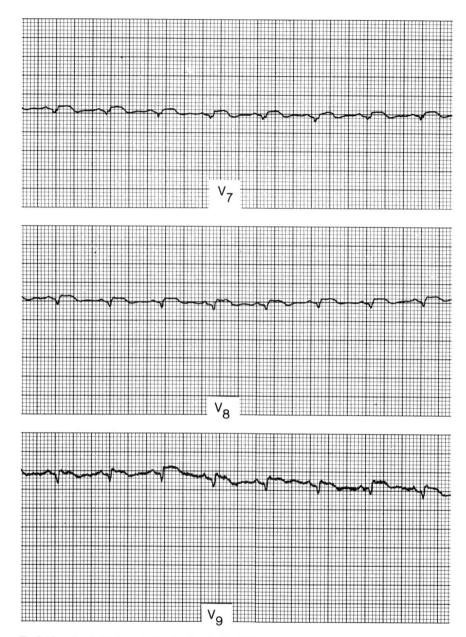

Fig 8-15c.—Leads V₇ through V₉ of patient in Fig 8-15a.

Conduction Defects in Acute Myocardial Infarction

Atrioventricular Blocks

Atrioventricular blocks are frequently seen during the acute stage of IWMI (Fig 8-16). They are usually due to delay or blockage in the AV nodal area and are generally transient and benign. The blocks associated with anterior wall infarctions, on the other hand, tend to be due to necrosis of the lower conduction system. They are usually permanent and an indication of a poor prognosis.[11]

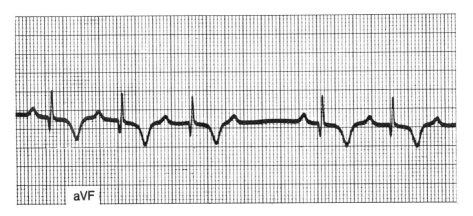

Fig 8-16.—Lead aVF, showing acute inferior wall infarction and 2° atrioventricular block type I (Wenckebach).

Bundle Branch Blocks

Left Bundle Branch Block

Various types of bundle branch blocks may be seen in conjunction with infarction. They may be due to the infarction, or may have been present prior to the disease, and they may be either transient or permanent.

Case Report. The tracing in Figure 8-17a, obtained in a 78-year-old man with chest pain, shows complete LBBB. In the ECG taken on the following day (Fig 8-17b), the QRS complexes are somewhat narrower, and the S-T segments and T waves reveal the classic changes associated with an acute ischemic process.

Right Bundle Branch Block

Myocardial infarction may also cause RBBB with or without associated hemiblock (Fig 8-18). The development of such intraventricular conduction defects is generally an unfavorable sign.

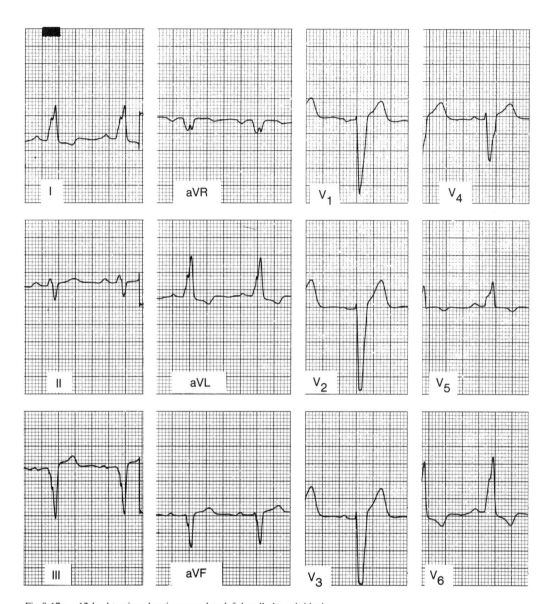

Fig 8-17a.—12-lead tracing showing complete left bundle branch block.

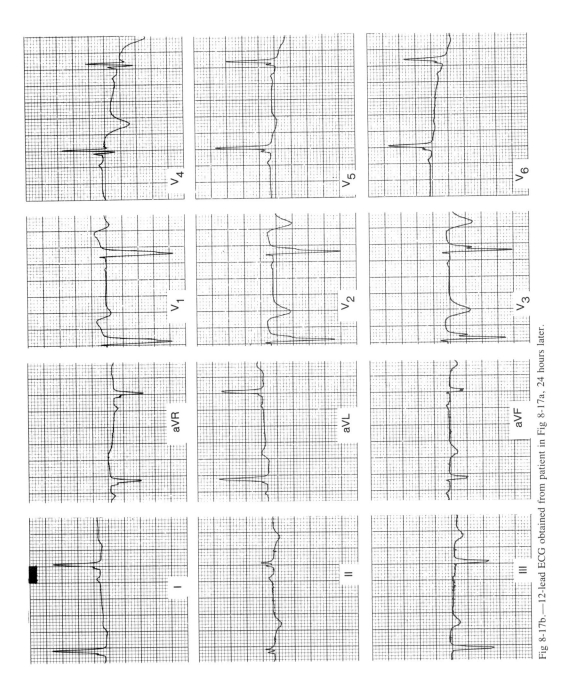

Fig 8-17b.—12-lead ECG obtained from patient in Fig 8-17a, 24 hours later.

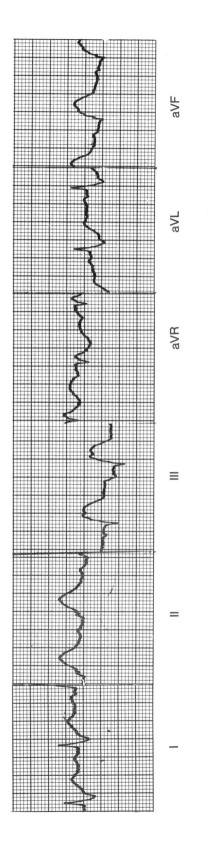

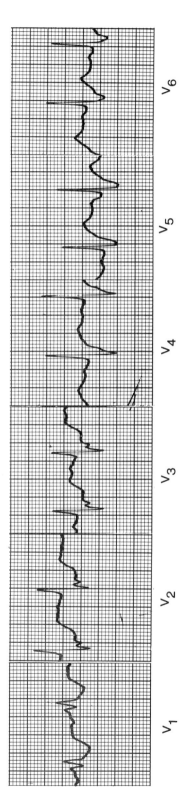

Fig 8-18.—Acute inferior wall infarction with right bundle branch block.

Recognition of acute MI in patients with preexisting bundle branch block is sometimes difficult, due to the distortion of the QRS complex and the abnormality of the T wave caused by the conduction defect. RBBB usually permits diagnosis of MI based on sequential S-T segment and T wave changes and on the appearance of Q waves, as shown in Figures 8-19a through d.

Case Report. The tracing in Figure 8-19a shows a recent inferoapical MI and an intraventricular conduction defect of the RBBB type in a 71-year-old man. It is possible that the configuration of lead V_1 is due to posterior wall involvement. Unfortunately, no posterior leads were obtained in this patient, so we cannot confirm this suspicion. The patient made an uneventful recovery and was discharged.

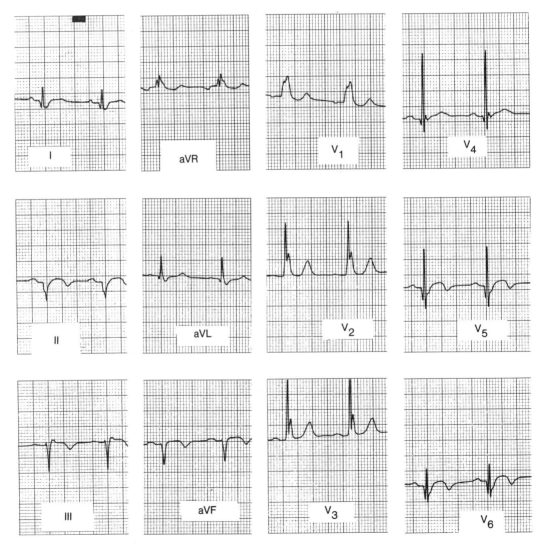

Fig 8-19a.—ECG of patient with recent inferoapical infarction and right bundle branch block.

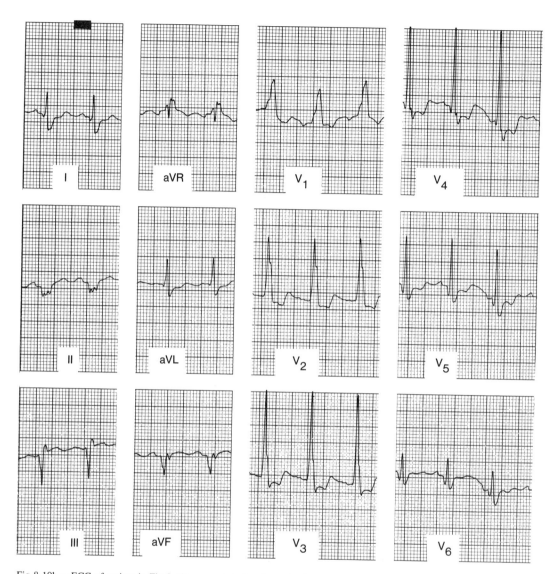

Fig 8-19b.—ECG of patient in Fig 8-19a on readmission 2 months later.

Approximately 2 months later, he was readmitted because of severe, acute chest pain. Pronounced S-T segment depressions in leads V_1 through V_4 of the admission ECG (Fig 8-19b) suggest anteroseptal ischemia.

Two days later, a current of injury pattern is apparent in leads V_2 through V_4 (Fig 8-19c), and further evolutionary changes, including the appearance of small Q waves in the affected leads, indicate that this patient has had an anteroseptal infarction (Fig 8-19d).

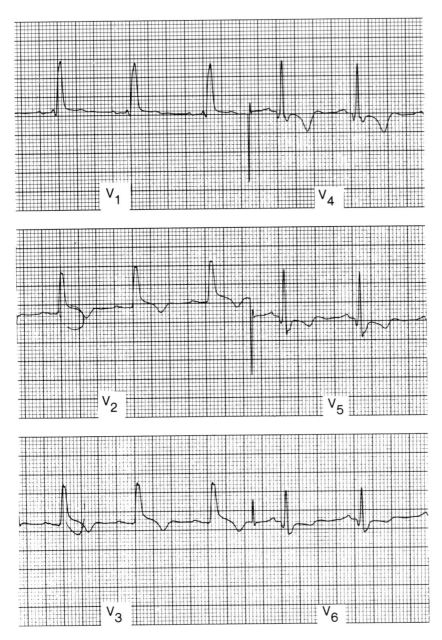

Fig 8-19c.—Precordial leads of patient in Fig 8-19a, 2 days later.

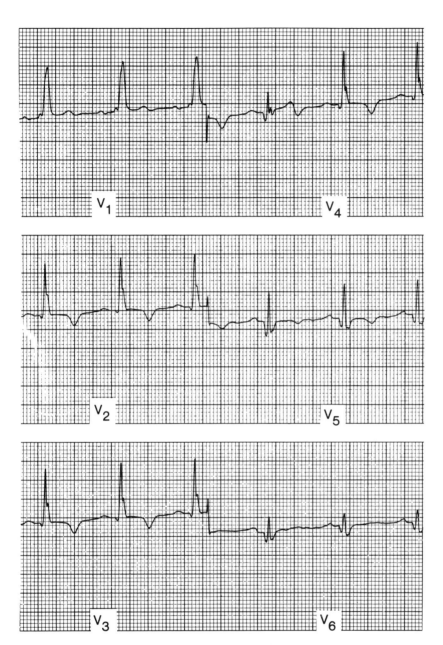

Fig 8-19d.—Precordial leads of patient in Fig 8-19a, after additional 24 hours.

Diagnosis

The presence of LBBB frequently obscures the ECG evidence of myocardial infarction. The diagnosis may be made on the basis of pathological Q waves and S-T and T wave changes occurring over time.[12] In complete LBBB, septal depolarization takes place from right to left, so the small septal Q waves normally seen in left ventricular leads are absent. Figure 8-20 shows significant Q waves in leads V_4 through V_6, as well as in leads I and aVL, as a sign of MI. Upward rounding of the T wave and apparent S-T elevation are frequently seen in the right precordial leads in LBBB, but these characteristics alone do not indicate MI. When they are combined with significant Q waves, as in Figure 8-20, however, the suspicion that MI has occurred is enhanced.

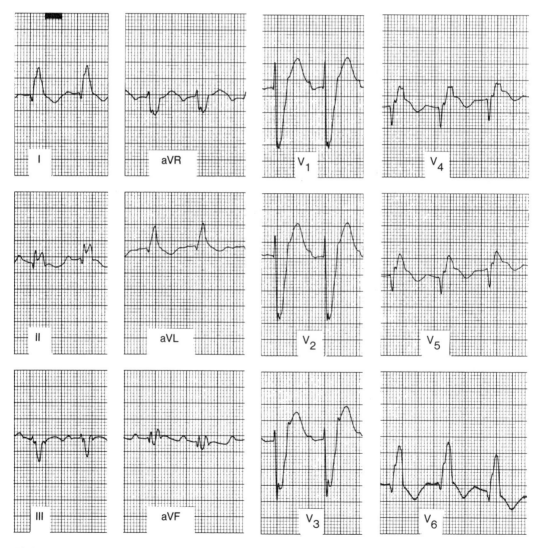

Fig 8-20.—Acute anterolateral infarction in the presence of complete left bundle branch block.

The significance of abnormal S-T segments in LBBB is best evaluated on the basis of serial ECGs obtained over a period of days. If these changes evolve as previously described, the diagnosis of MI is confirmed.

Peri-Infarction Block

Occasionally, a nonspecific intraventricular conduction defect appears at the time of MI and remains after the infarct has healed. This may occur if small areas of viable muscle within the infarct zone undergo late depolarization or if epicardial fibers remain viable in areas where the subendocardial Purkinje fibers have been destroyed.[13] ECG criteria for identification of this conduction defect include a QRS width of more than 0.11 second and significant pathological Q waves over the infarcted area. In peri-infarction block associated with anterolateral infarction, the QRS axis is about − 30°; whereas in IWMI, it may be directed toward the right, with late R waves in leads II, III, and aVF.[12,13] An example of peri-infarction block is shown in Figure 8-21.

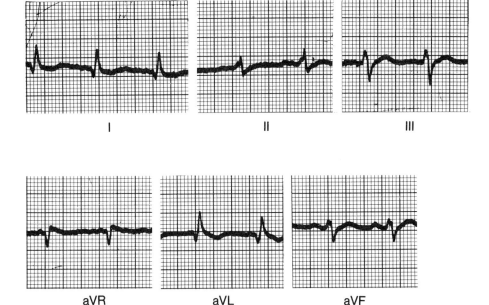

Fig 8-21.—Frontal plane leads showing nonrecent lateral wall infarction and intraventricular conduction delay.

Subendocardial Infarction

The diagnosis of subendocardial injury or infarction generally implies that the area of necrosis does not involve the entire thickness of the ventricular wall. Hence, such injuries are also often described as nontransmural.

The ECG evidence of such infarcts is somewhat controversial. Castellanos and Myerburg[3] state that "there is no characteristic ECG pattern for this type of infarction," while others[1(p142),2(p248)] list criteria for its diagnosis. Usually, the S-T segment is described as showing a depressed slope that merges imperceptibly with the deep, wide, symmetrically inverted T wave. These changes are usually widespread, indicating involvement of a large portion of the myocardium. The diagnosis is confirmed by clinical findings and the results of diagnostic studies, such as a characteristic rise in "cardiac" enzyme levels.

It would be a grave error to exercise less careful observation of these patients than is generally used in patients with MI. This is true for several reasons. Subendocardial infarctions tend to involve a large portion of the myocardium, and severe ischemia affecting a substantial area of the left ventricle can cause severe failure. In addition, an active ischemic process is more likely than a "complete" infarction to precipitate arrhythmias. Furthermore, the presence of subendocardial infarction is an indication of severe, widespread CAD and is frequently the forerunner of transmural infarction. The seriousness of this condition is well illustrated by the series of tracings shown in Figures 8-22a through d.

The first tracing (Fig 8-22a) shows some very minor changes in the S-T segments and might easily be interpreted as being within broad normal limits.

The second tracing (Fig 8-22b) shows changes that are compatible with sub-endocardial infarction involving the inferior as well as anterior portion of the left ventricle.

On the following day the patient had cardiac arrest, and the ECG obtained following resuscitation (Fig 8-22c) shows an acute AWMI as well as probable IWMI.

The last tracing (Fig 8-22d) was obtained shortly before death. It shows a renewed hyperacute injury pattern in the leads previously affected, and Q waves have appeared in lead aVL as well, indicating involvement of the lateral wall. This might well be described as a "paninfarction," ie, infarction of the entire left ventricle.

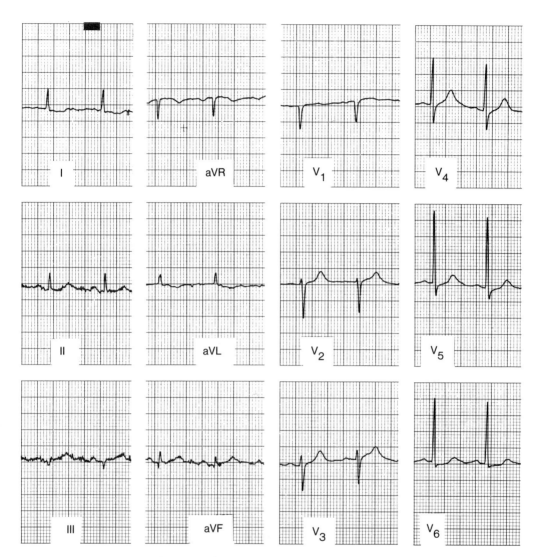

Fig 8-22a.—Admission ECG of 72-year-old woman with chest pain.

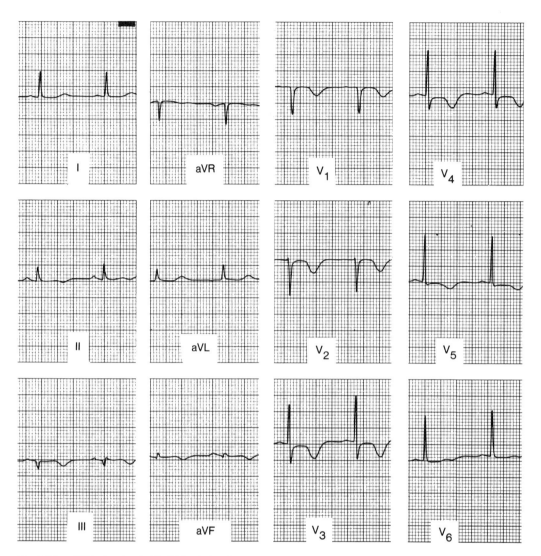

Fig 8-22b.—ECG of patient in Fig 8-22a, 3 days later.

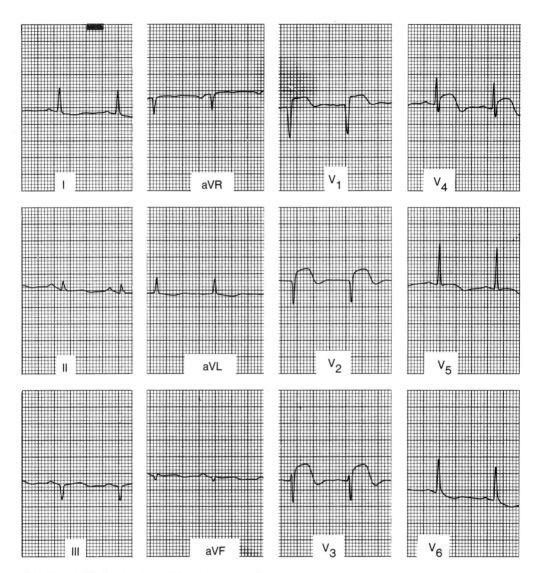

Fig 8-22c.—ECG of patient in Fig 8-22a following cardiac arrest.

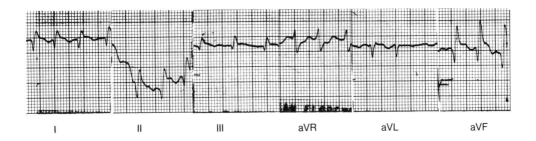

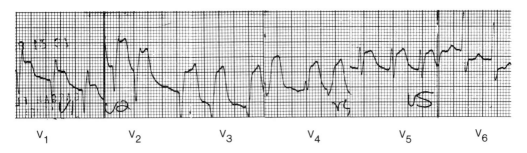

Fig 8-22d.—ECG of patient in Fig 8-22a shortly before death.

Subepicardial Injury

In subepicardial injury, the damage does not extend throughout the thickness of the ventricular wall. ECG evidence consists of an elevated and upward convex S-T segment and a symmetrically inverted T wave. The tracings shown in Figures 8-23a and b were obtained on successive days in a patient admitted because of severe, persistent chest pain. The S-T segments in leads V_2 through V_5 exhibit a characteristic current of injury pattern, but the typical Q waves of MI never appeared, suggesting that at least a portion of the affected ventricular myocardium remained viable.

Abnormal Evolution of Myocardial Infarction

At times the ECG fails to change in the characteristic evolutionary pattern. The most frequent variations are persistent S-T segment elevation and recurrence of S-T elevation.

Persistent S-T Segment Elevation

In the majority of patients, the S-T segment returns to its normal position within a few days following infarction. If the elevation persists for more than 2 weeks, it

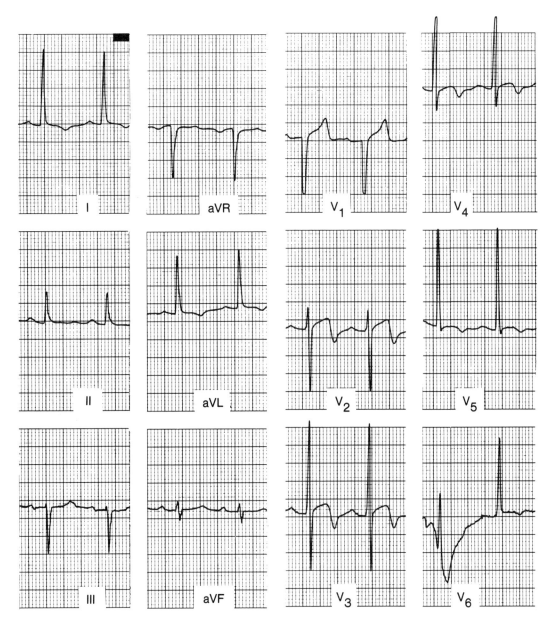

Fig 8-23a.—12-lead ECG of 55-year-old man with chest pain.

is usually permanent and is associated with asynergy of the affected area of the myocardium.[2(p239)] Persistent S-T segment elevation beyond the 2-week limit was found in 60% of patients who developed ventricular aneurysm following MI. This complication is most frequently associated with anteroseptal MI and should be suspected if deep Q waves persist, together with the S-T segment elevation.

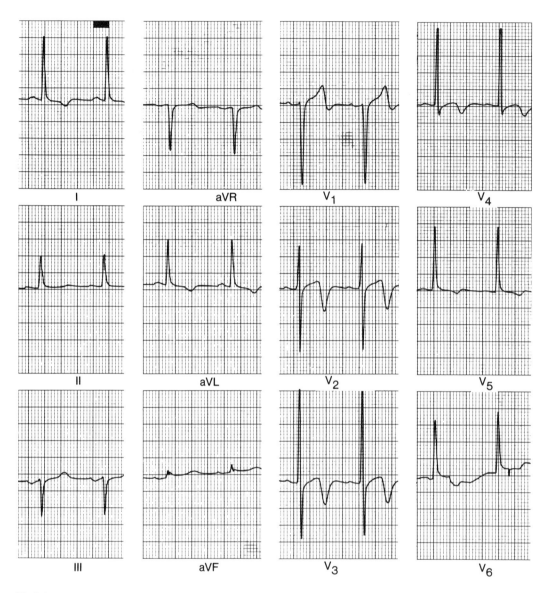

Fig 8-23b.—Tracing of patient in Fig 8-23a, 24 hours later.

Other causes of persistent S-T elevation include pericarditis, superimposed ischemia, and reinfarction, which can generally be verified clinically. The administration of digitalis may cause an upward rounding of the S-T segment in the leads that show the Q waves, but it does not usually cause the distinct upward displacement of the S-T segment seen in the patient with ventricular aneurysm (Fig 8-24).

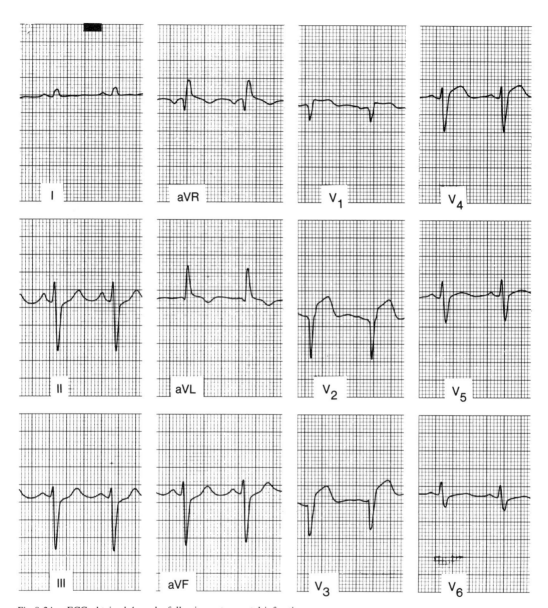

Fig 8-24.—ECG obtained 4 weeks following anteroseptal infarction.

Extension of Myocardial Infarction

The normal sequence of evolution may be interrupted by the appearance of a current of injury pattern in the leads adjacent to those originally affected. This may be accompanied by renewed elevation of the S-T segments that had returned to normal levels. Such a development usually reflects extension of the area of injury and infarction, as illustrated in Figures 8-25a and b.

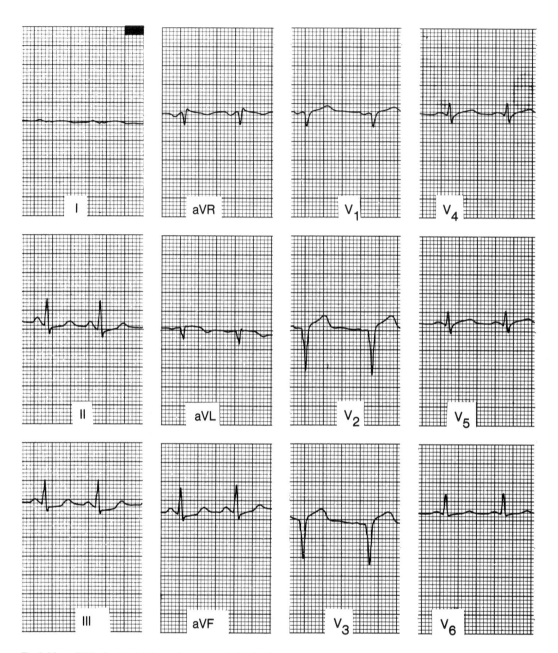

Fig 8-25a.—ECG of patient 2 days after myocardial infarction.

The tracing in Figure 8-25a shows an anteroseptal MI with distinct Q waves and S-T segments that have almost returned to the baseline. The ECG in Figure 8-25b, taken three days later, shows S-T elevation and formation of Q waves in leads V_4 through V_6, which had shown little or no prior involvement. An intraventricular conduction defect has also developed, and it masks the Q waves previously seen.

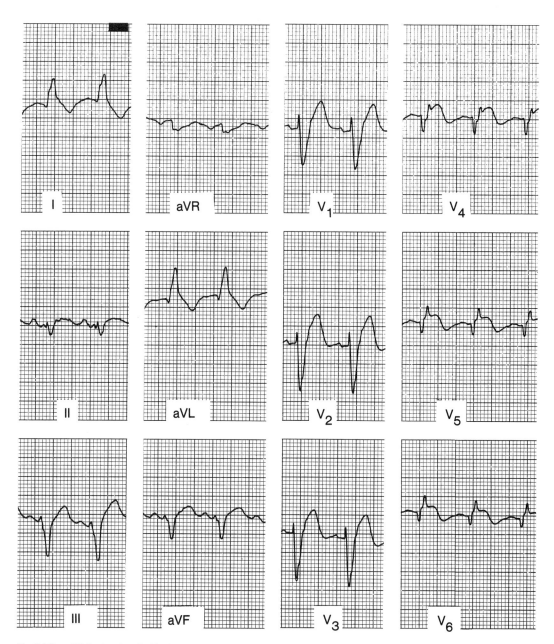

Fig 8-25b.—ECG of patient in Fig 8-25a, 2 days later.

Such a patient must be watched carefully because of the risk of arrhythmias and other complications of acute injury. Conversely, if a patient who was free from pain and apparently making a good recovery from MI suddenly complains of pain, the nurse should immediately obtain a 12-lead ECG and examine it for the changes described. The reflex administration of pain medication, without further examination of the patient and the ECG, may open the door to disaster.

Diagnostic Problems

Several conditions may mimic one or more of the ECG features of MI. Some of these are found in normal, healthy individuals, and care must be taken to avoid an erroneous diagnosis of MI. In other instances, the abnormality may be due to a clinical condition that requires appropriate treatment.

S-T Segment Elevation

In addition to the causes previously discussed, significant elevation of the S-T segment may be associated with pericarditis, mechanical injury, and vagotonia (Fig 8-26).

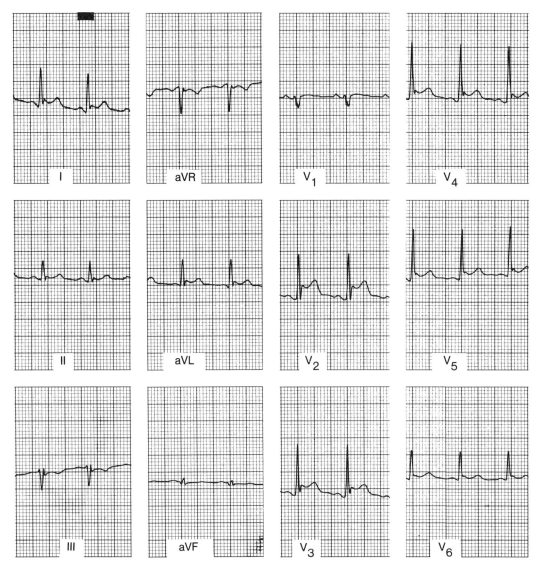

Fig 8-26.—ECG of patient with pericarditis, showing widespread S-T segment elevation.

In early *pericarditis,* the S-T segments are elevated in the leads overlying the affected area of the heart. In most cases, all leads, with the exception of aVR and V_1, are involved. These two leads frequently show S-T depression. The QRS complexes and T waves are usually normal, although the QRS voltage may be somewhat diminished.

In the later stages of the disease, the S-T segment returns to normal, and the T waves in the leads previously affected become inverted, while the T wave in lead aVR may become upright.

Mechanical injury may be caused transiently during surgery or when a needle is inserted to administer adrenalin or to withdraw fluid from the pericardial sac. In the latter case, the precordial electrode of an ECG recording device may be attached to the needle used for pericardiocentesis, and the appearance of a current of injury pattern is used to determine that the needle has reached the epicardium.[14]

Similarly, the contact between the tip of a pacing electrode and the endocardium is documented by S-T elevation, as shown in Figure 8-27.

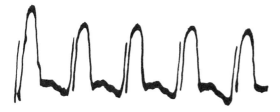

Fig 8-27.—Tracing recorded from pacing electrode, with electrode tip touching endocardium.

Contusion of the heart has been found in association with blunt chest trauma in 15%[15] to 76%[14] of cases. The ECG evidence of such injuries is often delayed and may appear as nonspecific S-T and T wave changes. At other times, a clear pattern resembling either pericarditis or acute injury current may be seen.[14]

Vagotonia is frequently seen in healthy, young athletic subjects. It is more common in males and is frequently seen in blacks.[1(p30)] These persons generally have S-T elevations, usually in the midprecordial and/or inferior leads, that are usually associated with very tall R waves (Fig 8-28). The condition has also been called early repolarization. It is associated with normal T waves, and in doubtful cases, the most significant finding is that the pattern does not evolve, ie, serial ECGs taken over a period of days will reveal no changes.

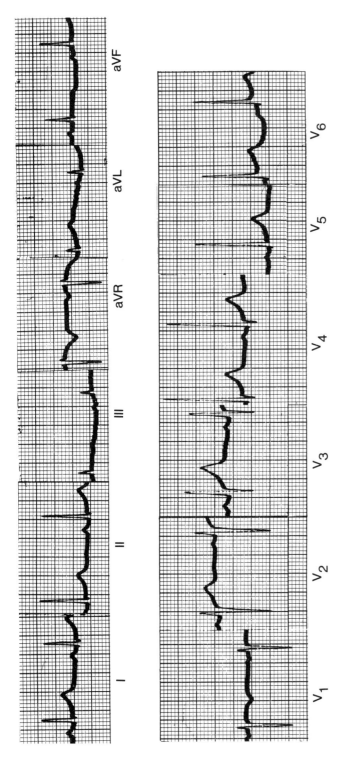

Fig 8-28.—ECG of healthy young man with minor S-T segment elevations in leads V_2 through V_6.

Q Waves and QS Complexes

Q waves are normally seen in the left ventricular leads, including aVL, V_5, and V_6, as a result of depolarization of the intraventricular septum. To be considered *significant* or *pathologic*, the Q wave must measure at least 0.04 second in width, and its depth must be at least equal to 25% of the R wave of the same complex, providing that the R wave is at least 5 mm tall. The width of the Q wave is considered to be the more significant of these two criteria.

Occasionally, a QS complex in lead V_1 or poor R wave progression in the precordial leads are misinterpreted as signs of AWMI. The lack of a small, initial R wave in V_1 is often seen in healthy persons, and is of no particular significance as an isolated finding. It is frequently caused by improper placement of the electrode.

The failure of the R wave to gain substantially in height from lead V_1 toward V_6 may be due to body build or position of the heart and is also seen when the precordial electrodes are improperly placed. The phenomenon may also be caused by pulmonary disease (chap 11).

Lead III frequently shows a Q wave and often shows an inverted T wave as well. Because this lead is greatly influenced by respiration, body position, and other factors, abnormalities of the QRS complex and T wave that are seen only in this lead can safely be ignored.

Missed Diagnosis

Patients should be admitted and treated on the basis of clinical findings, even if the ECG is normal. The patient is at greater risk of sudden death from arrhythmias during an acute episode of ischemia than he is later, when tissue necrosis has occurred. Significant ischemia may exist without producing ECG changes, at least initially. In rare instances, the ECG may not change at all, or it may show uncharacteristic signs, as shown in Figures 8-29a and b.

The tracing in Figure 8-29a shows tiny Q waves preceding the R wave in leads V_1 through V_4. These were considered abnormal and somewhat difficult to explain, since the S-T segments and T waves were not grossly abnormal. When the precordial electrodes were moved to the second intercostal space, the typical S-T elevation and T wave inversion of acute myocardial injury were recorded (Fig 8-29b).

The series of tracings in Figures 8-30a through g demonstrates the need to admit patients on the basis of clinical presentation. This series of tracings shows the entire spectrum of infarction, reinfarction, extension, and healing.

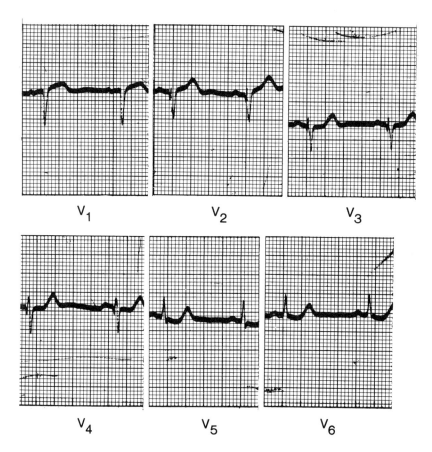

Fig 8-29a.—Precordial leads of patient with chest pain.

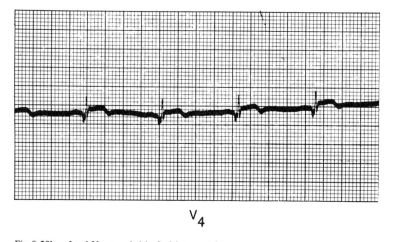

Fig 8-29b.—Lead V₄ recorded in 2nd intercostal space.

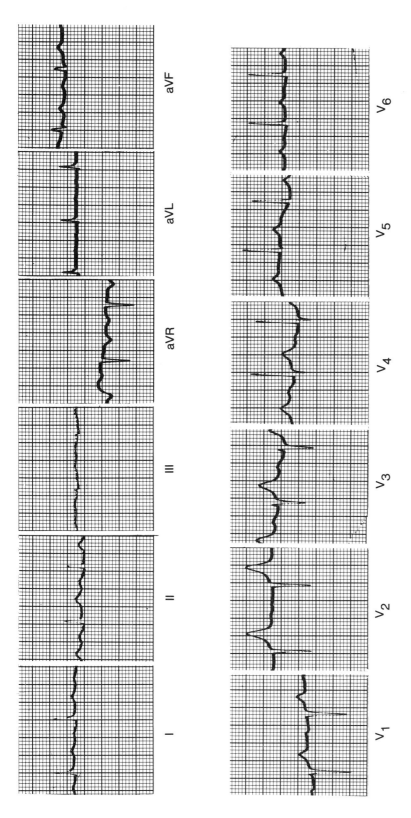

Fig 8-30a.—Admission ECG of 49-year-old man, 5/24/75.

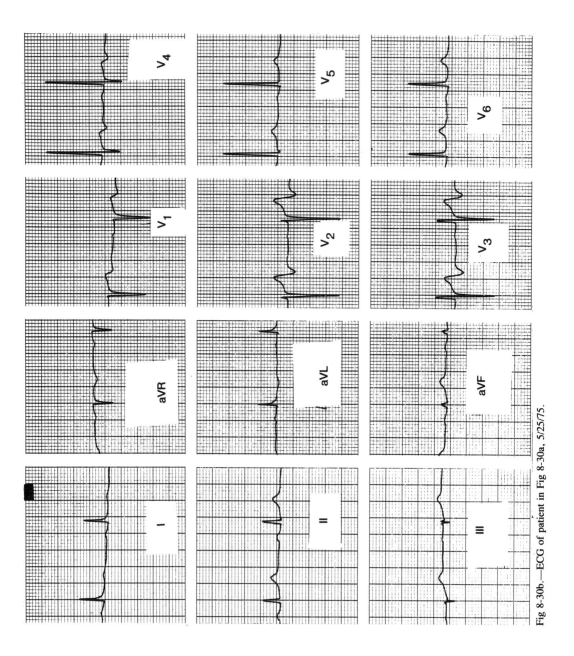

Fig 8-30b.—ECG of patient in Fig 8-30a, 5/25/75.

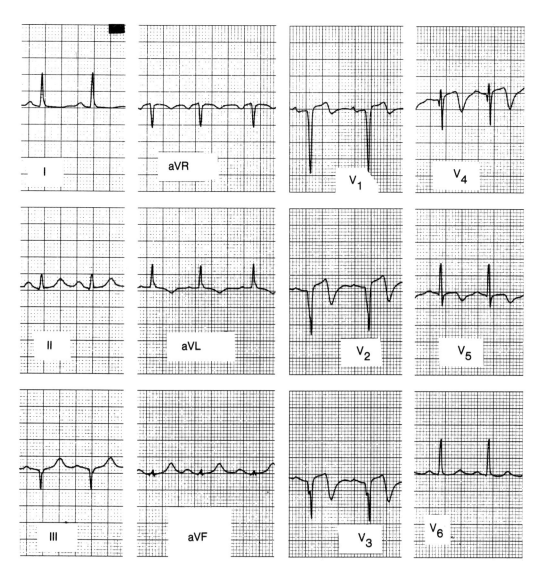

Fig 8-30c.—ECG of patient in Fig 8-30a, 5/26/75.

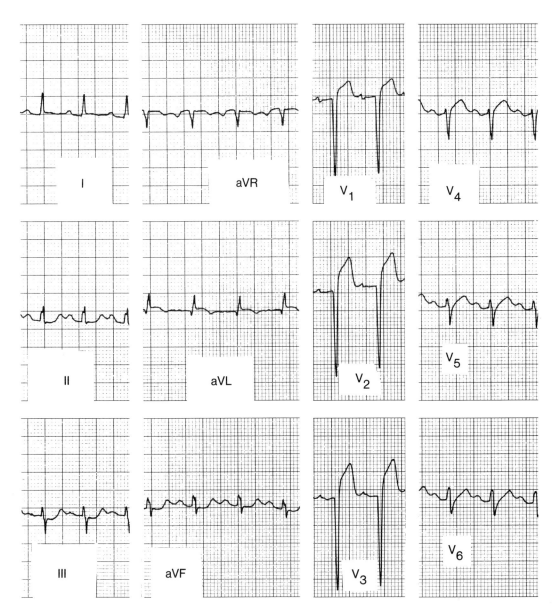

Fig 8-30d.—ECG of patient in Fig 8-30a, 5/29/75.

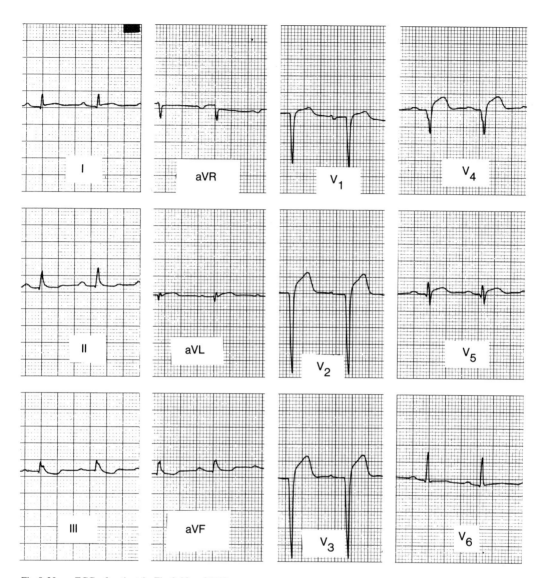

Fig 8-30e.—ECG of patient in Fig 8-30a, 6/3/75.

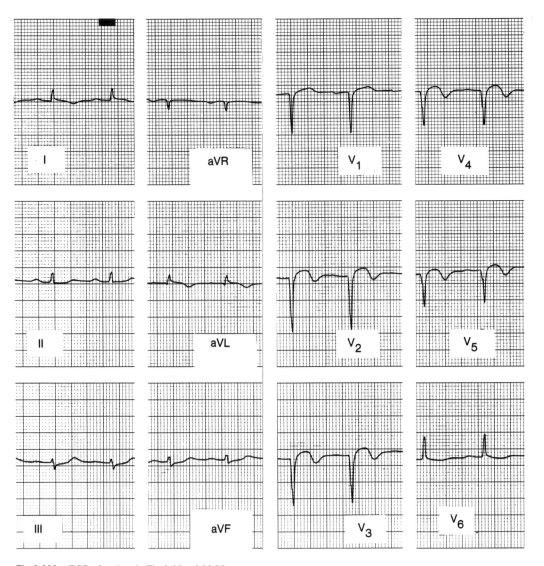

Fig 8-30f.—ECG of patient in Fig 8-30a, 6/25/75.

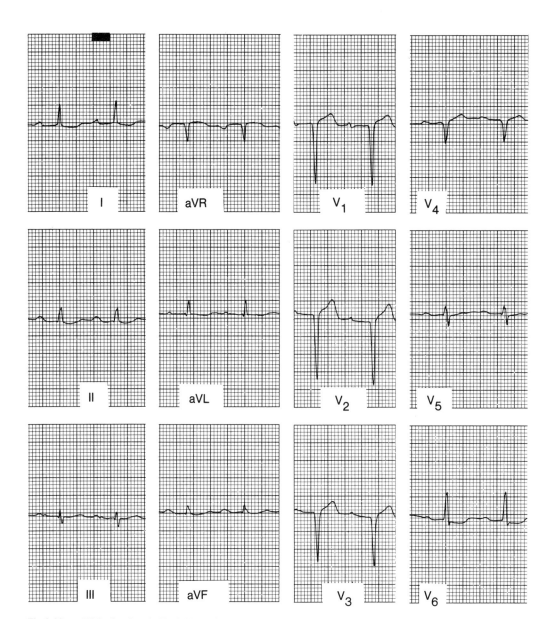

Fig 8-30g.—ECG of patient in Fig 8-30a, 4/30/78.

REFERENCES

1. Schamroth L: *The Electrocardiology of Coronary Artery Disease*. Oxford, England, Blackwell Scientific Publications, 1975.

2. Friedman HH: *Diagnostic Electrocardiography and Vectorcardiography,* ed 2. New York, McGraw-Hill Book Co, 1977.

3. Castellanos A, Myerburg RJ: The resting electrocardiogram, in Hurst JW (ed): *The Heart*. New York, McGraw-Hill Book Co, 1978, p 302.

4. Braunwald E, Maroko PR: The reduction of infarct size—an idea whose time (for testing) has come. *Circulation* 1974;50:206.

5. Page H: NIH study finds nitroglycerine beneficial in acute infarction. *Hospital Tribune*. April 1975, p 21.

6. Spence MI, Lemberg L: Glucose-insulin-potassium in acute myocardial infarction. *Heart Lung* 1980;9:905.

7. Goldman MJ: *Principles of Clinical Electrocardiography,* ed 7. Los Altos, Calif, Lange Medical Publications, 1970. Reprinted by permission.

8. Lewis BS, Schamroth L: The hyperacute phase of true posterior infarction. *Heart Lung* 1977;6:331.

9. Cohn JN: Right ventricular infarction revisited. *Am J Cardiol* 1979;43:666.

10. Sunquist JM, Mikell FL, Francis GS: Right ventricular infarction: Recognition, treatment, and nursing considerations. *Heart Lung* 1980;9:706.

11. Hurst JW, King SB, Walter PF: Atherosclerotic heart disease, in Hurst JW (ed); *The Heart*. New York, McGraw-Hill Book Co, 1982, pp 1124-1125.

12. Arcebal AG, Lemberg L: Acute myocardial infarction and left bundle branch block. *Heart Lung* 1981;10:532.

13. Lyon AF: The hemiblocks and peri-infarction blocks. *ECG Self-Reviews,* No. 4. Ardsley, NY, Maxon Davis, Inc, 1980.

14. Reynolds SF: Cardiac trauma and tamponade. *Crit Care Quart* 1981;4:27.

15. Torres-Mirabal P, Gruenberg JC, Brown RS: Spectrum of myocardial contusion. *Crit Care Med* 1981;9:154.

## Chapter 9

Pacemaker Function and Malfunction

Mechanical pacing of the heart has progressed tremendously since Zoll first reported successful resuscitation of a patient by external electrical stimulation in 1952.[1] The increased use of this technique was facilitated by the introduction of transvenous electrodes in the early 1960s,[2] sensing pacemakers in 1967,[3] and long-lasting power sources in the 1970s. This progress is illustrated by the increasing number of pacemakers used. In 1969, 1 of 5,000 persons in New Jersey had a pacemaker; the ratio was 1 in 1,300 persons in 1975.[2] These figures do not take into account the use of temporary pacing for various purposes.

General Considerations

Indications for Mechanical Pacing

Indications for the use of mechanical pacing, permanent or temporary, are numerous, and new applications of the technique are constantly being announced.

Indications for Mechanical Pacing

Permanent Pacing

1. Complete heart block due to fibrotic changes in the conduction system (most frequent indication)
2. Congenital or surgical heart block (rare)
3. Complete heart block following MI
4. Symptomatic bradyarrhythmias such as: sick sinus syndrome, sinus exit block, periods of sinus arrest, carotid sinus syncope, and intermittent blocks

---

Temporary Pacing

1. Cardiac arrest
2. Symptomatic bradycardias and AV blocks following MI
3. Suppression of supraventricular and ventricular arrhythmias[4,5]
4. Digitalis toxicity
5. Hyperkalemia
6. Diagnostic studies including electrophysiological studies (His bundle ECGs) to test effectiveness of drugs and to provide stress testing during cardiac catheterization
7. Precautionary measure, following open-heart surgery

Mixed Technique

A third technique, which represents a mixture of permanent and temporary pacing, uses an implanted pacemaker that is activated temporarily, either automatically or by the patient, when the need arises. This method has been used successfully to control recurrent supraventricular as well as ventricular arrhythmias[6] and to terminate reentry tachycardias in patients with preexcitation.[7]

Types of Pacemakers

In 1977 there were 44 different pulse generators available.[2] Since then the variety of pacing modalities has increased even further, and today there is a bewildering array of pacemaker models and methods, with new types being added constantly. Under these circumstances it is impossible to describe every existing pacemaker in detail, and only a few general facts will be discussed here, to facilitate understanding of pacemaker function.

Energy Sources

Lithium batteries are most widely used today. These batteries first became available in 1973 and have an expected longevity of 10 or more years.[3]

Nuclear-powered pacemakers were used for the first time in 1970.[8] Although pacemakers using plutonium as a power source have a potential life of 20 to 40 years, relatively few of them are in use. The reasons for this sparing use include: restrictive government regulations, high price, and the advanced age of most pacemaker recipients, which makes the use of this type of pacemaker impractical. Other energy sources no longer in use, or used only very rarely, include *mercury-zinc* batteries, *rechargeable* batteries, and *biogalvanic* batteries.

Programmable Pacemakers

The first pacemakers were set to deliver impulses at a specific, fixed rate and predetermined energy output, and no changes could be made once the unit had been implanted. Today it is possible to alter a number of variables noninvasively by magnetic switches.[3] Further reprogramming possibilities will no doubt become available in the future.

A number of pacemakers permit adjustment of the pulse per minute *rate* over a range of 25 to 125 pulses/minute. A heart rate of 70 beats/min is satisfactory for most patients; however, a higher rate may be more appropriate for some. On the other hand, a relatively slow rate of 50 to 60 beats/min may be advisable for persons with CAD, to reduce myocardial oxygen consumption.

The *electrical output* of a number of models can also be reprogrammed. About 4 months after implantation of a pacing electrode, the conditions in the tissues surrounding the electrode tip have generally stabilized, and it is possible to program the pacemaker to the smallest amount of voltage output that will produce myocardial capture. This procedure conserves energy and increases the longevity of the battery. A pacemaker that was functioning well at the time of implantation may suddenly fail to capture, due to an increase in threshold caused by tissue changes or a collection of fibrin in the area of the electrode tip. This problem can usually be resolved by increasing the electrical output of the pacemaker.

In some models the *pacing mode* can be changed. For example, some pacemakers can be reprogrammed from a demand mode into a fixed mode of pacing. Some of the newer, highly sophisticated pacemakers allow reprogramming of both atrial and ventricular pacing and sensing modes.

Sensitivity may be increased or decreased in some models, to meet the changing needs of the patient. Other variables that can be reprogrammed in some units include *refractory period, AV delay,* and *pulse width.*

Most reprogramming operations of pacemakers are performed through the intact skin, by use of units provided by the manufacturer. Such a unit is shown in Figure 9-1. This programmer can be used with all programmable pacemakers manufactured by the Cordis Corporation; it functions as follows.[9]

The unit is turned on, and the model number representing the patient's pacemaker is selected by pushing the appropriate button. The programmer then displays the programming capabilities of the particular pacing unit, and the user selects the desired parameters by using the push buttons and the visual display. Then the programmer is placed on the skin directly over the implanted pacemaker, and activation of the programmer transmits the desired changes to the pacer by a pulsating magnetic field.

The programmer has several other features such as a printout; these are clearly described in the manufacturer's instruction manual.[9]

Other companies also provide reprogrammers for their specific models. Such units are available from: CPI; Medtronics, Inc; Pace Setter; and Intermedics. The manufacturer's instructions should be followed carefully when these units are used.[10]

Pacemaker Nomenclature

The first pacing units delivered regularly timed stimuli to the ventricles and were easily described as fixed-rate ventricular pacemakers. Since then, a number of demand modes have been developed, and atria, as well as ventricles, are being paced. This has led to the use of a confusing variety of terms to describe

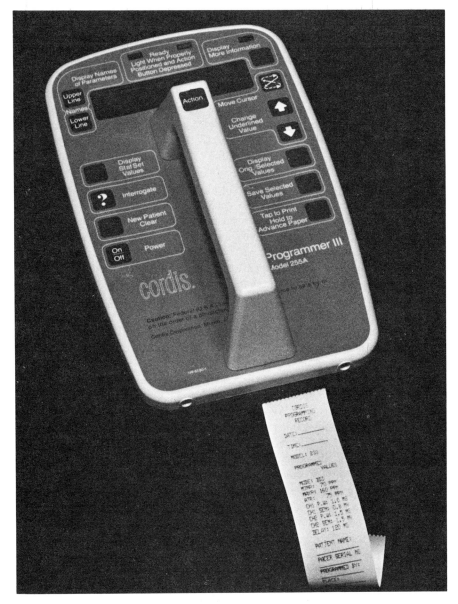

Fig 9-1.—Cordis Programmer III (model 255 A). Courtesy Cordis Corp.

pacemakers, and in 1974 a simple three-letter code was proposed that allows accurate, specific description of most models in use (Fig 9-2). The application of this code is demonstrated in Table 9-1.

More recently the addition of two letters has been suggested.[11] The first letter would be used to describe programming function and the second would indicate special tachyarrhythmia functions of the pacemaker. However, this addition to the code is not yet in general use.

THREE LETTER IDENTIFICATION CODE

1st LETTER	2nd LETTER	3rd LETTER
CHAMBER PACED	CHAMBER SENSED	MODE OF RESPONSE

V - VENTRICLE
A - ATRIUM
D - DOUBLE CHAMBER

I - INHIBITED
T - TRIGGERED
O - NOT APPLICABLE

First letter: The paced chamber is identified by V for ventricle, A for atrium, or D for double —both atrium and ventricle.

Second letter: The sensed chamber, if either, is again V for ventricle, A for atrium.

Third letter: The mode of response, if any, is either:
I for inhibited, a pacemaker whose output is *blocked* by a sensed signal, or
T for triggered, a unit whose output is *discharged* by a sensed signal.

The letter "O" indicates that a specific comment is not applicable.

Fig 9-2.—Reprinted from Parsonnett V, Furman S, Smyth NPD: Implantable cardiac pacemakers status report and resource guidelines. *Circulation* 1974;50:A-21. Used by permission of the American Heart Association, Inc.

Table 9-1.—Suggested Nomenclature Code for Implantable Cardiac Pacemakers*

Chamber paced	Chamber sensed	Mode of response	Generic description	Previously used designation
V	0	0	Ventricular pacing; no sensing function	Asynchronous; fixed rate; set rate
A	0	0	Atrial pacing; no sensing function	Atrial fixed rate; atrial asynchronous
D	0	0	Atrioventricular pacing; no sensing function	AV sequential fixed rate (asynchronous)
V	V	I	Ventricular pacing and sensing, inhibited mode	Ventricular inhibited; R inhibited; R blocking; R suppressed; noncompetitive inhibited; demand; standby
V	V	T	Ventricular pacing and sensing, triggered mode	Ventricular triggered; R triggered; R wave stimulated; noncompetitive triggered; following; R synchronous; demand; standby
A	A	I	Atrial pacing and sensing, inhibited mode	Atrial inhibited; P inhibited; P blocking; P suppressed
A	A	T	Atrial pacing and sensing, triggered mode	Atrial triggered; P triggered; P stimulated; P synchronous
V	A	T	Ventricular pacing, atrial sensing, triggered mode	Atrial synchronous, atrial synchronized, AV synchronous
D	V	I	Atrioventricular pacing, ventricular sensing, inhibited mode	Bifocal sequential demand, AV sequential

*Reprinted from Parsonnett V, Furman S, Smyth NPD: Implantable cardiac pacemakers status report and resource guidelines. *Circulation* 1974;50:A-22. Used by permission of the American Heart Association.

Evaluation of Pacemaker Function

Surveillance and evaluation of pacemaker function are important nursing responsibilities, extending from the time of implantation, through coronary care and telemetry units, to outpatient facilities. The first step in assessment of pacing function is to know the purpose of a particular unit.

Modes of Pacing

Asynchronous Ventricular Pacing (VOO)

In the asynchronous, or fixed, mode a pacemaker delivers a preset number of pulses per minute to the ventricles, without regard for spontaneous electrical activity in the patient. This mode is rarely used because most patients produce at least occasional intrinsic electrical activity and are exposed to the dangers of competition if a VOO pacemaker is used.

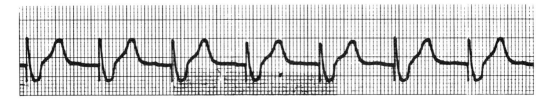

Fig 9-3.—Asynchronous ventricular pacing.

The rhythm strip in Figure 9-3 shows a paced rhythm at the rate of 74 beats/min. The pacing spikes are clearly visible and regular, and the QRS complexes are wide, since they originate from a ventricular focus. On the basis of this strip, it is impossible to determine whether the pacemaker is a VOO or a ventricular-inhibited (VVI) unit, in a patient who has no spontaneous beats.

Ventricular-Triggered Pacing (VVT)

The ventricular-triggered (VVT) pacemaker was the earliest widely used ventricular demand pacemaker. It senses spontaneous ventricular activity and fires immediately. If no spontaneous ventricular beat occurs within a preset period of time (escape interval), the pacemaker discharges at a regular rate corresponding to the escape interval.

The advantage of this mode is that the pacing artifact is always visible, making it easy to evaluate pacemaker function. These units are rarely used today, because the constant discharge of impulses hastens battery depletion and all QRS complexes are distorted by the pacemaker signal.

In the strip in Figure 9-4, the beats marked "E" (electrical) are paced at a fixed rate, corresponding to an escape interval of 820 ms (about 72 pulses/min). The complexes marked "S" (spontaneous) represent spontaneous ventricular depolarization. The pacing artifact occurs about 0.06 second after the beginning of the R wave and distorts the spontaneous QRS complex. There is a pause after each of the spontaneous beats, and the pacemaker emits a stimulus after elapse of the escape interval.

This type of pacing is not used very often, but it is important to be able to recognize correct VVT pacing, since some of these units may still be in use. Figure 9-5 shows another example of this pacing mode.

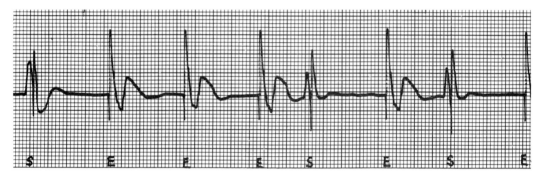

Fig 9-4.—Ventricular-triggered pacing. E = electrical and S = spontaneous.

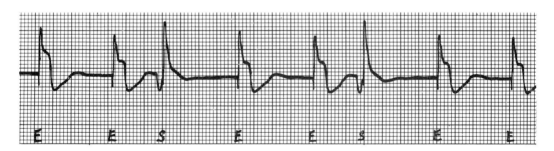

Fig 9-5.—Ventricular-triggered pacing. E = electrical and S = spontaneous.

Ventricular-Inhibited Pacing

Ventricular-inhibited (VVI) pacing is the most commonly used mode for temporary as well as permanent pacing. In this mode, spontaneous ventricular depolarization inhibits the discharge of the pacemaker and resets the escape interval (Fig 9-6).

While the patient is in sinus rhythm at a rate of 82 beats/min, there is no evidence of the pacemaker. The compensatory pause following a PVC causes the pacemaker to fire.

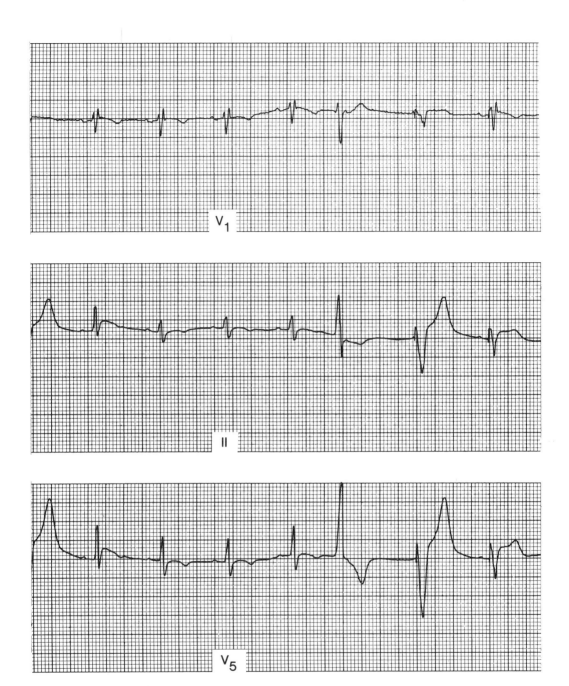

Fig 9-6.—Ventricular-inhibited pacing.

Atrial Synchronous Pacing

The atrial synchronous (VAT) mode was actually the first demand pacing method,[3] but it was rarely used because thoracotomy was required to place the electrodes. This pacing mode uses an atrial sensing electrode and a ventricular pacing electrode. The pacemaker functions as follows.

- At atrial rates ranging from 60 to about 140 beats/min, the pacemaker senses atrial depolarization, and after a delay corresponding to the normal P-R interval, paces the ventricle.
- When the spontaneous atrial rate falls below 60 beats/min, the pacemaker stimulates the ventricle at a rate of 60 pulses/min.
- At atrial rates above 140 to 150 beats/min, the pacer's refractory period prevents 1:1 conduction, and the paced ventricular rate is reduced to about 70 beats/min.

The function of a VAT pacemaker (Atricor, Cordis Corp) is illustrated in Figure 9-7. The patient exercised on a treadmill to increase the heart rate.

The top strip in Figure 9-7 shows a sinus rate of about 65 beats/min. The P waves are clearly seen. After a P-R interval of 0.17 second, there is a pacing artifact, followed by ventricular depolarization. Sinus arrhythmia is present, and it can be seen how well the pacemaker "follows" the atrial rhythm.

The P waves are not clearly visible in the middle strip of Figure 9-7; with the faster rate, they are hidden in the downstroke of the T wave. The ventricular rate is 130 beats/min.

The sinus rate is increased, until it approaches 150 beats/min in the bottom strip. There are two instances in which a P wave is not followed by a pacing artifact (arrow). This is not a malfunction of the pacemaker but represents a built-in mechanism designed to protect the ventricle from supraventricular tachyarrhythmias.

This mechanism is well illustrated in Figure 9-8. The pacemaker paces at a fixed rate of 60 pulses/min most of the time and never responds at an interval of less than 460 ms.

For patients with normal sinus function, this represents the ideal pacing mode, since it maintains synchronous, sequential depolarization of atria and ventricles over a physiological range of 60 to 140 beats/min. At the same time, a minimum rate of 60 beats/min is assured; if supraventricular tachyarrhythmias occur, a dangerously rapid ventricular response is prevented.

A number of electrodes that permit stable implantation in the right atrium by the pervenous route have recently become available.[12,13] This advance eliminates the major drawback to VAT pacing, and the use of these pacemakers will probably increase, especially in younger patients.

Atrioventricular Sequential Demand Pacing

With improvement in electrodes and the technique for transvenous insertion of atrial electrodes, dual-chamber pacing is being used with increasing frequency. Some physicians use a form of this technique in as many as 50% of their patients.[12]

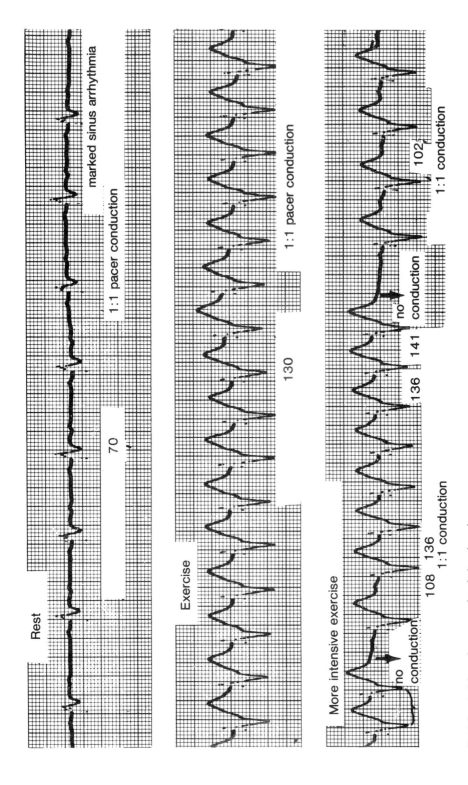

Fig 9-7.—Atrial synchronous pacing during slow sinus rate.

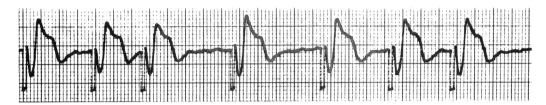

Fig 9-8.—Atrial synchronous pacing in atrial fibrillation. Courtesy Cordis Corp.

The method has been successful in suppressing tachyarrhythmias in patients with tachybradycardia syndrome[13] and is considered useful in patients with a history of congestive heart failure, who may require the "atrial kick" to improve cardiac output.

A variety of pacing modes is available for this purpose. In the DVI mode, both chambers are paced sequentially, with a programmed sensing and pacing interval of 0.16 to 0.20 second between atrial and ventricular pacing. Spontaneous ventricular depolarization, which occurs within this preset interval, is sensed and inhibits ventricular pacing (Figs 9-9, 9-10).

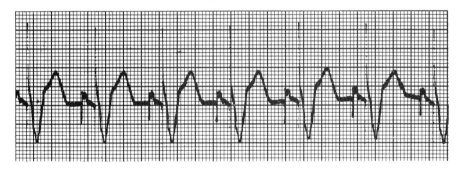

Fig 9-9.—DVI pacing. Courtesy Cordis Corp.

The pacemaker does not sense spontaneous atrial depolarization but continues to stimulate the atria at a fixed rate.

In the DDD mode, both chambers are sensed and paced, and pacing may be inhibited in either or both chambers. Most models that use the DDD mode follow the patient over a spontaneous rate ranging from 50 to 130 beats/min.

In the strip shown in Figure 9-11, the first two beats show both atrial and ventricular pacing, with an artificial P-R interval of 0.16 second. With a spontaneous atrial rate of 55 beats/min, atrial pacing is inhibited; however, ventricular pacing continues 0.16 second after the onset of each P wave.

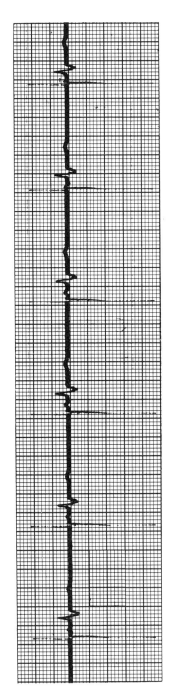

Fig 9-10.—DVI pacing. Courtesy Cordis Corp.

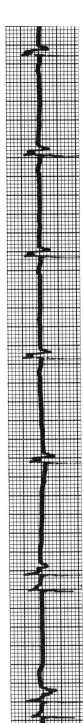

Fig 9-11.—DDD pacing. Courtesy Cordis Corp.

In Figure 9-12, the first three beats show atrial pacing at a rate of 60 pulses/min. The first and third ventricular beats are paced, and the second is a spontaneous beat, following within 0.16 second of the paced atrial beat. As the atrial rate increases, no further atrial pacing is seen, but ventricular beats are alternately spontaneous and paced.

In the strip in Figure 9-13, the first beat is entirely spontaneous, and thereafter, all atrial beats are paced. If the P-R intervals are measured carefully, a form of Wenckebach conduction is observed. The ventricular beats that follow closely after the paced atrial beats are spontaneous, but as the P-R interval lengthens, a fusion between spontaneous and pacer-induced ventricular depolarization occurs, and when the P-R interval lengthens to 0.20 second, the ventricular beat is paced.

In the VDD mode, both chambers are sensed, but only the ventricle is paced. In the strip shown in Figure 9-14, each spontaneous P wave is followed by ventricular pacing, after an interval of 0.16 second. Since this pacemaker has a preset fixed rate of about 60 pulses/min, a paced ventricular beat should have occurred after the fourth beat. However, the ventricular portion of the pacemaker functions in a dual role, that is, it is stimulated by atrial depolarization and inhibited by ventricular depolarization. The PVC, therefore, resets the ventricular escape interval.

Not only are pacing modes highly complex, but many of the newer pacemakers permit reprogramming into a different mode. To permit evaluation of pacemaker function, it is essential that patients carry information describing their particular pacemaker and that the information is appropriately updated each time parameters are reprogrammed.

Evaluation at Electrode Insertion

The initial evaluation of a pacing system takes place at the time of electrode insertion. It is not sufficient to determine that appropriate capture of the paced chamber occurs at this time. Capture and/or sensing may be lost within hours to weeks afterward, even if the electrode tip does not change its position, unless the necessary precautions are taken. The two most important parameters to be measured are stimulus threshold and intracardiac R wave potential.

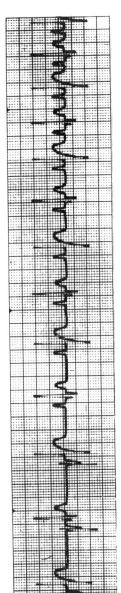

Fig 9-12.—DDD pacing, mechanically simulated. Courtesy Cordis Corp.

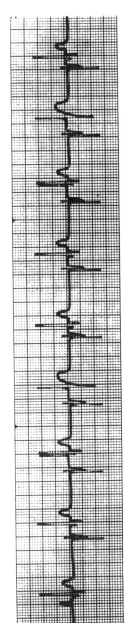

Fig 9-13.—DDD pacing, mechanically simulated. Courtesy Cordis Corp.

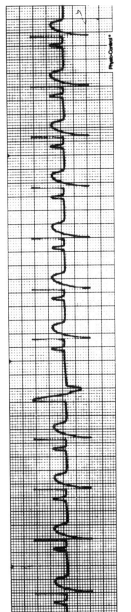

Fig 9-14.—VDD pacing, mechanically reproduced. Courtesy Cordis Corp.

Temporary System

Once satisfactory pacing has been established in a temporary system, tests for these two variables are performed.[10]

Evaluation of Pacing System

Test for Sensitivity (intracardiac R wave potential)

1. Reduce pacer rate to 10 beats/min below the patient's spontaneous rate. If patient has few or no spontaneous beats, sensitivity cannot be tested in this manner.
2. Slowly turn sensitivity dial counterclockwise from most sensitive position until pacemaker fires in spite of spontaneous depolarization.
3. Gradually turn sensitivity dial clockwise until pacer signal disappears.
4. Sensitivity threshold is represented by point shown on dial. Sensitivity of 6 mV is considered adequate.
5. Set sensitivity dial to lower (more sensitive) position than the one determined.

Test for Stimulation Threshold

1. Set pacemaker higher than patient's spontaneous rate to ensure continuous pacing.
2. Gradually decrease output (mA) until 1:1 capture is lost, that is, pacer signals are not followed by ventricular depolarization.
3. Gradually increase output, until 1:1 capture is established.
4. Point that has been reached on the mA dial represents threshold. Threshold of 1.0 mA or less is considered satisfactory.
5. Set mA dial at three to five increments above threshold that has been determined.

Permanent System

A number of methods can be used to test a permanent system. This is generally done in the cardiac catheterization laboratory.[10,14-16]

The method described for testing a temporary system may be adapted to check capture and sensing thresholds of an electrode inserted for permanent pacing. An external pacemaker is temporarily attached to the electrode, and the test is performed as for a temporary system.

Measurement of the *intracardiac R wave* determines the sensitivity threshold. The voltage of the R wave recorded from the surface of the body is not at all the same as the voltage of myocardial depolarization sensed by the pacing electrode.

The intracardiac R wave potential can be recorded by connecting the pacing electrode to a well-grounded ECG machine or an oscilloscope. At the same time a current of injury pattern that occurs when the electrode tip is in contact with the endocardium (Fig 8-27) can be recorded.

The safest, easiest, and most satisfactory method for testing a permanent system is to use a pacemaker systems analyzer (PSA) specifically designed for this purpose. This model (Fig 9-15) not only tests capture and sensitivity thresholds for both atrial and ventricular electrodes; it also functions as a temporary pacemaker and is also used to check the output and sensing capabilities of the pacing unit to be implanted. Detailed instructions for use are provided by the manufacturer.[14]

Systems for testing pacing parameters are available from a number of manufacturers of pacing equipment. The instructions for use should be carefully followed.

Position of Electrode Tip

The correct, stable position of the electrode tip is essential to ensure continued, effective pacing. The means used to ascertain the position include fluoroscopy, roentgenogram, and the 12-lead ECG.

Electrodes are usually inserted with fluoroscopic visualization, and this method may also be used to determine the position at a later time. Both posteroanterior and lateral roentgenograms are necessary to accurately determine the position of a pacing catheter.

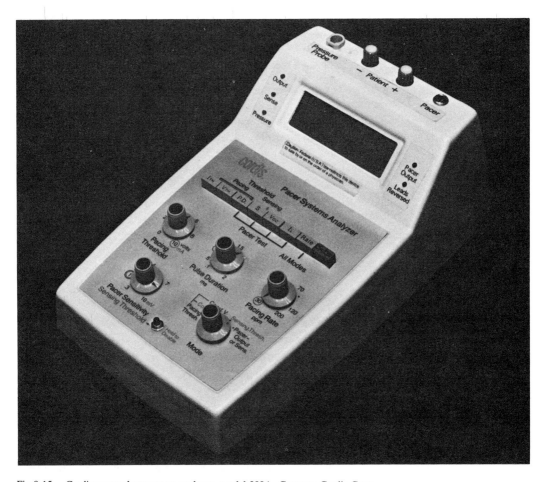

Fig 9-15.—Cordis pacemaker systems analyzer, model 209A. Courtesy Cordis Corp.

Evaluation Following Pacemaker Implantation

Patient Assessment

The *pulse rate, blood pressure, and signs of tissue perfusion* are always the *most important* variables to be monitored. No matter how perfect the system or the ECG, the pulse rate reflects actual myocardial contraction. It is, therefore, the most important criterion of the effectiveness of pacing.

Electrocardiogram

Continuous ECG monitoring is generally indicated for at least 24 hours following pacer implantation. Care must be taken to avoid some of the associated pitfalls.

The ECG in Figure 9-16 shows regular pacing spikes at a rate of 68 pulses/min; however, no ventricular capture occurs at any time. The apparent QRS complex represents the drift of the stylus back to the baseline following the pacing artifact. The danger of this problem is that the pacer artifacts are sensed by the monitor, so no alarm is activated. The lack of capture can be recognized by the absence of the QRS complex and the T waves and by the lack of palpable pulses.

At first glance, the rhythm strip in Figure 9-17 appears to show the same problem. There are pacing spikes, but no QRS complexes can be identified. However, T waves are present (arrow), and ventricular repolarization is only possible if depolarization has taken place. Taking the patient's pulse will confirm the presence of a regular ventricular rhythm at a rate of 75 beats/min.

Another occasional problem has been due to the filtering system of the monitor, which is designed to filter out both high- and low-frequency signals.[17] This may cause transient disappearance of the pacer signal and/or QRS complexes. A 12-lead ECG will confirm the presence of appropriate pacing, and the patient's pulse will reflect the actual ventricular rate.

The *12-lead ECG*, too, may occasionally cause a diagnostic problem. The ECG in Figure 9-18 shows regular QRS complexes at a rate of 75 beats/min. The complexes are wide and distorted, and no P waves can be seen. This patient's heart is paced at a rate of 75 pulses/min, but the pacer signal cannot be seen. This problem is occasionally encountered when bipolar electrodes are used.

Another rhythm strip (Fig 9-19) caused a great deal of confusion prior to diagnosis. The pacing spike is followed by large, square waves that bear no resemblance to QRS complexes. This apparent pacemaker malfunction was due to a protective mechanism built into a rather old-fashioned ECG machine. Whenever it sensed higher-than-normal voltages, the stylus went off the paper. A 12-lead tracing obtained with a modern machine demonstrated perfect pacemaker function.

Use of Magnet

Many patients with pacemakers have a spontaneous rhythm that is faster than the fixed rate of the pacemaker most of the time. If the heart is paced in the VVI mode, no evidence of pacing will be seen. It is, however, important to be able to determine whether capture will occur during pacing. In addition, many pacemakers are designed so that their fixed rate decreases with impending battery failure.

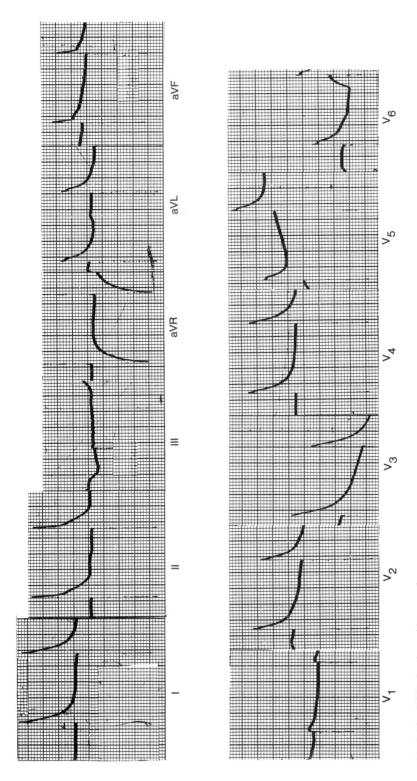

Fig 9-16.—ECG of patient with pacemaker.

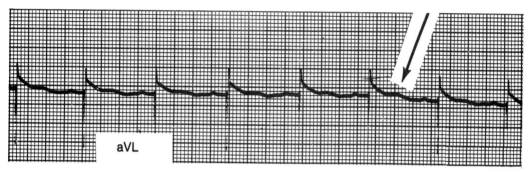

Fig 9-17.—Rhythm strip of patient with pacemaker; arrow shows T waves.

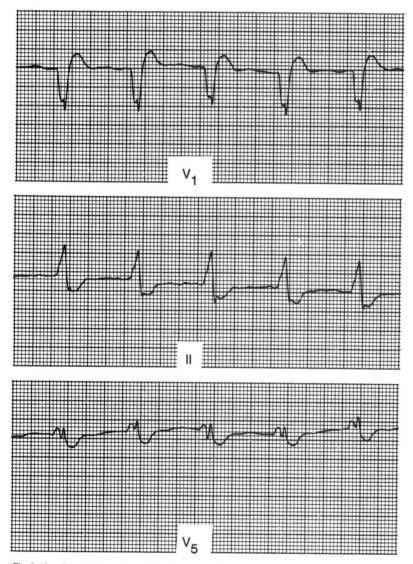

Fig 9-18.—Rhythm strip of patient with pacemaker.

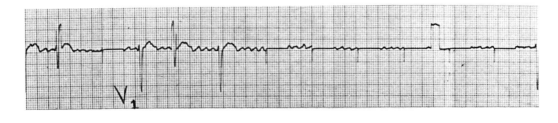

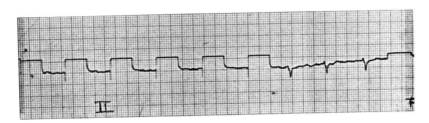

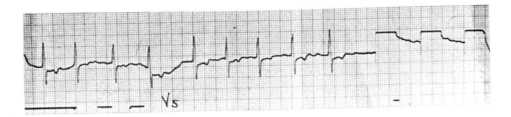

Fig 9-19.—Tracing for discussion.

For these reasons, a magnetically activated reed switch has been incorporated into all VVI pacing units. When a suitable magnet is applied to the skin above the implanted unit, the switch shuts off the sensing circuit, and the pacemaker is converted to the VOO mode. This function is illustrated in Figures 9-20a and b.

The tracing in Figure 9-20b shows pacing signals at a rate of 70 pulses/min. Capture occurs whenever the pacemaker stimulus does not fall within the refractory period following the preceding spontaneous beat.

With the increased use of programmable pacing units, this method is no longer considered satisfactory by some. Because our society is very mobile, patients with pacemakers are often visitors or newly moved to the area. A magnet rate of 60 pulses/min in such a patient may indicate the need for urgent replacement of the unit, or it may simply indicate that the pacemaker has been reprogrammed to that rate. Patients often do not know the answer, and in the absence of adequate information, unnecessary replacement of the pacemaker may be undertaken.

Consequently, some manufacturers have built units with characteristic "magnet rates" that differ from the fixed rate.

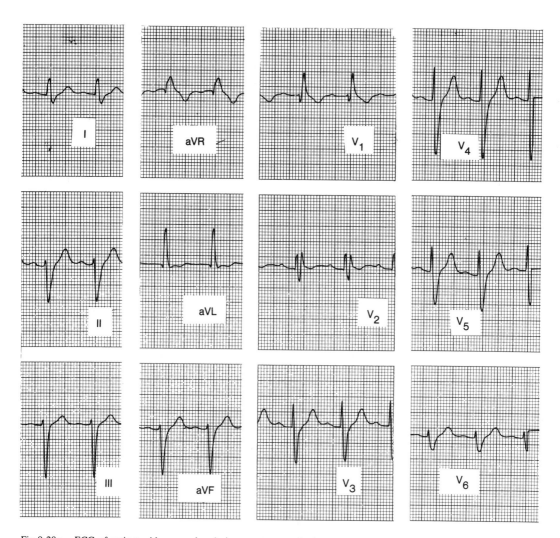

Fig 9-20a.—ECG of patient with pacemaker during spontaneous rhythm.

One example is the CPI Microlith pacemaker. When a suitable magnet is applied over this model, it will pace at a rate of 100 pulses/min. The first six beats following removal of the magnet will be paced at the asynchronous fixed rate. Thereafter the pacing unit will resume its VVI mode.

Many of the newer pacing models exhibit very characteristic behaviors when a magnet is applied.[16] It is important to be familiar with the patient's pacemaker, so the results of magnet application can be correctly interpreted.

Long-Term Evaluation

The most satisfactory means of long-term pacemaker surveillance is a periodic check at an organized center.[2] These centers usually provide physical examination, ECG evaluation, and electronic evaluation and recording of the pacer

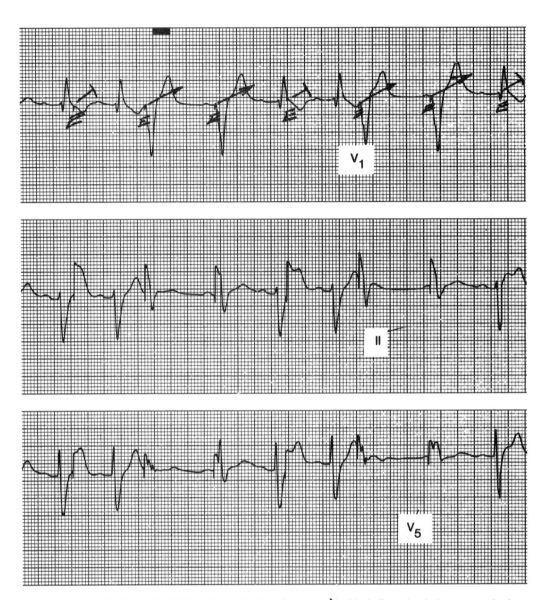

Fig 9-20b.—ECG of patient in Fig 9-20a during application of magnet. λ= block; E = electrical; ➔= conduction.

signal itself. The information obtained is computerized and readily available to other physicians, if the patient should travel. In addition, such centers or clinics often provide an excellent opportunity for patient education, as well as a social atmosphere that contributes to patient morale.

The pacemaker evaluation report (Fig 9-21) records all data necessary for pacemaker identification, reprogramming information, and a sample ECG. The photograph of the pacer signal's waveform permits analysis of pacer function. Relevant data concerning the patient's status are also included.

```
                  PACEMAKER EVALUATION REPORT

NAME:
NUMBER: JSMC00070 -03              MALE        BIRTHDATE: 9/29/1899
PACEMAKER TYPE: 039  (CORDIS 153B VOO, LOW)   PRESENT AGE:   78
ELECTRODE TYPE: 001  (CORDIS 6MM TV 322-261)
DIAGNOSIS: SINUS BRADY              IMPLANTS: FIRST    69  9/19/1969
REFERRED BY: DR(S).                          THIS # 03  75  4/22/1975
                                  TOTAL MONTHS PACED:   108
```

EVALUATION # 15 VISIT	MTHS IN	HEART RATE (BPM)	PULSE INTERVAL (MSEC)	PULSE WIDTH (MSEC)	PEAK AMP. (MV)	COMPE- TITION	1-1 CAP- TURE	1-1 SEN- SING	WAVE FORM
FIRST DATED 8/13/1975	4	69	868	1.0	140	NO	YES		1

```
                 COMPARISON WITH FIRST VISIT
              <- ABSOLUTE CHANGE ->  % CHANGE
```

#	MTHS	HEART RATE	PULSE INTERVAL	PULSE WIDTH	PEAK AMP.	COMPE- TITION	1-1 CAP- TURE	1-1 SEN- SING	WAVE FORM
# 2	8	+0	+0	+0.0	-36	NO		YES	1
# 3	12	+0	-1	+0.1	-26	NO		YES	1
# 4	15	+0	+0	+0.0	+14	NO		YES	1
# 5	18	+0	-2	+0.1	+25	NO		YES	1
# 6	21	+0	-2	+0.0	+19	NO		YES	1
# 7	24	+0	-3	+0.1	K7	NO		YES	1
# 8	27	+0	-2	+0.1	+7	NO		YES	1
# 9	29	+0	-2	+0.0	+21	YES		YES	1
# 10	31	+0	-2	+0.1	+7	NO		YES	1
# 11	33	+0	-2	+0.1	+7	NO		YES	1
# 12	35	+0	-1	+0.1	+10	NO		YES	1
# 13	37	+0	-1	+0.1	+7	YES		YES	1
# 14	39	+0	-2	+0.1	+6	NO		YES	1
THIS	41	+0	-1	+0.1	-43	NO		YES	1
DATED 9/14/1978		69	867	1.1	80				

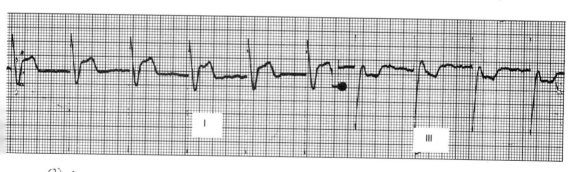

```
B.P. 9/(?)0                COMPLAINTS  U/C                    DR.
POCKET:      OK                                    HEARTSOUNDS:  ok
PACERFUNCTION: OK     RECOMMENDATIONS & Rx         MURMUR:  uo
  CAPTURE: OK                    Same              LUNGS:  clear
  SENSING: NA                                      EDEMA:  no
  BATTERIES: OK
PHONE CHECK:  NO   YES ✓

NEXT VISIT   2   MONTHS                                 1/(?)
```

Fig 9-21.—Pacemaker evaluation center report.

Pacemaker Malfunction

The most common causes of pacemaker malfunction include: battery depletion, electrode fracture, malposition of the electrode tip, and component failure. Inhibition of the pacemaker by external or internal sources is a much less common problem. Temporary systems may also malfunction because of disconnections and accidental changes in dial settings.

Determination of Electrode Position with 12-Lead ECG

Displacement of the electrode tip is one of the most frequent causes of pacemaker failure, especially immediately following implantation and in temporary systems. The nurse should, therefore, be able to evaluate the position of the electrode tip from the ECG.[18,19]

Correct Position of Transvenous Electrode

The correct position of the electrode tip for transvenous ventricular pacing is in the apex of the right ventricle, pointing forward (Fig 9-22). This position produces the following ECG characteristics in paced beats:

- left axis deviation in the frontal plane,
- LBBB pattern in lead V_1, and
- upright pacing spike in V_1.

Malposition of Pacing Electrode

The pacing spikes in Figure 9-23a are followed by P waves, implying that the tip of the electrode is in the atrium (Fig 9-23b). That would be acceptable if the object was atrial pacing. However, in this patient with acute IWMI, the electrode was inserted to permit temporary ventricular pacing during periods of symptomatic AV block. It is essential that the nurse recognize this malposition of the electrode before the patient has further episodes of AV block (Fig 9-24).

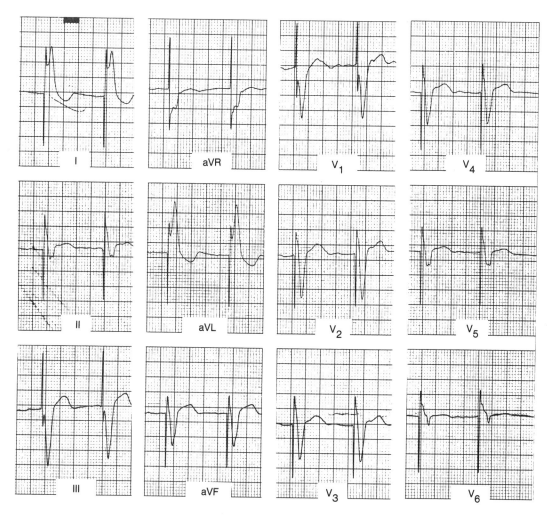

Fig 9-22.—ECG illustrating correct electrode position.

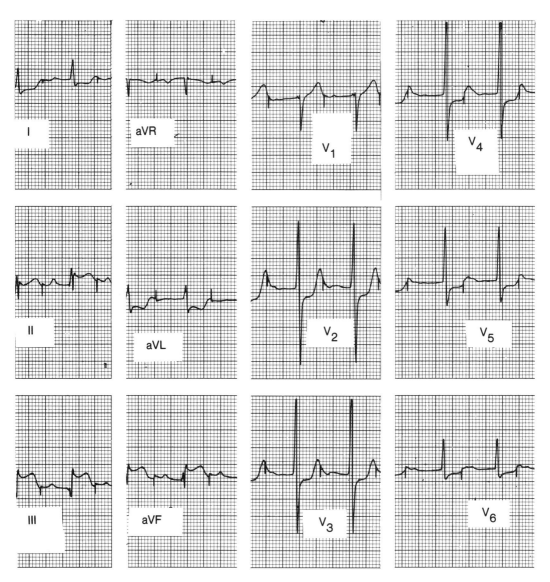

Fig 9-23a.—Tracing for discussion.

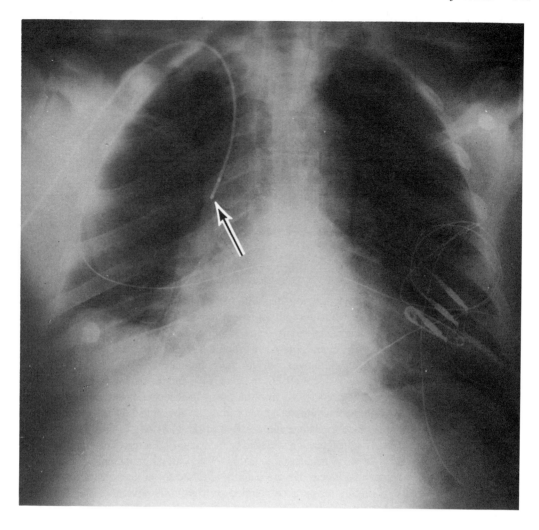

Fig 9-23b.—Chest X-ray of patient in Fig 9-23a. Arrow points to tip of electrode.

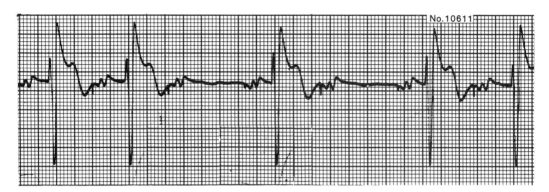

Fig 9-24.—Rhythm strip showing atrial pacing in presence of atrioventricular block.

Right axis deviation, together with LBBB configuration in lead V_1, results from pacing at or near the right ventricular outflow tract (Fig 9-25a). Electrodes inserted during emergencies are often "semi-floating" or "floating" and have a tendency to advance themselves. Again, this should be recognized, because pacing will be lost if the electrode moves out into the pulmonary artery.

In the tracing in Figure 9-26, the axis is 0^0, and the pacing spike is negative in lead V_1. An X-ray showed that the tip of the electrode was in the midcardiac region. Since pacing remained good and the tip appeared to be firmly anchored, no effort was made to change the position of the electrode.

An RBBB configuration of paced beats in lead V_1 indicates pacing from the left ventricle. In most instances this is due to myocardial implantation of electrodes, since epicardial electrodes are usually attached to the left ventricle. When the RBBB configuration is accompanied by right axis deviation, the electrode is attached to the lateral wall of the left ventricle (Figs 9-27a through c). Left axis deviation, on the other hand, reflects implantation near the apex of the left ventricle.

In the chest films shown in Figures 9-27b and c, the epicardial electrodes implanted in the lateral wall of the left ventricle can be clearly seen. A transvenous electrode, which was inserted when the pacemaker was exchanged, is also in place. Pacing via the transvenous electrode is shown in Figure 9-27d.

Apparent left ventricular pacing may also result when the tip of the electrode is in the coronary sinus or when it has perforated the wall of the right ventricle.[20]

Perforation of the thin wall of the right ventricle by a pacing electrode is not uncommon. Fortunately, the muscular wall of the ventricle generally acts "like a self-sealing tire,"[16] and cardiac tamponade rarely results. Nevertheless, the condition must be recognized and corrected, since it usually causes a loss of sensing and/or pacing. The ECG is much more sensitive in revealing this problem than the X-ray, since the displacement of the electrode tip by only a few millimeters may not be apparent on chest films, whereas the changes in the ECG are very noticeable.[16] Other signs include hiccoughs, due to stimulation of the diaphragm.

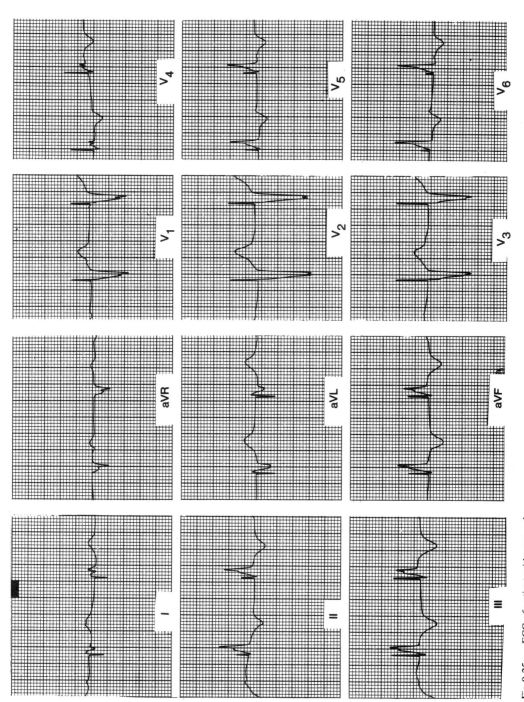

Fig 9-25a.—ECG of patient with pacemaker.

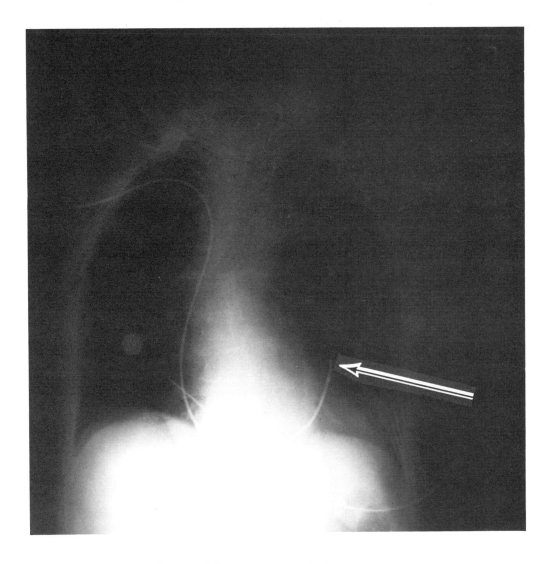

Fig 9-25b.—Chest X-ray of patient in Fig 9-25a. Arrow points to tip of electrode.

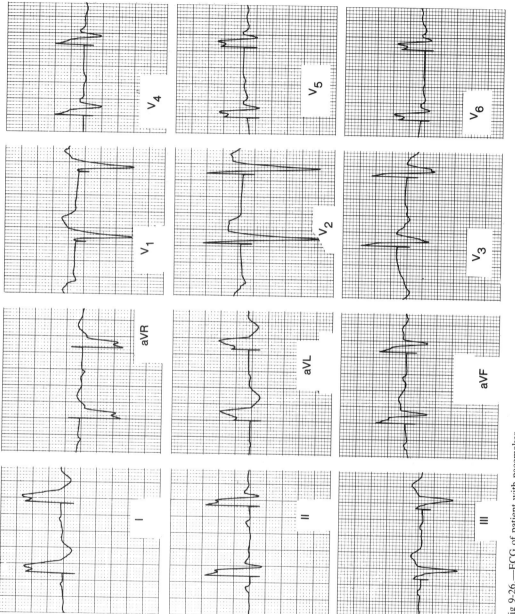

Fig 9-26.—ECG of patient with pacemaker.

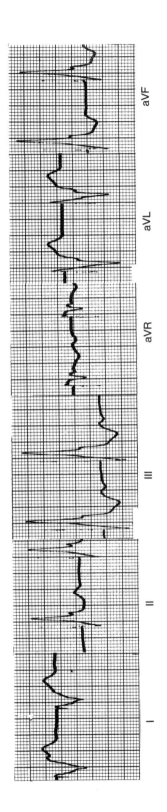

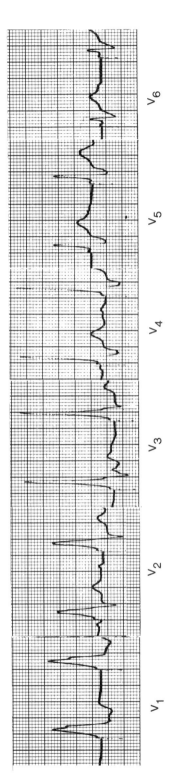

Fig 9-27a.—ECG of patient with pacemaker.

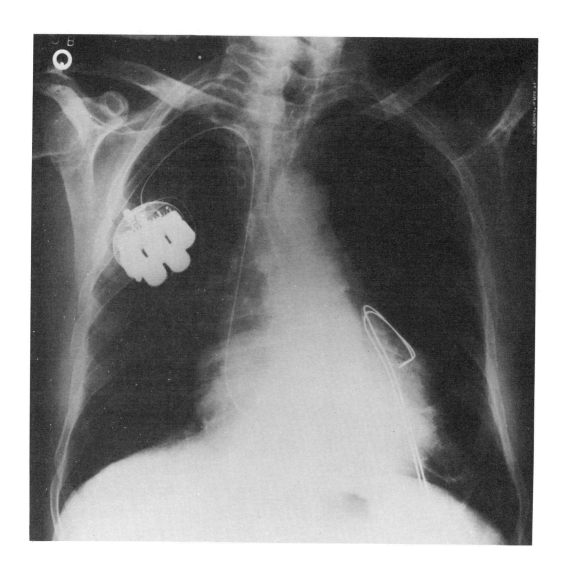

Fig 9-27b.—Posteroanterior X-ray of patient in Fig 9-27a.

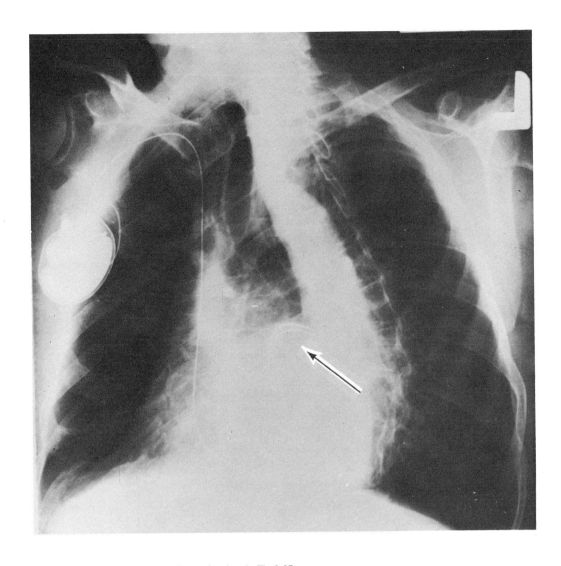

Fig 9-27c.—Left anterior oblique X-ray of patient in Fig 9-27a.

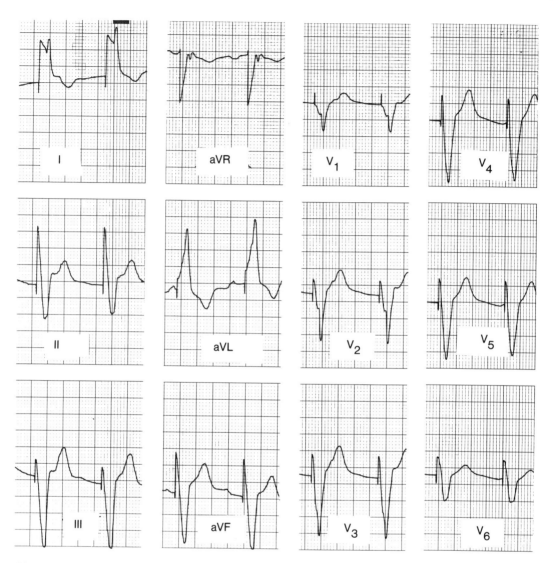

Fig 9-27d.—ECG of patient in Fig 9-27a paced via transvenous electrode.

The 77-year-old woman whose ECGs are shown in Figure 9-28a began complaining of a ''jumping'' sensation in the epigastric area shortly after implantation of her pacemaker. The ECG shows an RBBB configuration in lead V_1, and one instance of failure to capture. The paced rate is 100 beats/min, since this is a CPI pacemaker, and a magnet was applied while the tracing was taken.

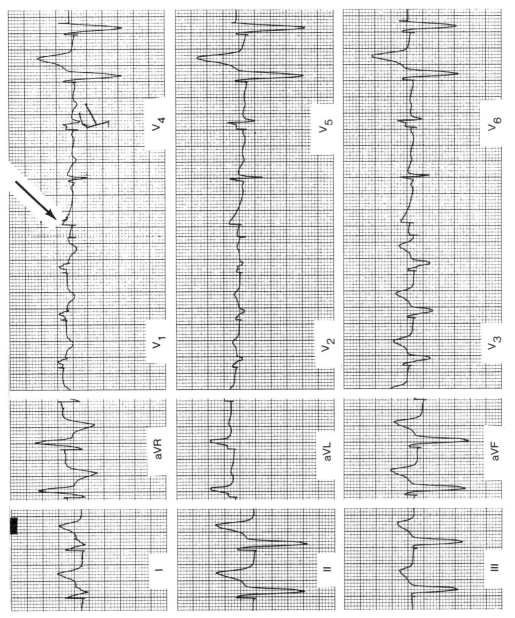

Fig 9-28a.—ECG of patient with pacemaker.

A rhythm strip obtained with a magnet on the following day shows only one captured beat (Fig 9-28b). The electrode was repositioned, and Figure 9-28c shows correct VVI pacing. The two paced beats have an LBBB configuration in lead V_1. Chest X-rays did not provide evidence of perforation of the right ventricle, but the jumping sensation disappeared after correction of the electrode position.

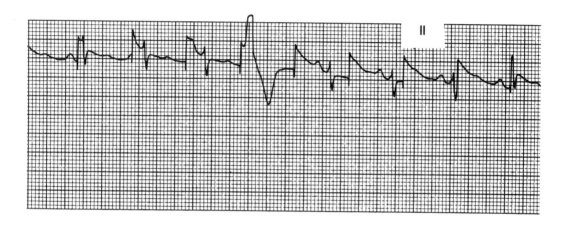

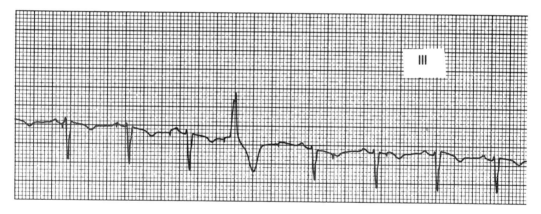

Fig 9-28b.—ECG of patient in Fig 9-28a on following day, showing one captured beat.

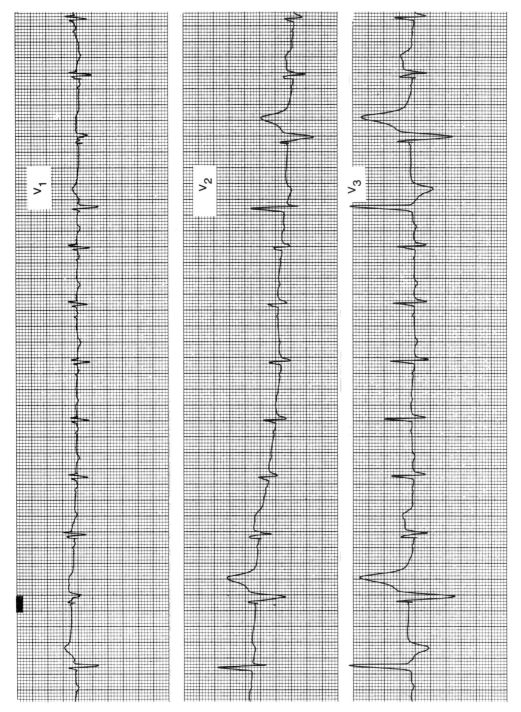

Fig 9-28c.—ECG of patient in Fig 9-28a following repositioning of electrode.

ECG Evidence of Pacemaker Malfunction

The most common ECG signs of pacemaker malfunction are failure to pace, failure to capture, and failure to sense. These problems may be transient or permanent and may occur singly or in combination.

Failure to Pace

Failure to pace is characterized by the absence of pacing artifacts when the spontaneous heart rate is slower than the pacemaker's fixed rate.

When lack of pacing is seen with *external pacemakers*, the battery, dial settings, and connections should be checked. The connections were the cause of the failure to pace in the tracing shown in Figure 9-29; a wire had come loose during a dressing change.

Causes of Failure to Pace

1. Battery depletion
2. Pacemaker component failure
3. Electrode fracture
4. Inhibition of demand pacemaker by intrinsic or extrinsic signals
5. Loose connections or accidental changes in dial settings in external pacemaker

---

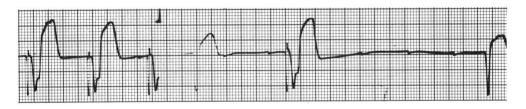

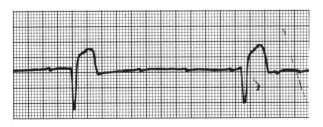

Fig 9-29.—Continuous rhythm strip showing loss of pacing.

Most of the problems that occur with *implanted pacemakers* cannot be corrected by the nurse, but there are some exceptions, as shown in Figures 9-30a and b.

In Figure 9-30a (top), the patient is paced at a rate of 72 beats/min. Pacing suddenly stops (middle), and with the exception of a single ventricular escape beat, ventricular asystole ensues (bottom). This episode occurred when the patient was turned to her left side, and precipitated a syncopal attack. When the nurse returned the patient to the supine position to start cardiopulmonary resuscitation, pacing immediately resumed.

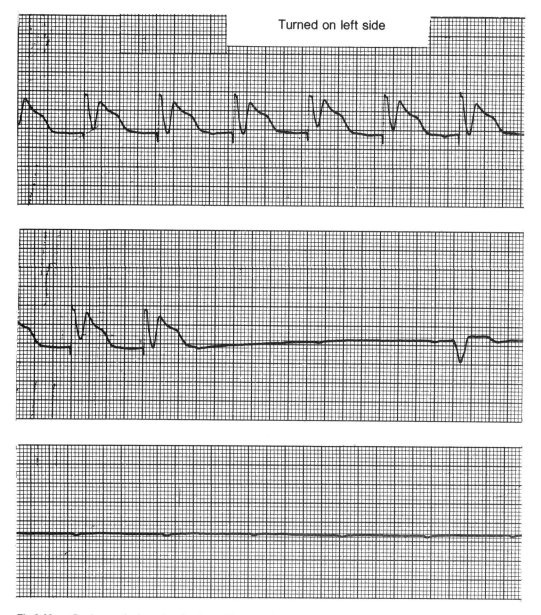

Fig 9-30a.—Continuous rhythm strip of patient with pacemaker.

On the basis of this information, the nurse should try to arrive at an answer to the problem through a process of elimination.

- Battery failure is not likely, since pacing was resumed.
- Transient displacement of the electrode tip is unlikely, because this may cause loss of capture, but pacer signals are usually seen.
- Transient failure of pacemaker components is possible but not likely.
- Electrode fracture is a distinct possibility. The patient's movement might have pulled the ends of a broken electrode wire far enough apart to prevent transmission of electrical impulses.
- Inhibition of the demand pacemaker by intrinsic or extrinsic signals is a possibility.

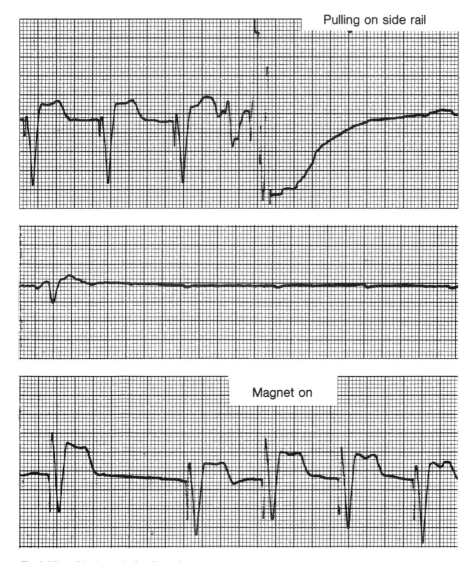

Fig 9-30b.—Rhythm strip for discussion.

The rhythm strip in Figure 9-30b shows how the problem was resolved. When the patient was allowed once again to pull on the side rail and turn herself, the pacing stopped. A magnet was applied over the pacemaker, with immediate results: pacing was resumed.

The isometric exercise of pulling on the rail apparently had produced sufficient electrical potential in the muscle overlying the pacemaker to inhibit its function.

Myopotential inhibition of demand pacemakers is frequently reported in the literature.[20] This problem is readily diagnosed by the procedure described here. If the patient does not have an adequate spontaneous rhythm and has a programmable pacemaker, it is best to reprogram it to a fixed mode of pacing until the problem can be resolved.

Electromagnetic inhibition of demand pacemakers is almost never seen with the newer models, since they are very resistant to interference. Even the fear of exposure to microwave ovens appears unnecessary because the Food and Drug Administration stated in 1976 that warnings near microwave ovens in public places are not necessary.[21] Continuous monitoring is still used when electric cautery and other medical devices are employed in the care of patients with pacemakers, but problems are rarely seen.

Failure to Capture

Failure to capture is characterized by the presence of one or more pacing artifacts that are not followed by myocardial depolarization. Failure to capture may be intermittent or constant.

Causes of Failure to Capture

1. Battery depletion
2. Component failure
3. Electrode fracture
4. Displacement of electrode tip
5. Increase in threshold
6. Inability of myocardium to depolarize
7. Loose connections or accidental change in dial settings with external pacemaker

---

Battery depletion is usually signaled by preceding slowing of the fixed rate and is revealed by a change in the pacer signal, seen with appropriate electronic devices.

Sudden *component failure* can generally be evaluated only after the unit has been replaced.

The rhythm strip in Figure 9-31 shows that the pacemaker is sensing correctly but the pacing impulses do not cause ventricular depolarization. The escape interval corresponds to the preset rate of 70 pulses/min, so battery depletion is not likely to be the cause of the problem.

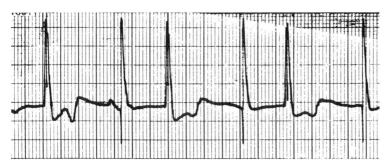

Fig 9-31.—Rhythm strip of ventricular-triggered pacemaker.

Electrode fracture is usually recognized on X-ray. It also causes a characteristic change in the pacer signal seen with appropriate electronic devices. Alteration in the voltage of the pacemaker signals has also been reported as a sign of electrode fracture.[16]

Most of the pacing artifacts in the strip in Figure 9-32 do not produce ventricular depolarization. The only pacemaker stimuli followed by a QRS complex (arrow) are those that fall on the T wave of the PVC that follows each spontaneous beat. In this patient, pressure applied to the anterior chest wall caused a resumption of pacing. Chest X-rays revealed a broken pacing electrode. Apparently, pacing resulted when the broken ends were brought into contact by pressure applied over the area. It is more difficult to explain the captures that occur when the pacing signal falls on the T wave of the PVC. The most likely explanation is that a weak signal is transmitted through the broken wire and is conducted when it falls in the supernormal period following the PVC. Another less likely explanation is Wedensky facilitation (chap 2).

Increase in stimulation threshold occurs soon after electrode implantation, due to tissue changes and fibrin deposits in the area of the endocardium that is in contact with the tip of the electrode. This is generally not a problem, since the output of the pacemaker is much greater than the stimulation threshold determined at the time of implantation.

A few patients have abnormal increases in threshold that exceed the output of the pacemaker. If such a patient has a programmable pacemaker, the output can be increased, as shown in Figures 9-33a and b. If not, repositioning of the electrode or implantation of a high-output pacemaker may be required.

In the tracing in Figure 9-33a, which was obtained with a magnet in place, only one pacemaker artifact is followed by ventricular depolarization. The rhythm strip in Figure 9-33b was recorded from the same patient after the output of the pacemaker was reprogrammed. It shows 1:1 capture and a larger pacing signal, reflecting the increased voltage output of the pacemaker.

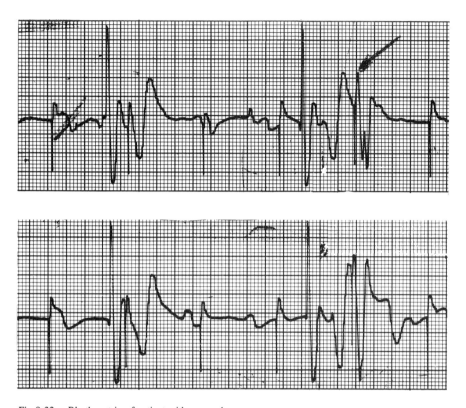

Fig 9-32.—Rhythm strip of patient with pacemaker.

When the ventricular myocardium is unable to depolarize, even the best pacing system cannot help (Fig 9-16).

Loose connections on an external pacemaker may cause loss of capture and/or sensing (Fig 9-34, top). Figure 9-34 (bottom) shows a rhythm strip of the same patient after the problem was corrected.

Failure to Sense

Failure to sense is characterized by the fact that the pacemaker fires following a preceding spontaneous beat, before the elapse of the escape interval. The combination of failure to capture and failure to sense is most frequently seen with component failure, but may also occur with electrode deviation.

The tracing shown in Figure 9-35 represents an intermittent failure of the sensing mechanism. This is a VVT unit, as indicated by the pacing artifacts transposed on the first three spontaneous QRS complexes at a rate of 94 beats/min. Then the pacing artifacts are seen at a fixed rate of 70 pulses/min, and capture occurs, except when the pacer signal is transposed into the refractory period of the preceding spontaneous beat. The last beat of the strip is once again sensed. This particular problem was due to a component failure and necessitated an exchange of the unit.

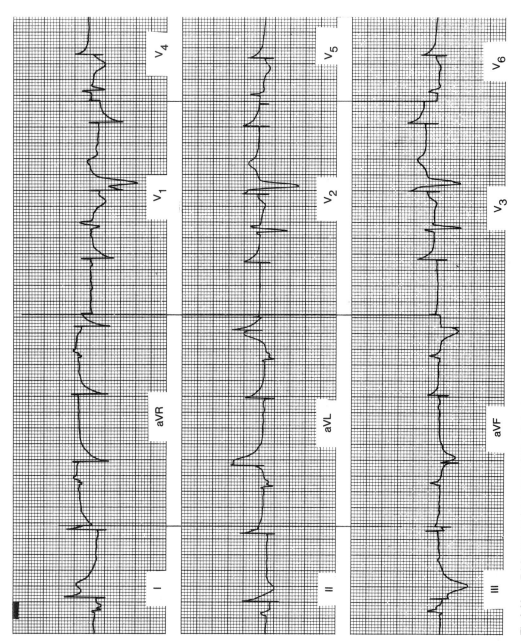

Fig 9-33a.—ECG showing intermittent failure to capture.

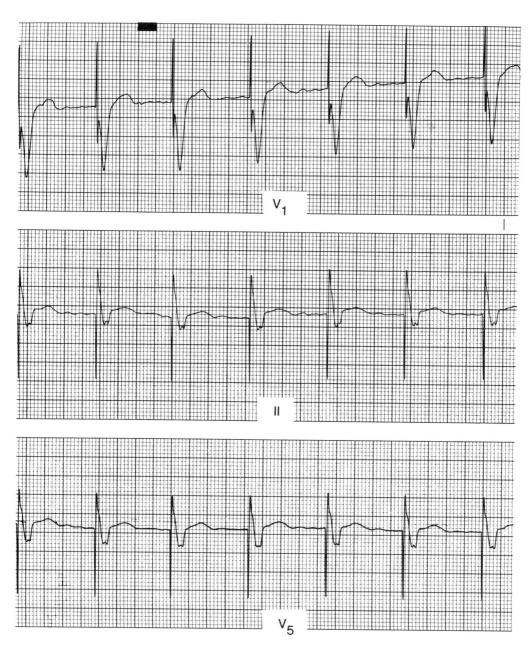

Fig 9-33b.—Rhythm strip of patient in Fig 9-33a, following reprogramming.

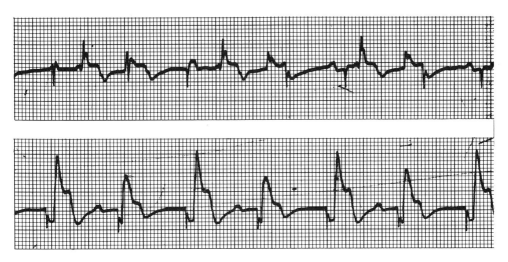

Fig 9-34.—Rhythm strip showing loss of capture and intermittent failure to sense (top) as well as appropriate pacing (bottom) after connections were tightened.

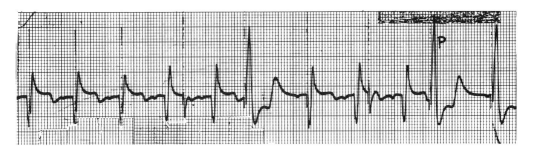

Fig 9-35.—Rhythm strip of patient with VVT pacemaker. P = paced.

Causes of Failure to Sense

1. Component failure
2. Improper setting of external pacemaker
3. Change in voltage in intracardiac R wave

The pacemaker's ability to sense spontaneous depolarization of the sensed chamber depends primarily on the *voltage of the depolarizing current* within the chamber. For example, the VAT pacemaker shown in Fig 9-8 is unable to sense the current produced by atrial fibrillatory waves, and it functions, therefore, in a fixed mode. The voltage of the intraventricular R wave may be diminished by extensive myocardial infarction, widespread fibrosis, or diffuse cardiac myopathy.[19]

Another factor that affects the pacer's ability to sense spontaneous depolarization is the *slew rate* (change in voltage with respect to time) of the intracardiac R wave. Pacers are designed to sense currents that are propagated rapidly, such as QRS complexes, rather than those that move more slowly, such as T waves. Changes in electrolytes or pH may change the slew rate of the intracardiac R wave and may cause a loss of sensing.[16] This factor may account for a pacemaker's inability to sense PVCs, which is occasionally encountered.

The pacing unit's failure to sense the PVCs (Fig 9-36) might be due to these factors. There is, however, another more likely explanation. All pacemakers have a built-in *refractory period,* which prevents them from either sensing or emitting stimuli for about 300 to 400 ms after they have either sensed or fired. In the tracing shown, the PVCs occur 280 ms after the preceding QRS. In each instance, the pacemaker has sensed the normal QRS and is, therefore, unable to "see" the PVC, so it fires after an appropriate escape interval of 820 ms.

The tracing in Figure 9-37 illustrates the effect of pacer refractory period. Spontaneous beats occurring 240 to 280 ms after the pacer signal are not sensed, whereas those that occur later reset the pacemaker's escape interval.

There are no captures in this tracing. Absence of capture, with appropriate sensing, may be seen with increases in threshold or with displacement of the electrode tip.

The series of tracings in Figure 9-38 illustrates the problems that may be encountered in identifying pacemaker malfunction. From observation of the first two beats in Figure 9-38 (top), it must be assumed that there is appropriate pacing. A QRS complex is not apparent, but there is a T wave, so ventricular depolarization must have taken place. There is a small, negative deflection immediately after the pacing artifact, which becomes more noticeable with each beat and can be seen clearly in lead aVF. It becomes apparent that this deflection is the patient's spontaneous QRS complex and the source of the T wave. The patient's spontaneous heart rate is almost identical to the rate of the pacer, so the pacer signal and the QRS complexes sometimes coincide.

Figure 9-38 (bottom) shows an apparent bigeminal rhythm. Because this is a VVT pacemaker, the early beats are sensed and cause immediate discharge of the pacemaker. Since there is a QRS complex hidden in the pacing signal, these beats are followed by T waves. The late beats correspond to the pacemaker's escape interval. They are not followed by T waves, since they do not capture the ventricle, so this unit senses but fails to capture.

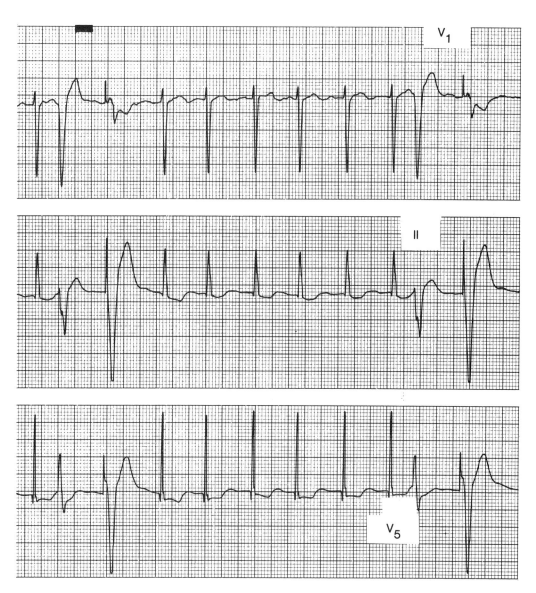

Fig 9-36.—Pacemaker with intermittent failure to sense.

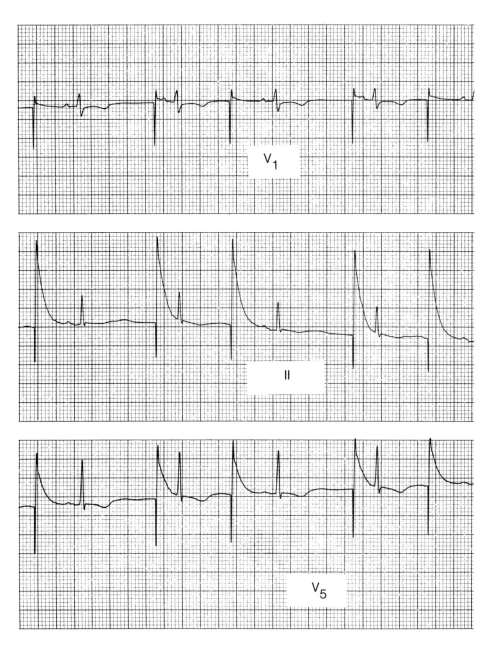

Fig 9-37.—Simultaneous rhythm strips of patient with pacemaker.

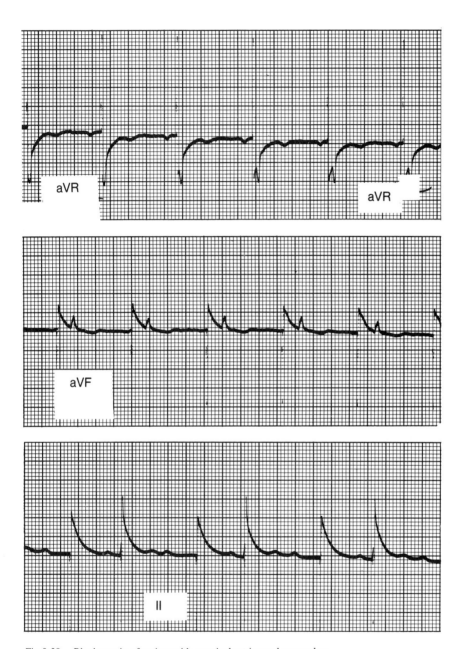

Fig 9-38.—Rhythm strip of patient with ventricular-triggered pacemaker.

Competition

Failure to sense exposes the patient to the danger of various arrhythmias.

In the tracing in Figure 9-39, the pacemaker fires at a rate of 78 pulses/min. It fails to sense the interpolated spontaneous beats, which occur at the same rate, and the patient's resulting ventricular rate is 156 beats/min, a very uncomfortable and potentially detrimental tachycardia.

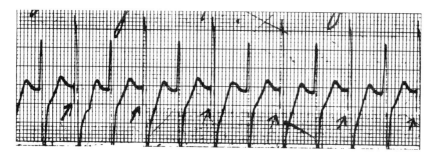

Fig 9-39.—Pacemaker bigeminy; ✔ = pacing artifact.

The VVT unit in Figure 9-40 fails to sense most of the spontaneous ventricular beats and fires mainly at a fixed rate. A dangerous arrhythmia is prevented because most of the pacer impulses do not capture the ventricle.

Ventricular tachycardia and fibrillation may result from a paced beat being transposed on the vulnerable portion of the preceding T wave (Fig 9-41).[16,19] This is not usually the case in stable patients undergoing long-term pacemaker therapy. It is, however, a real danger in patients with acute MI or ischemia and in those suffering from metabolic derangements or digitalis toxicity.

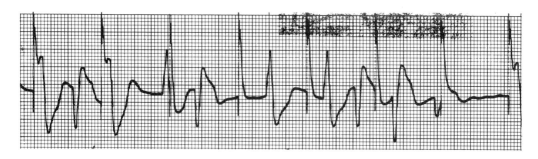

Fig 9-40.—Ventricular-triggered pacemaker with competition.

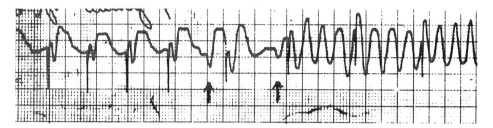

Fig 9-41.—Start of torsade de pointes by paced beat falling on preceding T wave; arrows indicate spontaneous beats. Reprinted by permission from Sweetwood HM, *The Patient in the Coronary Care Unit.* Springer Publishing Co, 1976, p 185.

Diagnosis of Myocardial Infarction in Patients with Pacemakers

In the patient whose heart is continuously paced, the ECG diagnosis of cardiac disorders such as MI becomes very difficult. Characteristic changes of the S-T segments and T waves are shown in the tracings in Figures 9-42a through c.

The tracing in Figure 9-42b shows elevation of the S-T segment in lead V_4 and inversion of the previously upright T waves in leads V_4 through V_6. There is also considerable loss of voltage in these leads, and the QRS complexes have become upright in lead V_1.

An ECG obtained on the following day (Fig 9-42c) shows further extension of this anterolateral myocardial infarction, with S-T elevation and T wave inversion in leads V_2 and V_3.

At times these changes are fairly subtle and can only be interpreted if previous tracings are available for comparison. This is illustrated in Figure 9-43a; "suggestive" configurations of the S-T segment and T wave are seen in leads II, III, and aVF, as well as in the left precordial leads. These changes become much more impressive when the tracing is compared with an ECG obtained while the patient was in good health (Fig 9-43b).

The diagnosis of MI is confirmed by clinical signs and laboratory studies. At times the ECG evidence of abnormalities is not as clear as it is in the tracings in Figures 9-43a and b. In these cases, other procedures have to be used to facilitate diagnosis.

If the patient has a programmable pacemaker, it may be possible to reduce the pacer's output to the point at which capture is lost, in the hope that a spontaneous rhythm will occur. With other units, the fixed rate may have to be reduced for the same purpose.

In patients whose pacemakers do not permit reprogramming, the permanent unit may be shut off temporarily with the use of an external pacer. In all of these cases the nurse must be prepared to reinstitute pacing promptly if asystole should result.

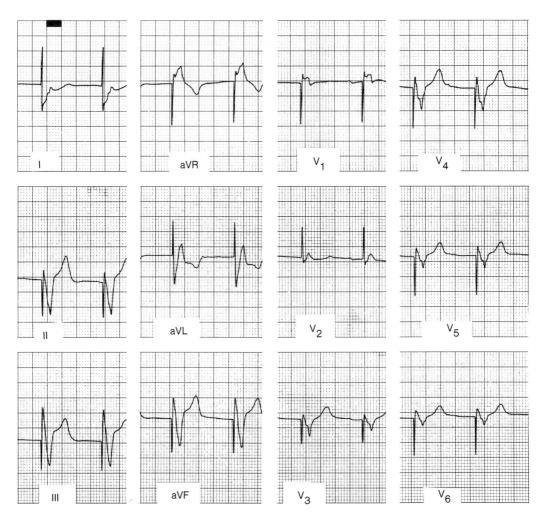

Fig 9-42a.—ECG showing continuous pacing.

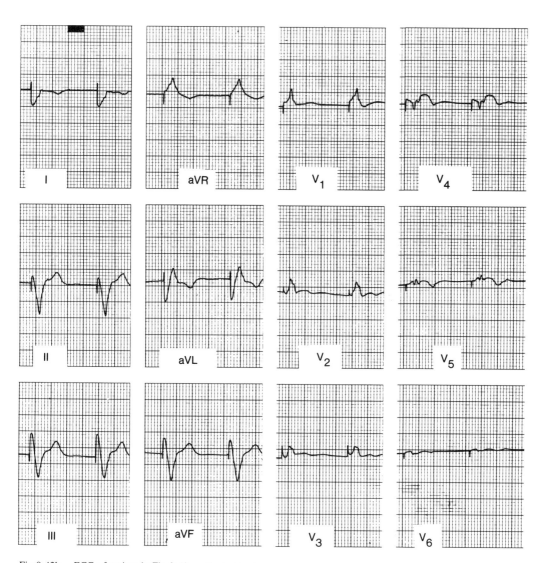

Fig 9-42b.—ECG of patient in Fig 9-42a with chest pain.

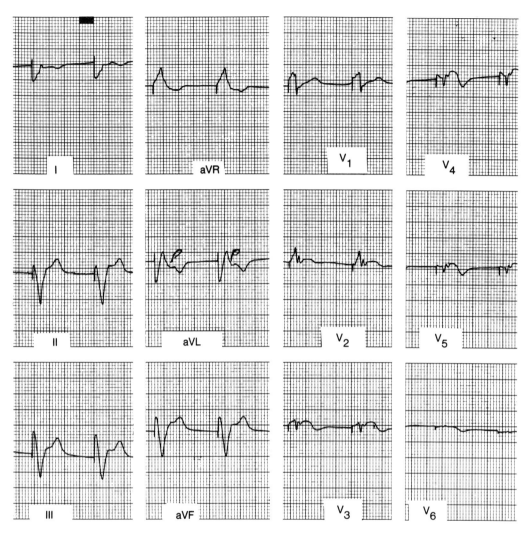

Fig 9-42c.—ECG of patient in Fig 9-42a on following day. P = P wave.

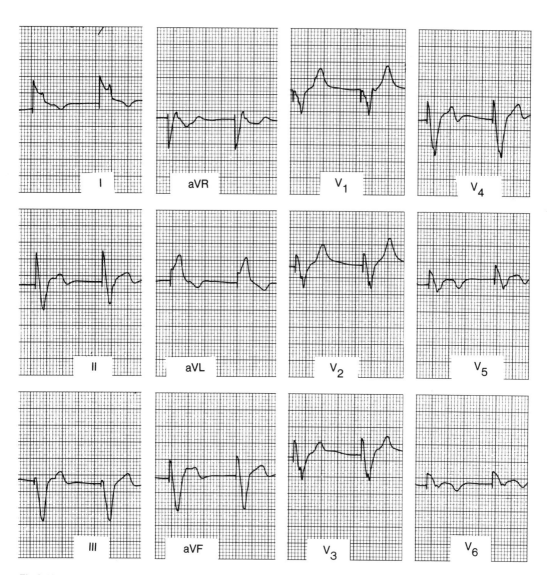

Fig 9-43a.—ECG of pacemaker patient with chest pain.

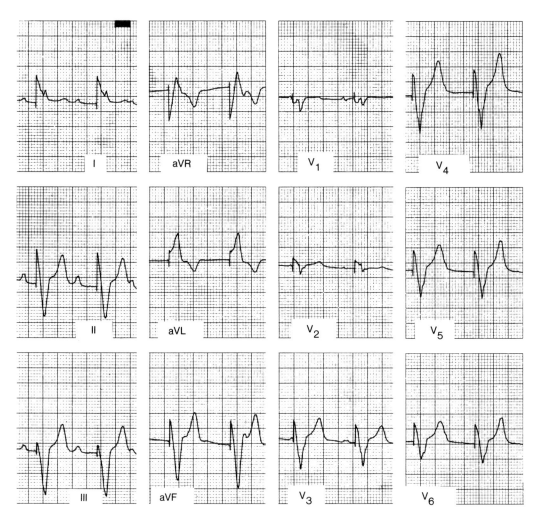

Fig 9-43b.—Previous ECG of patient in Fig 9-43a.

How to Use External Pacemaker[10]

1. Place suction cups or electrode pasties as follows.
   a. With unipolar electrodes, place one suction cup over the implanted unit, and the other over the apex area (over tip of electrode).
   b. With bipolar system, place one suction cup over the apex area, and the other 1 inch higher and to the right.
2. Connect extension cable to the external pacemaker and to the suction cups, with the positive clip attached to the suction cup over the pacing unit (or proximal ring of bipolar system) and negative clip attached to the suction cup over the apex (distal pole).
3. Turn pacemaker to a rate higher than the patient's permanent unit.
4. Be prepared to shut off the external unit if asystole or symptomatic bradycardia occurs.

In Figure 9-44 (top), the patient's implanted unit functions at a rate of 69 pulses/min. When the external pacer is turned on (Fig 9-44 bottom, first arrow), pacing artifacts are seen at a rate of 82 pulses/min. The external pacemaker applied in this manner is not able to capture the ventricles.

However, the implanted unit senses the output of the external pacer and is inhibited by it. This allows the patient's intrinsic rhythm to be recorded. In the strip in Figure 9-44, bottom, the spontaneous rate is 65 beats/min, and all characteristics of the QRS complex and T wave can readily be evaluated. Pacing is promptly resumed when the external unit is shut off (second arrow).

This method is only useful with ventricular inhibited pacemakers and would not succeed with VOO or VAT units.

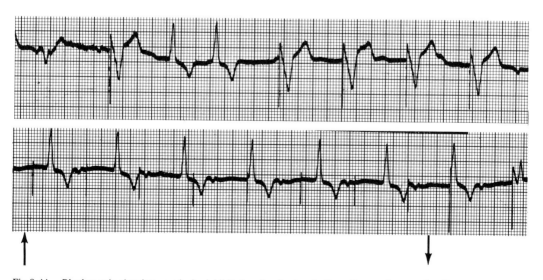

Fig 9-44.—Rhythm strip showing ventricular-inhibited pacing (top) and effect of external pacemaker (bottom).

Troubleshooting the Pacemaker

The most common forms of pacer malfunction, as well as suitable nursing interventions, are shown in the following tables. In most of these instances, cardiopulmonary resuscitation (CPR) and/or antiarrhythmic therapy may be required and may take precedence over attempts to correct pacer malfunction.

Problem: no pacing artifact seen, although patient's rate is below preset pacer rate

Conclusion: failure to pace

Table 9-2.—Troubleshooting the Pacemaker

Possible Cause	Check	Nursing Intervention
Permanent pacemaker		
Pacing spikes may be present, but difficult to see	Is patient's rate same as known pacer rate? Does QRS configuration suggest paced beats? Take 12-lead ECG and look for pacer artifacts.	Normal function - May occur with bi-polar electrode, or monitor may "filter" artifact
Myopotential inhibition	Does application of magnet restore pacing?	Ask patient to avoid the actions that precipitate the problem
Inhibition by extrinsic signals (very rare)	Does application of magnet restore pacing?	Remove/replace suspect electrical equipment
Electrode fracture	Obtain chest X-ray and look for electrode fracture	Electrode must be spliced/replaced
Pacemaker failure	Do none of the above apply?	Pacemaker must be replaced
Temporary pacemaker		
Patient's rate faster than pacemaker rate	Patient's rate faster than rate set on pacemaker?	Normal function - Increase pacer rate if desirable
Battery failure	Pace-sense indicator needle not moving?	Replace battery
Pacemaker malfunction	Pace-sense needle not moving after replacement of battery?	Replace pacemaker
Loose connections	Are there any loose connections?	Tighten all connections
Inhibition by extrinsic electrical signals	Set pacemaker sensitivity dial on 'F' and observe for evidence of pacing	Remove suspect electrical equipment from patient area, or leave pacer on fixed (VOO) mode, while electrical surroundings are checked

Problem: pacing artifacts seen but not always followed by ventricular depolarization

Conclusion: failure to capture

Table 9-3.—Failure to Capture in Permanent Pacemaker

Possible Cause	Check	Nursing Intervention
Insufficient output	Is this a programmable pacer?	Increase output
Increased threshold	May be checked as discussed	Notify physician; may have to change to high-output pacer or try steroids
Ischemia, MI	Patient's condition and ECG	Notify physician
Electrolyte imbalance, especially hyperkalemia	Serum electrolytes	Emergency treatment needed
Pacer stimulus falls into refractory period of preceding beat	Is this a sensing pacemaker? Is it programmable? Is it a V00 pacemaker?	May require increase in sensitivity, replacement of pacer, or elimination of spontaneous beats with drugs
Deviation of electrode tip (rare later than 1-2 wk after implantation)	Does change in position facilitate pacing? Changes in paced QRS morphology Stimulation of diaphragm? Chest roentgenogram	Leave in position that permits pacing Notify physician
Electrode fracture (not uncommon)	Variation in amplitude of pacer artifact? Chest roentgenogram	Notify physician
Dying heart	Patient's condition	Notify physician, CPR
Pacemaker malfunction	If none of the above Is rate of artifacts slower than preset rate?	Notify physician

Table 9-4.—Failure to Capture in Temporary Pacemaker

Possible Cause	Check	Nursing Intervention
Insufficient output	Turn up output (mA) and check for capture	Leave dial set at output setting slightly above point at which capture occurs
Acute increase in threshold due to— Collection of fibrin	As above If unsuccessful, threshold may be tested as described	As above If unsuccessful, call physician; wire may be repositioned, or administration of steroids may be tried
Ischemia, MI	Patient condition and ECG	Notify physician
Hyperkalemia	Serum potassium	Notify physician
Pacer stimulus falls into refractory period preceding spontaneous beat	ECG	Increase sensitivity
Deviation of electrode tip (common)	Does change in patient's position affect capture?	Leave patient in position that facilitates capture
	Do occasional paced beats show changed morphology?	Notify physician
	Does patient exhibit hiccoughs or other signs of penetration of right ventricular wall? Chest roentgenogram	Electrode will have to be repositioned
Poor electrode connection	Check all connections	Tighten all connections
Electrode fracture (rare)	Do pacer signals show changes in height? Chest roentgenogram	Notify physician
Dying heart	Patient's general condition	Notify physician, CPR
Mechanical malfunction	If none of the above	Exchange pacemaker

Problem: pacing artifacts occur after spontaneous beats, within less than the preset escape interval

Conclusion: failure to sense

Table 9-5.—Failure to Sense in Permanent Pacemaker

Possible Cause	Check	Nursing Intervention
V00 pacemaker	Patient's pacemaker identification card	Notify physician
Pacemaker programmed to V00 mode	Patient's records	Reprogram pacer to VVI
Spontaneous beats occur within 0.4 s after paced beat	ECG	Notify physician; some pacers permit reprogramming of refractory period
Pacemaker cannot sense PVCs	Does failure to sense occur only after PVCs, acute MI, or ischemia?	Treat PVCs, if indicated Notify physician
Reduced intracardiac voltages	Electrolyte imbalance	Notify physician; some pacers permit reprogramming of sensitivity
Electromagnetic interference (rare)	Electrical environment	Remove suspected equipment
Pacer malfunction	If none of the above	Notify physician

Table 9-6.—Failure to Sense in Temporary Pacemaker

Possible Cause	Check	Nursing Intervention
Sensitivity set too low	Sensitivity setting	Increase sensitivity
Spontaneous beats occur— within 0.4 s after pacer discharge	ECG	Normal pacer function Notify physician, who may increase pacer rate or decrease spontaneous rate with drugs
within 0.4 s after previous spontaneous beat	Is pacer rate above 75 beats/min?	Reduce pacer rate below 70 beats/min and notify physician
Pacemaker cannot sense PVCs	Does failure to sense occur only after PVCs, acute MI, or ischemia?	Treat PVCs with lidocaine if appropriate (eg, acute MI) and notify physician
Intracardiac potential too low to sense	Electrolyte imbalance?	Notify physician; increase sensitivity setting
Mechanical failure	None of the above?	Replace pacemaker

Problem: pacemaker impulses occur more rapidly than the set rate
Conclusion: ''runaway'' pacemaker[22,23]

Table 9-7.—Runaway Pacemaker

Possible Cause	Check	Nursing Intervention
Temporary pacemaker		
Component failure	Paced rate faster than preset rate, up to 600 beats/min	Replace pacemaker immediately
Permanent pacemaker		
Battery failure, component failure, leakage of tissue fluids, or electrical interference	Paced rate faster than preset rate, up to 600 beats/min	Notify physician immediately Apply magnet; try to reprogram rate, reprogram mA to stop pacing, shut off with external pacer Be prepared for immediate removal and replacement

REFERENCES

1. Zoll PM: Resuscitation of the heart in ventricular standstill by external electrical stimulation. *N Engl J Med* 1952;247:768.

2. Parsonnett V, Manhardt M: Permanent pacing of the heart: 1952-1976. *Am J Cardiol* 1977;39:250.

3. Furman S: Recent developments in cardiac pacing. *Heart Lung* 1978;7:813.

4. Preston TA: The use of pacemaking for the treatment of acute arrhythmias. *Heart Lung* 1977;6:249.

5. Spence MI, Lemberg L: Cardiac pacemakers. III: Pacemakers in the management of reciprocating tachycardia. *Heart Lung* 1975;4:128.

6. Moss AJ, Rivers RJ: Termination and inhibition of recurrent tachycardias by implanted pervenous pacemaker. *Circulation* 1975;50:942.

7. Curry PVL, Rowland E, Krikler DM: Dual-demand pacing for refractory atrioventricular re-entry tachycardia. *PACE* 1979;2:137.

8. Strumpfer G: History of the nuclear demand pacemaker. *Media Fact Sheet.* Minneapolis, Medtronic, Inc, 1973.

9. *Programmer III, Instructions for Use.* Miami, Cordis Corporation, 1981.

10. Millar S, Sampson LK, Soukup N, et al: *Methods in Critical Care.* Philadelphia, WB Saunders, 1980.

11. Parsonnett V, Furman S, Smyth NPD: A revised code for pacemaker identification. *Circulation* 1981;64:60A.

12. Parsonnett V: Routine implantation of permanent pacemaker electrodes in both chambers: A technique whose time has come. *PACE* 1981;4:109.

13. Levy S, Gerard R, Jausseran JM, et al: Long-term results of permanent atrioventricular sequential demand pacing. *PACE* 1979;2:175.

14. *The Cordis Pacer Systems Analyzer*. Miami, Cordis Corp, 1976.

15. Widman WD, Edoga JK, Thomas L, et al: Pitfalls in measuring R waves in pacemaker dependent patients. *PACE* 1979;2:186.

16. Levine PA: *Pacemaker Puzzles*. Sylmar, Calif, Pacesetter Systems, Inc, 1978.

17. Boincey P, Zellinger A, Levine PA: *Pacesetter Puzzles*. Sylmar, Calif, Pacesetter Systems, Inc, 1981.

18. Lemberg L, Vinsant M: Pacer electrode location. Read before the National Teaching Institute, American Association of Critical Care Nurses, New Orleans, 1974.

19. Vera Z, Awan NA, Amsterdam E: Cardiac pacemakers: Indications and complications. *Heart Lung* 1975;4:444.

20. El Gamal M, Van Gelder B: Suppression of an external demand pacemaker by diaphragmatic myopotentials: A sign of electrode perforation? *PACE* 1979;2:191.

21. Villforth C: *Policy Statement: Cardiac Pacemaker Warning Signs Near Microwave Ovens*. US Food and Drug Administration, Washington, DC, September 1976.

22. Kallenbach J, Millar RN, Obel JPW: Runaway temporary pacemaker. *Heart Lung* 1977;6:517.

23. Odabashian HC, Brown DF: "Runaway" in a modern generation pacemaker. *PACE* 1979;2:152.

## Chapter 10

Chamber Enlargement

The size of a cardiac chamber may be increased either by hypertrophy (the thickening of its muscular walls) or by dilation. This distinction is easily made in echocardiography but cannot always be made in electrocardiography. By convention, the term hypertrophy generally applies to ventricular enlargement, whereas the term abnormality is preferred for description of changes affecting the atria.

Atrial Abnormalities

The ECG evidence of atrial abnormalities is readily understood, if one remembers the sequence of atrial depolarization and the placement of the positive electrode in various leads.

Normal P Wave

Since the sinus node is in the right atrium, this chamber is depolarized slightly before the left atrium. The beginning of the P wave, therefore, represents right atrial depolarization, and depolarization of the left atrium continues the curve of the P wave as shown in Figure 10-1. This produces the smooth, slightly rounded P waves normally seen in leads II, III, and aVF.

In the precordial leads, the P wave is normally best seen in lead V_1, since the V_1 electrode is generally placed over the junction between the right atrium and right ventricle. Right atrial depolarization proceeds toward lead V_1, producing an initial upright deflection. The depolarization currents of the left atrium move away from V_1, so the terminal portion of the P wave may be slightly negative, but this negative portion should not exceed 0.04 millimeter-second (Fig 10-2).

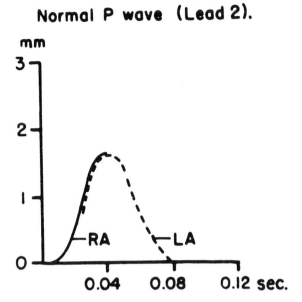

Fig 10-1.—Normal P wave. RA = right atrium and LA = left atrium. Reprinted from Chou T-C, Helm RA: The pseudo P pulmonale. *Circulation* 1965;32:96. Used by permission of the American Heart Association, Inc.[1(p128)]

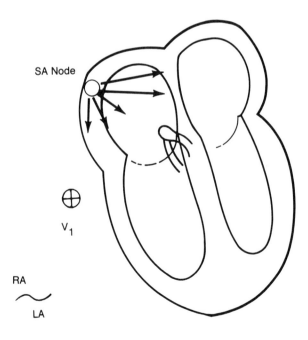

Fig 10-2.—Normal P wave in lead V₁. SA = sinoatrial node. RA = right atrium and LA = left atrium.

ECG characteristics[1](p86)

- P wave upright in leads I, II, and aVF
- P axis generally around $+50°$ to $+60°$
- P wave diphasic in lead V_1, with terminal force less than 0.04 milli-meter-second
- duration in adult 0.10 second or less
- height 2.5 mm or less in leads II, III, and aVF

Right Atrial Abnormality

In right atrial abnormality (RAA), a greater than normal amount of current is generated by the right atrium. This is superimposed on the left atrial curve and produces a tall, sharply pointed P wave (P pulmonale), as seen in Figure 10-3.

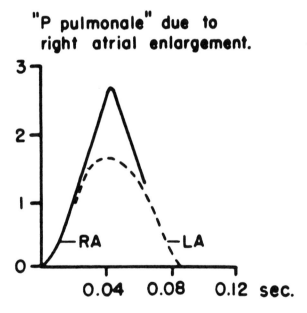

Fig 10-3.—Inscription of P wave in right atrial abnormality. RA = right atrium and LA = left atrium. Reprinted from Chou T-C, Helm RA: The pseudo P pulmonale. *Circulation* 1965;32:96. Used by permission of the American Heart Association, Inc.[1](p128)

Causes

- pulmonary disease (most common cause)
- congenital heart disease such as atrial septal defect
- Ebstein's anomaly, producing extremely tall, pointed P waves

ECG characteristics

- P wave taller than 2.5 mm in leads II, III, and aVF
- P wave narrow-based and pointed or peaked
- P wave duration generally less than 0.11 second
- right precordial leads showing diphasic P wave with increased voltage of the initial component
- initial Q wave possible in lead V_1[2]
- terminal portion or entire P wave negative in lead V_1 (in emphysema)
- in acquired RAA, axis shifted toward +90° (P pulmonale), usually due to pulmonary problems
- in congenital heart disease, axis generally more normal and about +60° (P congenitale)[3]

The criteria for RAA must be applied with caution, since a number of factors such as tachycardia may cause tall, pointed P waves to appear in the tracings of healthy subjects. In addition, left atrial abnormality (LAA) may at times produce some of the findings cited above.

The tracing in Figure 10-4 illustrates the tall, pointed P waves of P congenitale in a child with congenital heart disease (probably an ostium primum defect).

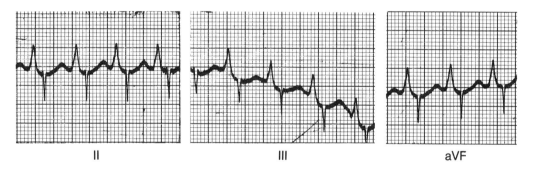

II   III   aVF

Fig 10-4.—Leads II, III, and aVF in child with congenital heart disease.

The tracing in Figure 10-5, showing P pulmonale, suggests acquired pulmonary disease. The P wave axis is close to +90°, and the ECG shows other signs of pulmonary disease (chap 11).

Figure 10-6 also shows P pulmonale. The axis in the frontal plane is +90°. In V_1 the P wave is mainly negative. This negativity of the P wave in V_1, seen in combination with P pulmonale, is usually a sign of emphysema.

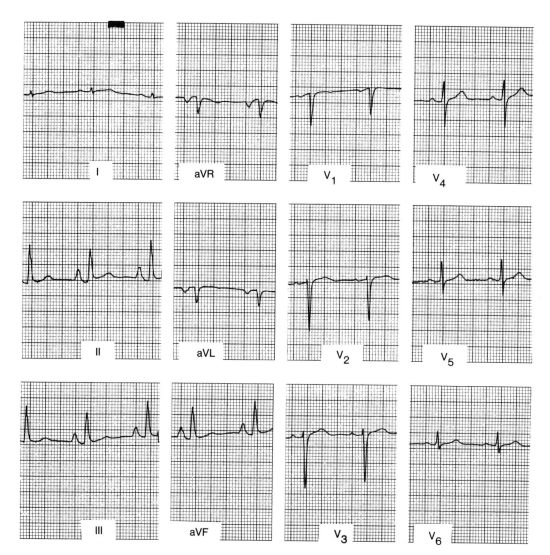

Fig 10-5.—ECG of adult with P pulmonale.

Left Atrial Abnormality

In left atrial abnormality, the initial curve produced by right atrial depolarization is followed by an increased, prolonged left atrial curve. This produces a double-peaked P wave (P mitrale), as shown in Figure 10-7.

In lead V_1, the prolonged depolarization of the left atrium produces a P terminal force greater than 0.04 millimeter-second. The measurement of the P terminal force is illustrated in Figure 10-8.

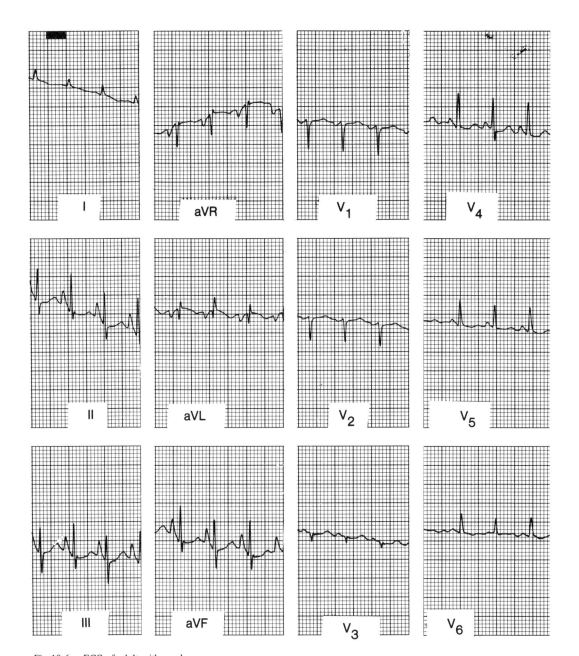

Fig 10-6.—ECG of adult with emphysema.

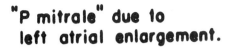

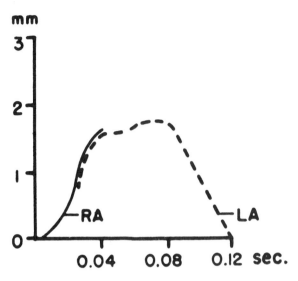

Fig 10-7.—Inscription of P wave in left atrial abnormality. Reprinted from Chou T-C, Helm RA: The pseudo P pulmonale. *Circulation* 1965;32:96. Used by permission of the American Heart Association, Inc.[1(p128)]

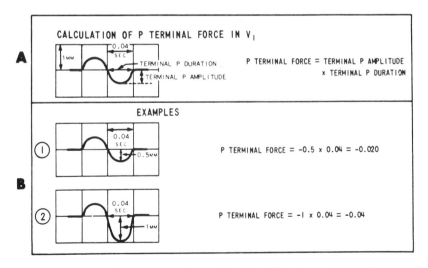

Fig 10-8.—Measurement of the P terminal force in lead V_1. *(A)* The P wave is divided into initial and terminal portions. The duration (in seconds) and the amplitude (in millimeters) of the terminal component are measured. The P terminal force is the algebraic product of these two values and is expressed in milimeter-seconds. *(B)* Examples: (1) Normal P terminal force; (2) Abnormal P terminal force. Modified after Morris JJ, Estes EH Jr, Whalen RF, et al: P wave analysis in valvular heart disease. *Circulation* 1964;29:242. Used by permission of the American Heart Association, Inc.[1(p59)]

The duration of normal and abnormal P waves may also be measured by the Macruz index (Fig 10-9), which relates the duration of the P wave to the length of the P-R interval. The increased duration of the P wave in LAA may increase the P-R interval, producing apparent 1° AV block.

MACRUZ INDEX

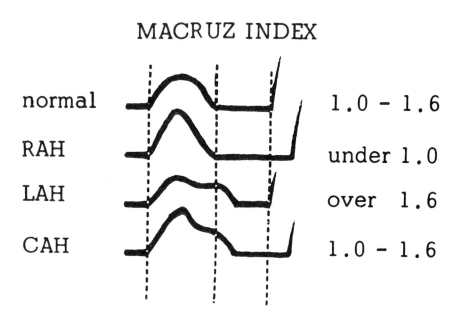

normal	1.0 - 1.6
RAH	under 1.0
LAH	over 1.6
CAH	1.0 - 1.6

Fig 10-9.—Macruz index. RAH = right atrial hypertrophy. LAH = left atrial hypertrophy, and CAH = combined atrial hypertrophy (from Marriott[3(p89)]).

Causes

- mitral valve disease (most frequent cause; hence the term P mitrale)
- left ventricular hypertrophy from any cause
- left ventricular failure from any cause

ECG characteristics

- duration of the P wave more than 2.5 mm
- double-peaked P waves with distance between peaks 0.04 second or more
- mean electrical P wave axis to left of $+45°$
- P terminal force more than 0.04 millimeter-second in lead V_1
- coarse atrial fibrillation, with fibrillatory waves more than 1 mm in height in lead V_1
- left axis deviation of terminal portion of P wave[3]

The mere presence of a notched P wave is not sufficient to establish the diagnosis of LAA unless the peaks of the P wave are more than 0.04 second apart. Also, a negative terminal P in lead V_1, as an isolated abnormality, is not sufficient to label a tracing abnormal. The ECG diagnosis of LAA is best made when other abnormalities are present as well.

The tracing in Figure 10-10 demonstrates the classic "M" shape of the P wave in P mitrale, both in the frontal and the precordial leads. The P wave axis is close to $+30°$, and the negative terminal portion of the P wave in lead V_1 is prolonged.

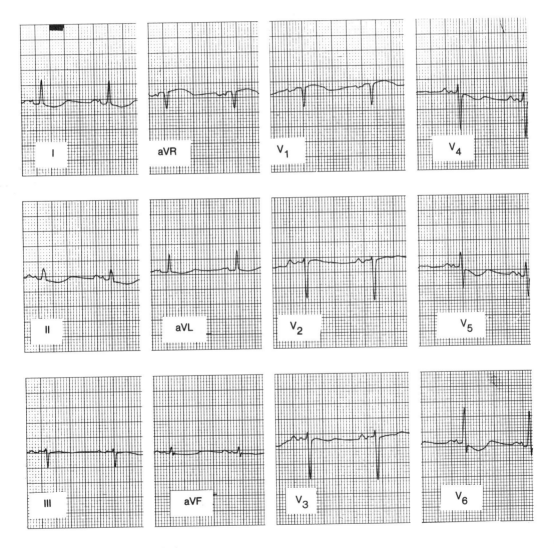

Fig 10-10.—ECG showing P mitrale.

The major sign of LAA in Figure 10-11 is the P wave in lead V_1, which is almost completely negative.

The ECG in Figure 10-12 shows several signs of LAA, including a slight negativity of the P wave in lead aVF, as well as left ventricular hypertrophy.

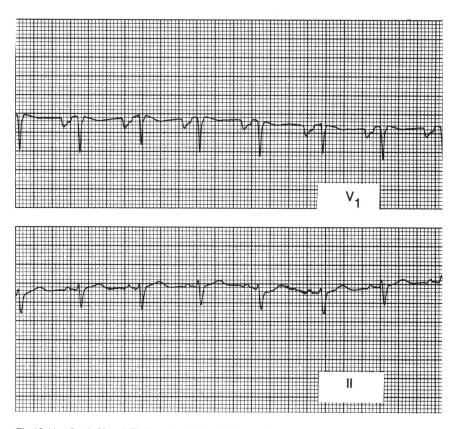

Fig 10-11.—Leads V_1 and II, illustrating left atrial abnormality.

Biatrial Hypertrophy

When both atria are enlarged, as may be the case in severe mitral stenosis with pulmonary hypertension, biatrial abnormality may be seen. This is usually reflected in an increase in the height and width of the P wave. Lead V_1 in Figure 10-13 suggests possible biatrial abnormality.

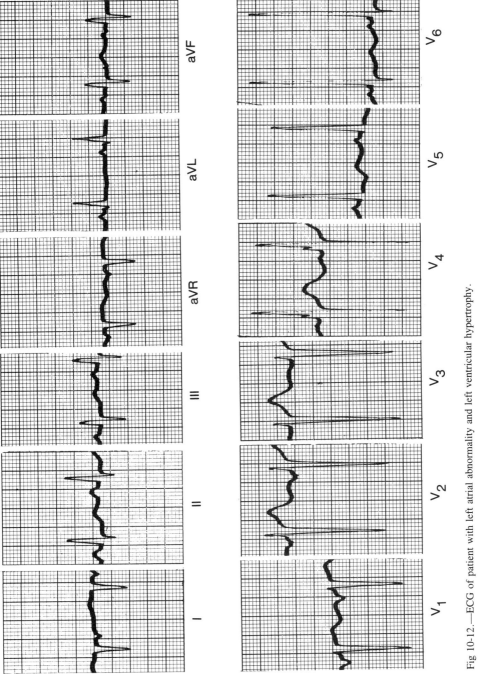

Fig 10-12.—ECG of patient with left atrial abnormality and left ventricular hypertrophy.

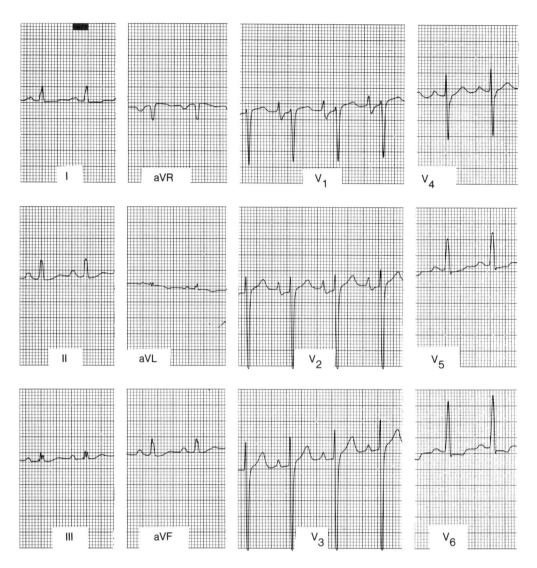

Fig 10-13.—ECG suggesting biatrial abnormality.

Left Ventricular Hypertrophy

The nomenclature used to describe left ventricular hypertrophy (LVH) is not very precise. The term hypertrophy is generally used, although the problem may be due to diastolic or volume overloading of the chamber (dilation), as well as to a systolic or pressure overload (muscular hypertrophy). There is also a distinction between concentric and eccentric hypertrophy.[4] In the former, there is an increase in wall thickness but not in the diameter of the chamber. This may be seen, for example, in pure aortic stenosis. In eccentric hypertrophy, on the other hand, there is an increase in muscle mass, as well as dilation of the ventricle. The patient with mitral regurgitation usually has eccentric hypertrophy.

Causes

- Systolic overload: aortic stenosis, coarctation of the aorta, chronic hypertension, and coronary artery disease
- Diastolic overload: patent ductus arteriosus, ventricular septal defect, and aortic insufficiency

ECG Criteria

The major criteria of LVH are summarized in the Estes score card (Table 10-1). The purpose of the score card is to emphasize that the presence of more than one criterion is required to diagnose LVH.

Voltage Criteria

The voltage criteria discussed here are applicable only to individuals over age 40, since normal younger persons tend to produce large voltages.[5] Increased voltage is often a sign of LVH, but LVH may be present even if the voltages recorded are normal or low.[6]

Voltage criteria for adults over age 40

- R wave greater than 25 mm in any lead
- R wave in leads V_5 or V_6 plus S wave in V_1 or V_2 35 mm or more
- R wave 13 mm or more in lead aVL (horizontal heart)
- R wave 20 mm or more in aVF (vertical heart)
- R wave in V_6 greater than R wave in V_5
- S wave greater than 25 mm in V_1 or V_2

Table 10-1.—LVE: Estes' Score Card*

1. R or S in limb lead:	20 mm or more ⎫	
S in V_1, V_2, or V_3:	25 mm or more ⎬ 3	
R in V_4, V_5, or V_6:	25 mm or more ⎭	
2. Any ST shift (without digitalis)		3
Typical "strain" ST-T (with digitalis)		1
3. LAD: $-15°$ or more		2
4. QRS interval: 0.09 sec or more		1
5. ID in V_{5-6}: 0.04 sec or more		1

(5 = LVE; 4 = probable LVE)

*LVE = left ventricular enlargement, LAD = left axis deviation, and ID = intrinsicoid deflection (from Marriott[3(p94)]).

The tracing in Figure 10-14 was obtained in an 81-year-old patient and meets the voltage criteria for LVH in leads V_4 and V_5. There is also left axis deviation and LAA, and there are characteristic S-T and T wave changes in the left precordial and left lateral leads (I and aVL).

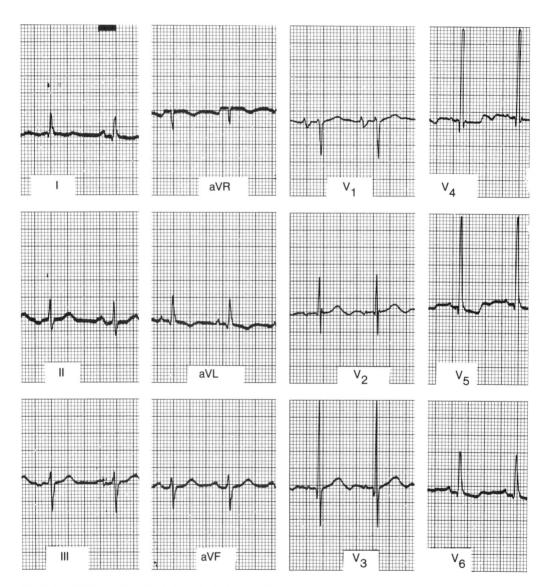

Fig 10-14.—ECG of patient with left ventricular hypertrophy.

The tracing in Figure 10-15 was obtained in a 91-year-old woman; it meets the voltage criteria for LVH in leads I and aVL. There are also S-T and T wave changes in these leads, as well as left axis deviation.

The voltage criteria for LVH were also met in Figures 10-12 and 10-14.

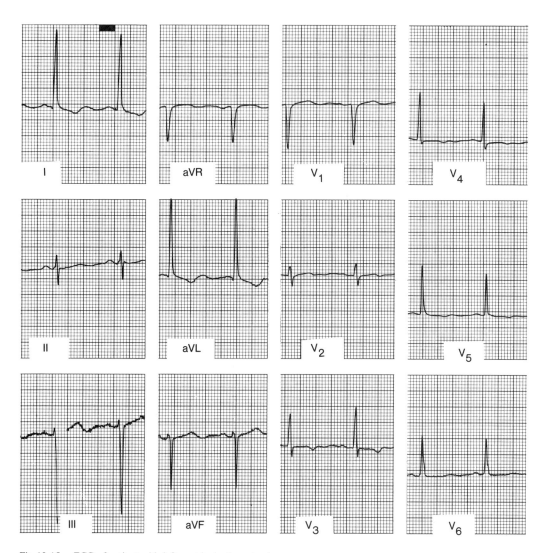

Fig 10-15.—ECG of patient with left ventricular hypertrophy.

S-T and T Wave Abnormalities

In the normal heart, the QRS and T vectors should be similar in most leads. Pronounced divergence of these vectors, especially in the left ventricular leads (V_4 through V_6), is always a sign of an abnormality. The pathological change of the T wave vector is seen as an inversion of the T wave and is illustrated in leads V_5 and V_6 of Figure 10-14 and in leads I and aVL of Figure 10-15. The pattern is again demonstrated in Figure 10-16.

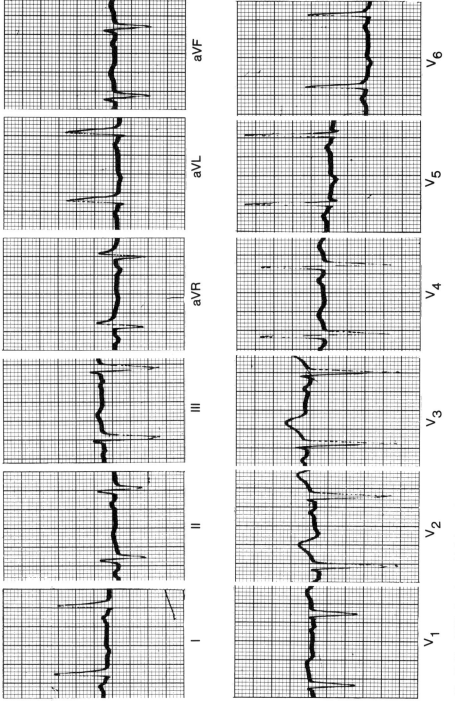

Fig 10-16.—ECG of patient with left ventricular hypertrophy.

When the T wave is deeply inverted and the S-T segment is depressed 0.5 mm or more it is often referred to as a left ventricular strain pattern. An extreme example of left ventricular strain is shown in Figure 10-17. Initially, it was believed that the patient had CAD; however, diagnostic studies negated this diagnosis, and echocardiography revealed severe concentric hypertrophy of the left ventricle and idiopathic hypertrophic subaortic stenosis (IHSS). The cause of this strain pattern, which closely resembles the ischemic changes seen with CAD, is not definitely known.[1(p140)]

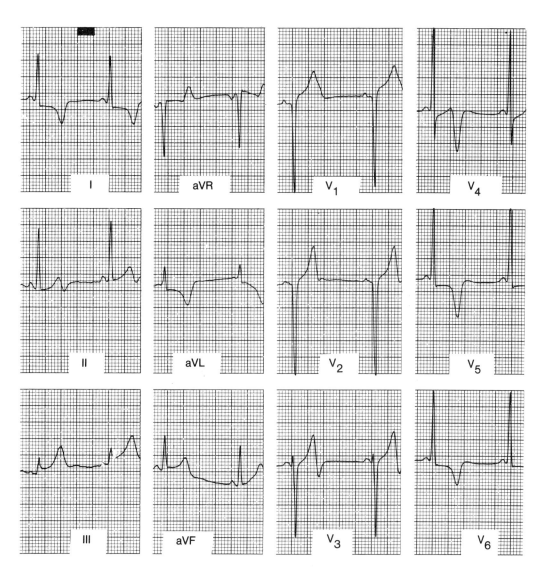

Fig 10-17.—ECG of patient with pronounced strain pattern.

Left Axis Deviation

Left axis deviation (LAD) is frequently seen in LVH, as illustrated by most of the tracings shown. It must be remembered, however, that most of these ECGs were obtained from elderly patients, so this axis deviation may be due to age rather than to LVH. Recent studies have shown that LVH per se does not cause LAD.[6] Certainly LVH may be seen in combination with a normal axis, and LAD alone does not prove that an abnormality is present.

Widening of QRS Complex

The QRS complex frequently widens to 0.09 second or more in LVH. This is not a specific sign but contributes to the diagnosis when other criteria are present. The diagnosis of LVH in the presence of complete LBBB is somewhat controversial. In clinical practice, however, it is not uncommon to observe a gradual widening of the QRS complex in patients with LVH over a period of years, until complete LBBB develops. Thus, it can be safely assumed that there is a connection between LVH and LBBB in this patient group.

The peculiar tracing in Figure 10-18 meets voltage criteria for LVH (leads V_2 and V_3); there is also an intraventricular conduction delay.

Intrinsicoid Deflection

The intrinsicoid deflection (ID), also called ventricular activation time, is measured from the onset of the ventricular complex to the peak of the R wave. This period of time may be increased to 0.04 second or more when the ventricle is enlarged. An example of prolonged ventricular activation time is shown in lead V_5 of Figure 10-19. The phenomenon may be related to the generalized widening of the QRS complex described above.

Other Criteria

The diagnosis of LVH tends to be substantiated by the presence of LAA. An R wave in lead V_6 that is taller than the R wave in lead V_5 also suggests the presence of LVH.

Left ventricular hypertrophy may also be present in patients with RBBB. This problem should be suspected when the R wave measures 20 mm or more in leads V_5 and/or V_6 in the presence of RBBB.

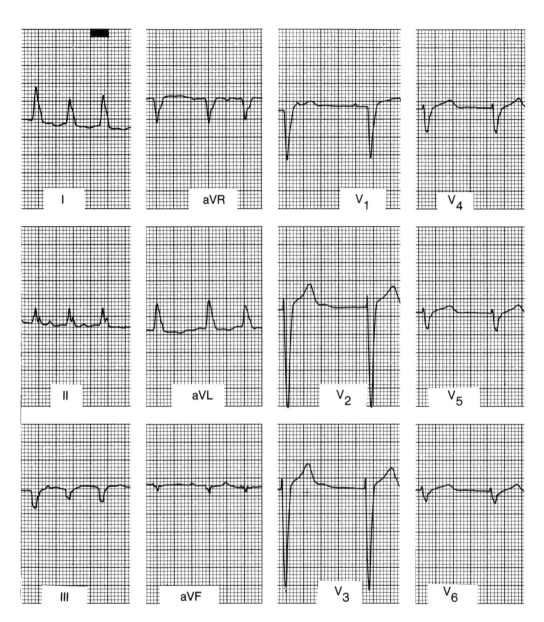

Fig 10-18.—ECG showing left ventricular hypertrophy.

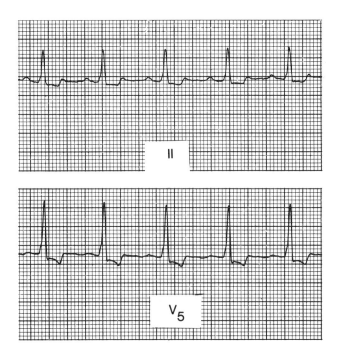

Fig 10-19.—Tracing showing prolonged ventricular activation time.

Right Ventricular Hypertrophy

Right ventricular hypertrophy (RVH) is seen less frequently than LVH. The ECG diagnosis of this abnormality is less specific and more complex than that of LVH.

Causes

- mitral valve disease
- chronic obstructive lung disease with cor pulmonale
- congenital heart disease (Fallot's tetralogy, pulmonic stenosis, Eisenmenger's syndrome)
- acute right ventricular overload (pulmonary embolism)

ECG characteristics for adults older than 35 years

- right axis deviation (RAD) greater than $+90°$
- an R/S ratio greater than 1 in lead V_1, or S/R ratio greater than 1 in lead V_6

The ECG in Figure 10-20 of a patient with mitral valve disease shows an axis of $+135°$ and a predominantly positive QRS complex in lead V_1. The rhythm is atrial fibrillation, a common finding in patients with mitral valve disease.

The criteria for axis deviation must be assessed in light of the patient's age. In adults under 35, an axis up to $+110°$ may be normal, whereas the axis may be as far right as $+135°$ in the healthy newborn.[7]

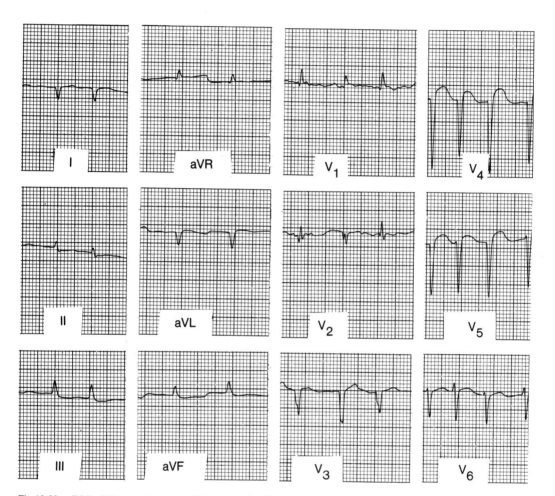

Fig 10-20.—ECG of 70-year-old patient with mitral valve disease.

Voltage criteria

- R wave with height of 7 mm or more in lead V_1
- R wave in V_1 plus S wave in V_5 or V_6 equals 10 mm or more

These criteria are illustrated in Figure 10-21.

The tracing in Figure 10-21 was obtained in a 30-year-old woman with severe pulmonary artery hypertension (Eisenmenger's syndrome) due to an uncorrected, and now inoperable, septal defect. There is also pronounced P pulmonale and RAD.

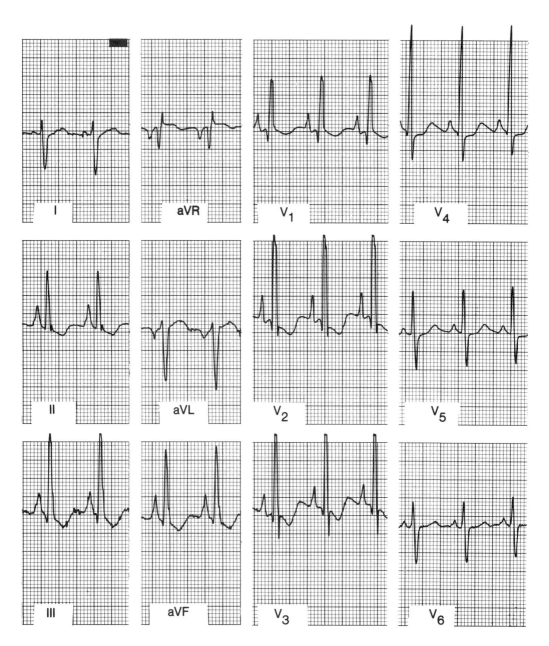

Fig 10-21.—ECG of 30-year-old woman with RVH.

Incomplete RBBB

Incomplete RBBB is not a specific sign of RVH, since it may also occur in normal individuals. It is often normal if the R wave in V_1 measures less than 8 mm, the R′ wave measures less than 6 mm, and the R/S ratio is less than 1. The taller the R′ wave, the greater is the likelihood that RVH is present.[1(p160)] Incomplete RBBB is frequently seen in mitral stenosis and atrial septal defects (Fig 10-22).

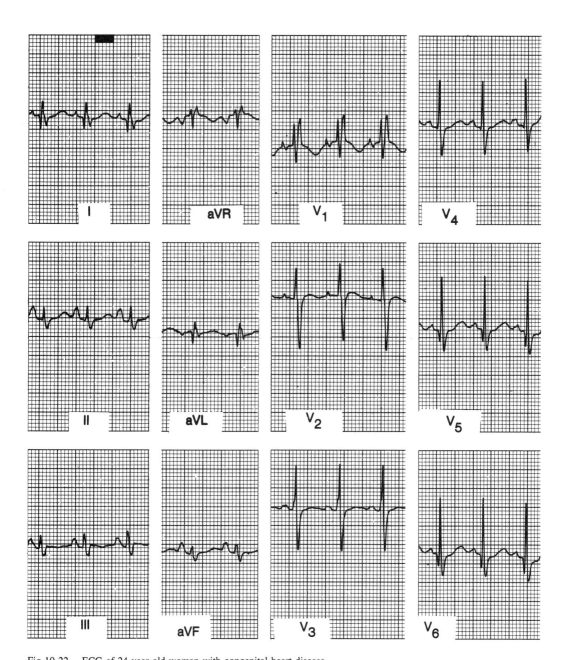

Fig 10-22.—ECG of 24-year-old woman with congenital heart disease.

Suggestive ECG Criteria

The following criteria suggest RVH but are not diagnostic

- S-T depression and T wave inversion in right precordial leads, also seen in leads II, III, and aVF as a right ventricular strain pattern (Fig 10-21)

- small R wave and deep S wave (rS complex) in all precordial leads
- pronounced S waves in leads I, II, and III (S_1 S_2 S_3 pattern) particularly suggestive of RVH in children

Some authors[1(p162),3] distinguish between right ventricular pressure (systolic) overload and volume (diastolic) overload. Pressure overloads may occur with pulmonic stenosis, Fallot's tetralogy, mitral stenosis, cor pulmonale, and pulmonary hypertension.

ECG characteristics of right ventricular systolic overload

- RAD
- tall R wave in lead V_1
- right ventricular strain pattern in right precordial leads and often in leads II, III, and aVF

The pattern of right ventricular systolic overload is well illustrated in Figure 10-21.

Cause

- ostium secundum defect
- anomalous pulmonary venous drainage
- tricuspid insufficiency

ECG characteristics of right ventricular diastolic overload

- R' complex in V_1 associated with RAD
- delayed ID and QRS of normal or increased duration
- presence of R' complex, together with LAD, suggesting an ostium primum defect

Biventricular Hypertrophy

The diagnosis of biventricular hypertrophy is not always easy to make, since the ECG frequently reflects the enlargement of only one chamber.

ECG characteristics

- precordial leads showing voltage criteria for both RVH and LVH
- midprecordial and limb leads showing large, equiphasic complexes that "go off the paper" when the ECG is taken at full standard (Katz-Wachtel sign; Fig 10-23b).

The tracing in Figure 10-23a was obtained in a 30-year-old woman who had had mitral valve replacement years earlier. The ECG meets the voltage criteria for LVH for a person of her age group (S wave in V_1 plus R wave in V_6 greater than 50 mm).

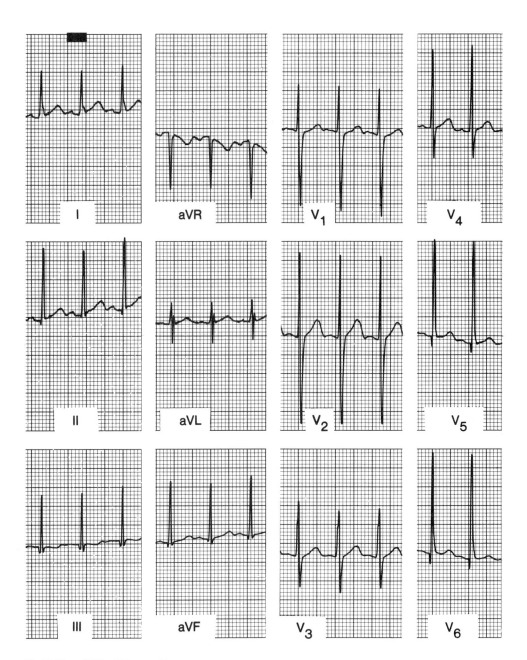

Fig 10-23a.—ECG of 30-year-old woman.

Figure 10-23b was obtained in the woman 2 years later. This tracing shows the Katz-Wachtel sign, as well as a left ventricular strain pattern. Echocardiography demonstrated the presence of large tumors in both the right and left ventricles. The tumors were identified as leiomyosarcoma during attempted surgery, but unfortunately the patient died of her disease.

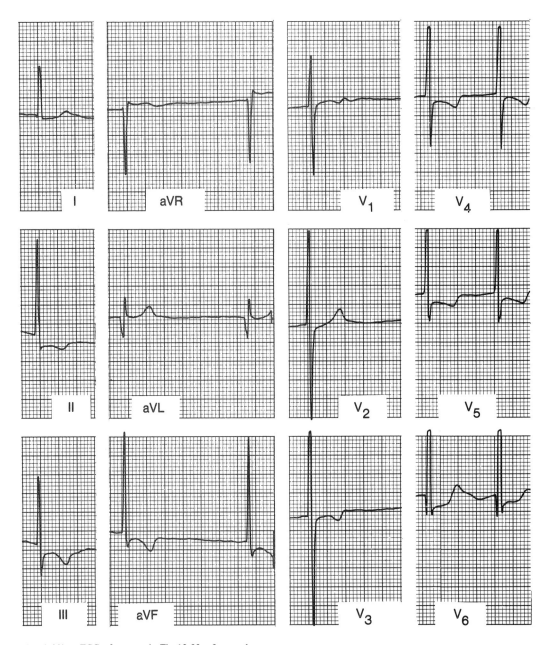

Fig 10-23b.—ECG of woman in Fig 10-23a, 2 years later.

Septal Hypertrophy

In most hearts the septum is part of the left ventricular chamber and increases in size in proportion to the free wall of the left ventricle. There are, however, several exceptions to this rule.

Idiopathic Hypertrophic Subaortic Stenosis

In idiopathic hypertrophic subaortic stenosis, the intraventricular septum enlarges in an asymmetrical fashion, so the affected portion of the septum is up to one third thicker than the opposed free wall of the left ventricle. The characteristic ECG evidence of this disorder is the presence of deep, broad Q waves, usually seen in leads II, III, and aVF and over the left precordium.[8] These may easily lead to the erroneous diagnosis of myocardial infarction.

Septal Hypertrophy Due to Right Ventricular Hypertrophy

In severe RVH, the ventricular septum may enlarge, together with the free wall of the right ventricle. This problem is illustrated in Figure 10-24. The most striking abnormality in this tracing is the depth of the Q waves in leads V_5 and V_6.

Mitral Valve Disease

Mitral valve disease deserves special emphasis, since it causes substantial morbidity and mortality. Although rheumatic fever, the chief cause of both mitral stenosis and mitral regurgitation, is on the decline in this country, there are still many patients who have valvular damage due to this disease.

Mitral Stenosis

Causes

- rheumatic fever, in more than 50% of cases[9]
- accumulation of calcium
- congenital (very rare)[10]

ECG characteristics

- left artial abnormality (P mitrale)
- RVH
- atrial fibrillation frequently seen

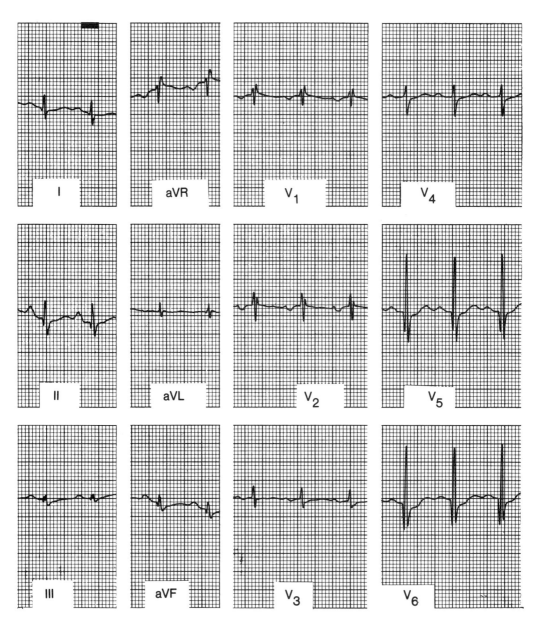

Fig 10-24.—ECG of 52-year-old woman with mitral stenosis.

The young woman whose ECG is shown in Figure 10-25 was admitted with severe heart failure. The tracing shows the classic signs of mitral stenosis: the P wave is double-peaked in many leads and has a pronounced negative component in lead V_1, and the P axis is $+30°$; there is a tall R wave in lead V_1, and a right ventricular strain pattern is seen in leads V_1 to V_3. The young lady is enjoying a normal, happy life, following mitral valve surgery.

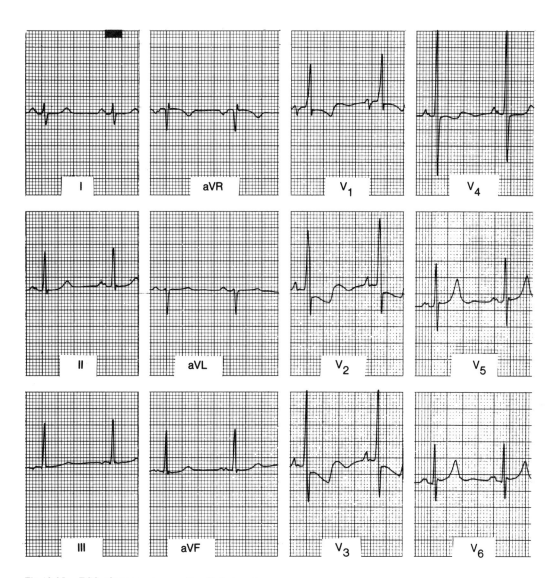

Fig 10-25.—ECG of young woman with mitral stenosis.

Mitral Regurgitation

Insufficiency of the mitral valve may be acute or chronic.[9]

Causes

Chronic

- mitral leaflet prolapse
- CAD
- left ventricular dilatation

- calcification of mitral annulus
- papillary muscle dysfunction
- rheumatic fever
- congenital heart disease[10]

Acute

- mitral insufficiency may occur following myocardial infarction, due to dysfunction or rupture of chordae tendineae or papillary muscles

ECG characteristics

- P mitrale
- LVH
- coarse atrial fibrillation possible

These signs are not diagnostic, since they may also be seen with other problems. The ECG of a 55-year-old man (Fig 10-26) shows the classic P mitrale pattern of LAA. The tracing also exhibits voltage criteria for LVH.

Combined Mitral Stenosis and Regurgitation

A combination of these abnormalities may be seen as a result of rheumatic fever, when the scarred leaflets of the mitral valve fail to open fully during ventricular diastole and are unable to close completely during systole. The ECG may provide evidence of the relative severity of the respective problems, that is, it shows RVH if stenosis predominates and LVH if the regurgitation is the more serious problem.[9]

The young man whose ECG is shown in Fig 10-27 was diagnosed as having mitral regurgitation at age 5, and corrective surgery was undertaken at that time. Some years later, mitral stenosis developed, and he had surgery again. He has been doing well following mitral valve replacement. The ECG shows the tall R wave and strain pattern of RVH, but the size of the QRS complexes in the midprecordial leads suggests that LVH may be present as well.

Mitral Valve Prolapse

With the increased use of echocardiography, mitral valve prolapse has become the most frequently diagnosed valvular abnormality.[11] Pathological causes of this problem include: myxomatous degeneration of the valve, thinning and elongation of the chordae tendineae, excessive valve tissue, and rheumatic endocarditis.[12]

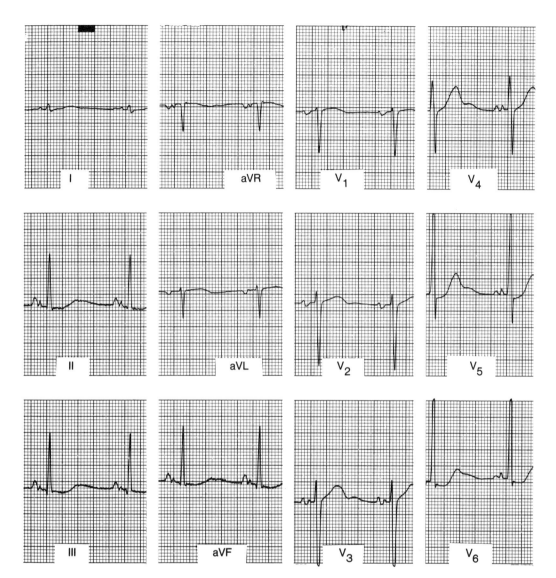

Fig 10-26.—ECG of patient with mitral regurgitation.

The condition is generally benign and may be found, often more or less accidentally, in 6% to 10% of healthy, asymptomatic young women.[11] Nevertheless, the patient deserves careful examination, and a thorough history should be taken because the disorder may cause mitral regurgitation, chest pain, or cardiac arrhythmias and because sudden death has been reported.[13] Antibiotic prophylaxis prior to dental work has been recommended to prevent bacterial endocarditis, as is the practice in treating many patients with valvular problems.

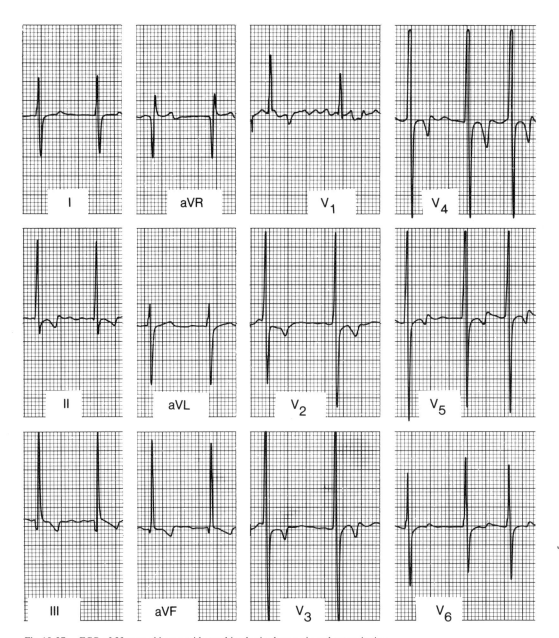

Fig 10-27.—ECG of 23-year-old man with combined mitral stenosis and regurgitation.

ECG characteristics

- T wave inversion in leads II, III, and aVF and at times in leads V_4 through V_6
- S-T segments usually normal but may be slightly depressed
- possibility of prolonged Q-T interval

These changes are not seen in all patients and may not be constant in a patient who has them (Figs 10-28a and b).

The ECG shown in Figure 10-28a is that of a 44-year-old woman who was referred for an exercise stress test because of a "feeling of fullness in the chest and palpitations." The resting tracing is perfectly normal. After six minutes of exercise, however, slight S-T segment depression and inversion of the T wave appeared in leads II, III, and aVF, as well as in leads V_5 and V_6. These persisted well into the recovery period and are still visible in Figure 10-28b, which was taken five minutes after termination of exercise.

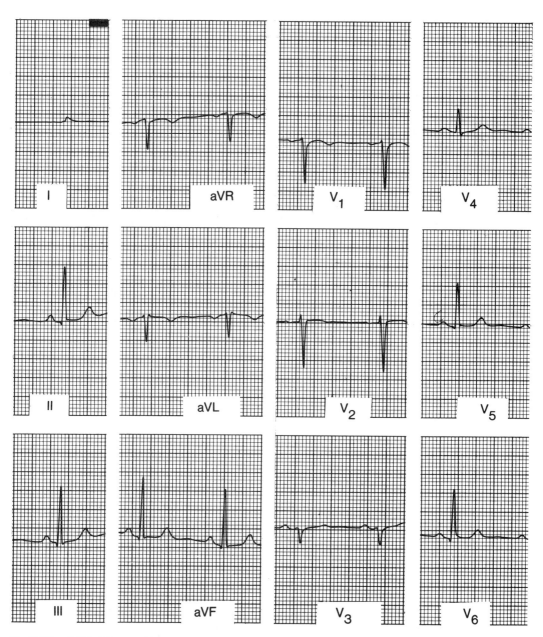

Fig 10-28a.—ECG of 44-year-old woman at rest.

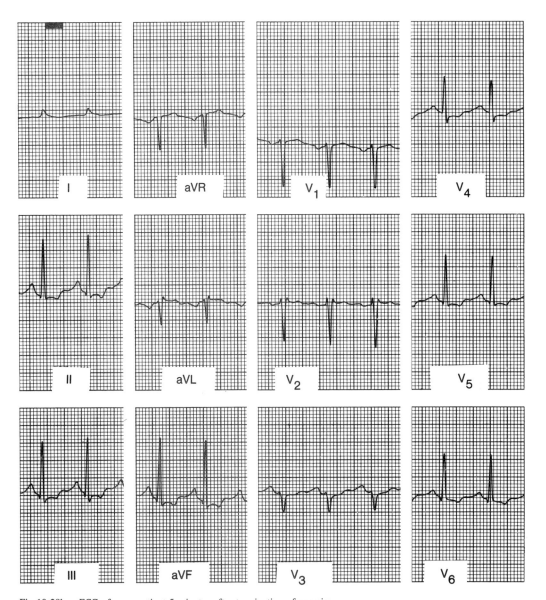

Fig 10-28b.—ECG of same patient 5 minutes after termination of exercise.

In view of the equivocal history and stress test results, coronary angiography was performed and revealed normal coronary arteries. An echocardiogram showed prolapse of a mitral leaflet, which is probably the cause of her symptoms, as well as of the ECG changes.

The rhythm strip in Figure 10-29 shows an example of the arrhythmias that may occur in some patients with this disorder. The frequent PVCs were not only uncomfortable for the patient but certainly appear to be dangerous. Therefore, although this condition is usually benign, each individual patient deserves careful evaluation.

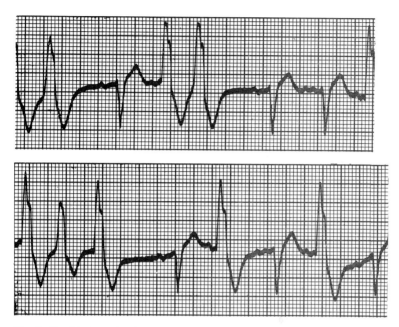

Fig 10-29.—Rhythm strip of young man with mitral leaflet prolapse.

REFERENCES

1. Friedman HH: *Diagnostic Electrocardiography and Vectorcardiography,* ed 2. New York, McGraw-Hill Book Co, 1977.

2. Schamroth L: *Electrocardiographic Excursions.* Oxford, England, Blackwell Scientific Publications, 1975, p 16.

3. Marriott HJL: *Workshop in Electrocardiography.* Tarpon Springs, Fla, Tampa Tracings, 1972. Reprinted by permission.

4. Hudson RB: The pathology of heart failure, in Hurst JW (ed): *The Heart,* ed 4. New York, McGraw-Hill Book Co, 1978, p 536.

5. Bachman S, Sparrow D, Smith KL: Effect of aging on the electrocardiogram. *Am J Cardiol* 1981;48:513.

6. Castellanos A, Myerburg RJ: The resting electrocardiogram, in Hurst JW (ed): *The Heart,* ed 4. New York, McGraw-Hill Book Co, 1978, p 308.

7. Lyon AF: Right ventricular hypertrophy. *ECG Self-Reviews,* No. 6. Ardsley, NY, Maxon Davis, Inc, 1980.

8. Braunwald E: Idiopathic hypertrophic subaortic stenosis, in Hurst JW (ed): *The Heart,* ed 4. New York, McGraw-Hill Book Co, 1978, p 1560.

9. Rackley CE, Edwards JE, Karp RB, et al: Mitral valve disease, in Hurst JW (ed): *The Heart,* ed 5. New York, McGraw-Hill Book Co, 1982, p 892.

10. Keith JD, Rowe RD, Vlad P: *Heart Disease in Infancy and Childhood.* New York, Macmillan Co, 1958, p 577.

11. Kannel WB: Incidence, prevalence and mortality of cardiovascular disease, in Hurst JW (ed): *The Heart,* ed 5. New York, McGraw-Hill Book Co, 1982, p 627.

12. Crawley IS, Morris DC, Silverman BD: Valvular heart disease, in Hurst JW (ed): *The Heart,* ed 4. New York, McGraw-Hill Book Co, 1978, p 1015.

13. Zipes DP, Noble JD: Assessment of electrical abnormalities, in Hurst JW (ed): *The Heart,* ed 5. New York, McGraw-Hill Book Co, 1982, p 337.

## Chapter 11

Electrocardiography in Pulmonary Disease

The ECG is used as a primary tool in the diagnosis and management of cardiac disorders. To follow the patient's progress, ECGs are taken frequently, occasionally too frequently, and monitoring in various forms is freely used to facilitate early detection of potentially detrimental arrhythmias. It is the author's belief that the ECG is of equal importance in cases of severe pulmonary disorders, but it does not always receive the attention it merits.

The work by Ayers and Grace[1] and Ayers and Mueller[2] clearly indicates the deadly consequences of the hypoxia and acid-base and electrolyte disturbances that frequently accompany serious pulmonary problems. The effect of hypoxia and acid-base disturbances on cardiac rhythm in non-MI patients has been demonstrated.[3] A more recent study reports that "ventricular arrhythmias in patients with chronic obstructive pulmonary disease (COPD) resemble, both in frequency and severity, those recorded in patients recovering from myocardial infarction."[4] The report stresses the importance of continuous ECG monitoring in this patient group.

In addition to revealing potentially life-threatening arrhythmias, the ECG can also be helpful in assessing the severity of a pulmonary disease, for instance, the presence of cor pulmonale, and can be useful in detecting problems that arise suddenly, such as pulmonary embolism and pneumothorax.

Arrhythmias in Pulmonary Disease

Both supraventricular and ventricular arrhythmias are frequently seen in patients with clinically stable and well-compensated chronic pulmonary disease. They tend to become more severe with respiratory failure and with mechanical ventilation. Complex ventricular arrhythmias and multifocal atrial tachycardia are very serious prognostic indicators in this patient category. An in-hospital mortality of 30% to 50% has been reported for patients with lung disease and multifocal atrial tachycardia.[4]

The tracings in Figures 11-1a through c illustrate this fact. They were obtained from a 64-year-old male patient with COPD, over a period of three days.

Figure 11-1a shows sinus tachycardia with very frequent PACs. The evidence of pulmonary disease consists of P pulmonale, RAD, incomplete RBBB, and low voltage.

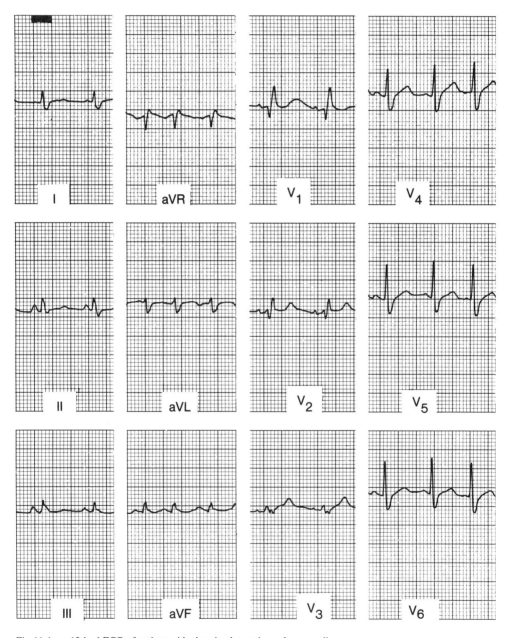

Fig 11-1a.—12-lead ECG of patient with chronic obstructive pulmonary disease.

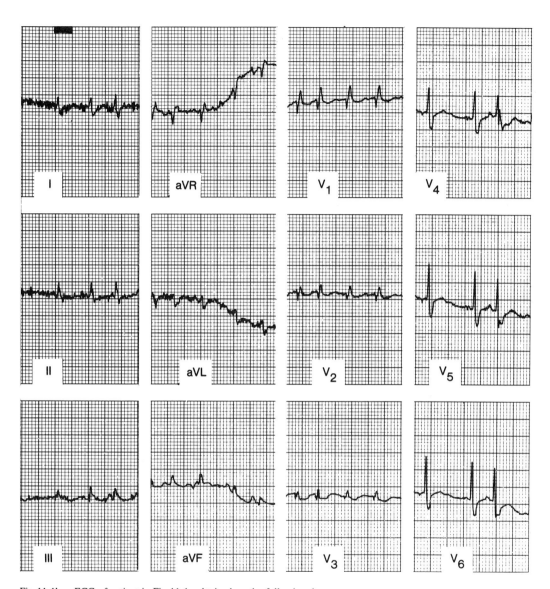

Fig 11-1b.—ECG of patient in Fig 11-1a obtained on the following day.

The ECG in Figure 11-1b shows multifocal (chaotic) atrial tachycardia with an average ventricular rate of 185 beats/min. The tracing in Figure 11-1c is incomplete, since ventricular tachycardia and fibrillation occurred while the ECG was being taken.

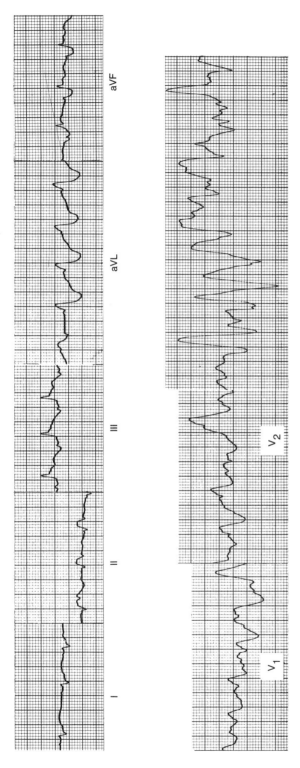

Fig 11-1c.—Portions of ECG of patient in Figure 11-1a.

ECG Diagnosis of Chronic Pulmonary Disease

The criteria for ECG diagnosis for chronic pulmonary disease are not nearly as clear-cut as they are for many other disorders. A high index of suspicion is often required to detect the signs of lung disease. In some patients, the classic evidence of right ventricular overload (chap 10) can be seen. In others, the signs are more subtle and the diagnosis is made by considering a combination of several abnormalities, each of which, taken by itself, would not be a definite sign of disease.

ECG characteristics

- P pulmonale, often seen in combination with significant negativity of P wave in lead V_1
- RAD or an indeterminate axis, in which all QRS complexes in frontal plane are equiphasic
- pseudo-LAD of pulmonary disease[5]
- low voltage of extremity and precordial leads
- isoelectric configuration of the P, QRS, and T waves in lead I[6]
- clockwise rotation of the heart (poor R wave progression and persistence of significant S waves across precordium)
- T wave inversion in right precordial leads
- S waves in leads I, II, and III (S_1 S_2 S_3)
- nonspecific T wave abnormalities and rather flat T waves often seen

Some authors suggest that a right ventricular overload pattern is usually seen in chronic pulmonary disease complicated by pulmonary hypertension,[5] whereas the most significant signs of "pure" emphysema are low voltage, pseudo-LAD and the isoelectric P, QRS, and T waves in lead I.[5,6]

These abnormalities may be difficult to recognize and remember, but they are well worth mastering, since a recent study[7] found the ECG to be more reliable than the chest X-ray in detecting right ventricular disease caused by obstructive lung disease.

The tracing in Figure 11-2 illustrates sinus tachycardia; P pulmonale with apparent LAA in lead V_1; an indeterminate axis; P, QRS, and T isoelectric in lead I (S_1 S_2 S_3); and clockwise rotation of the precordial leads.

The ECG in Figure 11-3 meets the criteria for P pulmonale. Although the P wave is not particularly pointed or tall, it does have an axis of $+90°$. This ECG also shows indeterminate axis, low voltage, lack of R wave progression, and S-T and T wave abnormalities. There are frequent PACs as well as PVCs, a common finding in patients with COPD.

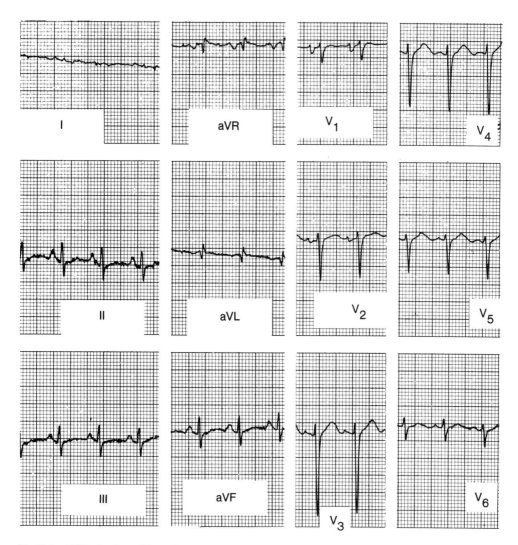

Fig 11-2.—ECG of patient with emphysema.

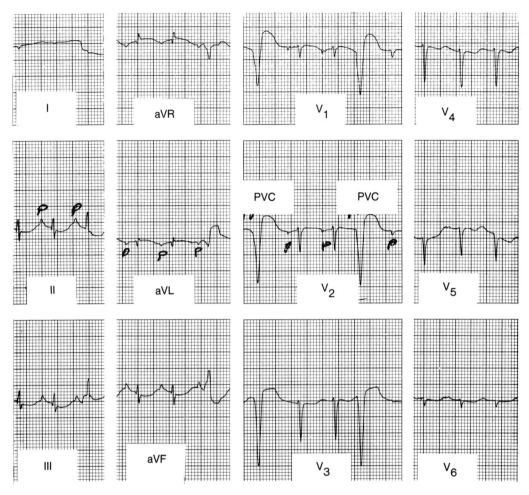

Fig 11-3.—ECG of patient with chronic obstructive pulmonary disease. PVC = premature ventricular contraction, P = P wave.

At first glance the tracing in Figure 11-4 looks normal. Closer examination shows sinus tachycardia, and the P waves are slightly pointed, with an axis close to + 80°. The ventricular vector of + 70° is more to the right than would be expected in a patient who is 60 years old. There is also a pronounced R wave in lead V_1, together with inversion of the T wave in that lead. This is not enough to establish the diagnosis of pulmonary disease, but it should lead to careful assessment of the patient's respiratory system.

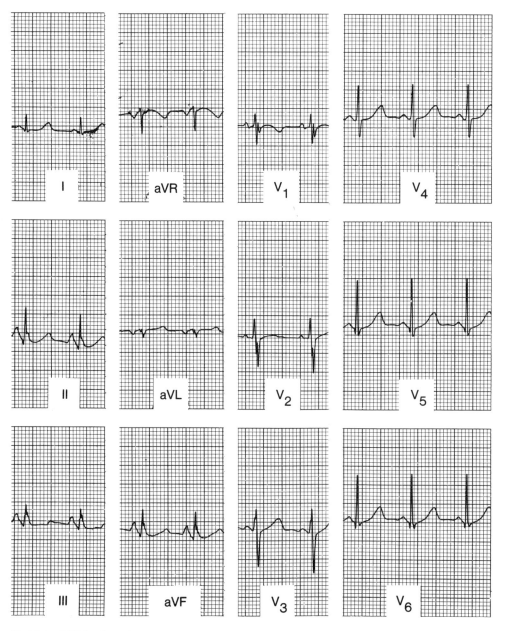

Fig 11-4.—ECG for discussion.

There can be little doubt of the abnormality of the ECG in Figure 11-5. If this were a young patient, a congenital cardiac problem would be suspected, but that is not likely in a 76-year-old man. The RVH shown in this tracing is due to severe pulmonary hypertension caused by chronic lung disease.

Another tracing of a patient with chronic lung disease (Fig 11-6) shows a nearly isoelectric lead I with LAD. There is relatively low voltage and poor R wave progression.

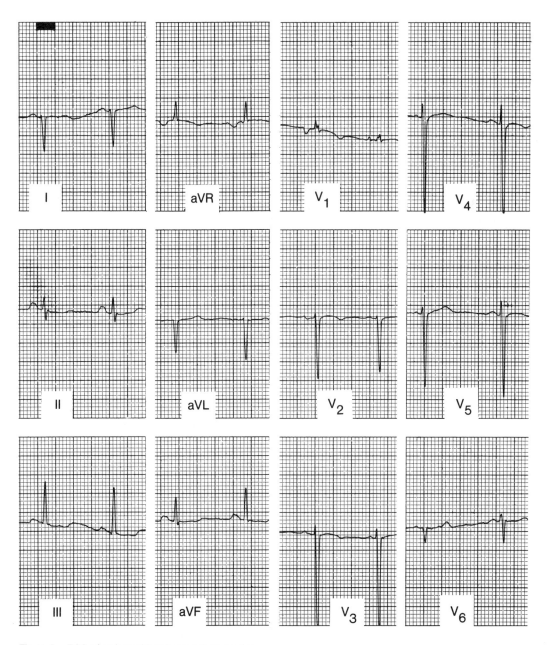

Fig 11-5.—ECG of patient with pulmonary hypertension.

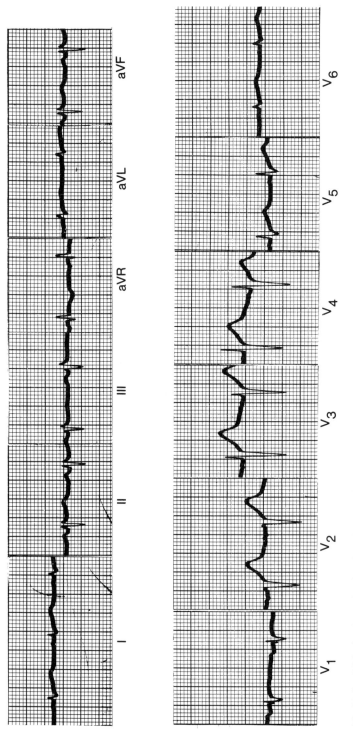

Fig 11-6.—ECG of patient with chronic pulmonary disease.

Cor Pulmonale

Cor pulmonale is caused by right ventricular overload due to pulmonary disease. The most common cause of acute cor pulmonale is pulmonary embolism, but it may also be precipitated by acute respiratory failure due to COPD, asthma, or other causes. Chronic cor pulmonale may be seen in patients with severe COPD. It is not usually possible to tell the cause of this problem by examining the ECG, but the sudden appearance of certain ECG characteristics should give warning of a serious condition.[8-10]

Pulmonary Embolism

Rhythm Changes

The changes due to pulmonary embolism may be transient, so the nurse must be alert to recognize them. The arrhythmias are usually supraventricular. One study[11] reported supraventricular tachycardia in 75% of cases. In my experience, tachycardia has almost always been present, at least transiently, and its absence casts doubt on the diagnosis of pulmonary embolism.

ECG characteristics

The axis may shift to the right or, more frequently, to the left.[8]
The most *suggestive characteristics* are [8-10]

- S wave in lead I, Q wave in lead III, and inverted T wave in lead III ($S_1 Q_3 T_3$)
- S wave in lead I and inverted T wave in lead III and in right precordial leads ($S_1 T_3$)
- an $S_1 Q_3 T_3$ pattern, together with RBBB

If these characteristics appear suddenly, they are strongly suggestive, although not diagnostic, of pulmonary embolism. Since these changes occur in only 10% to 35% of cases,[8,9] their absence does not preclude the possibility that the patient has had a pulmonary embolism.

The most *frequently seen pattern* consists of nonspecific changes of the S-T segment and T waves.[8,9] These changes are not diagnostic, since they may be caused by a great variety of diseases and conditions.

Other Patterns

All of the ECG abnormalities described under chronic lung disease may be seen in patients with pulmonary embolism.

The ECG in Figure 11-7 was obtained in a 37-year-old man; it strongly supports the diagnosis of pulmonary embolism. It shows sinus tachycardia, $S_1 Q_3$ pattern, and incomplete RBBB. When such abnormalities occur suddenly, they should definitely lead to further appropriate diagnostic studies.

ECG changes that are not very specific or dramatic may gain significance and importance when they are viewed in the light of previous tracings in the same patient.

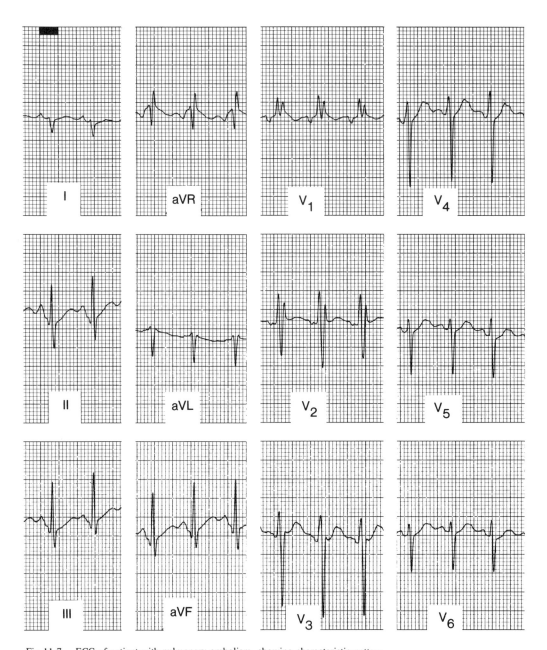

Fig 11-7.—ECG of patient with pulmonary embolism, showing characteristic pattern.

The ECG in Figure 11-8a was obtained during routine follow-up examination of a 55-year-old man. Except for the minimal remaining evidence of an IWMI that he had several years previously, the tracing is normal. The second tracing (Fig 11-8b) was taken on hospital admission for chest pain. It shows sinus tachycardia, a shift in axis from $-15°$ to $+90°$, S-T and T wave changes in the frontal plane, the appearance of an R wave in lead V_1, and T wave inversion, especially in the right precordial leads. These changes are suggestive of pulmonary embolism, although other possibilities, such as true posterior infarction, must also be considered.

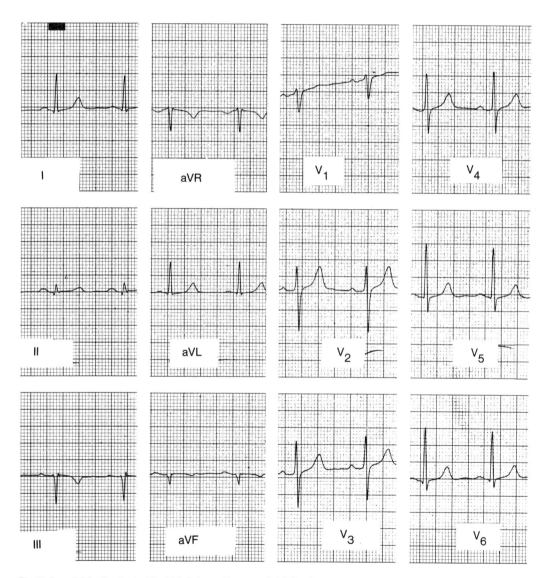

Fig 11-8a.—ECG of patient with old inferior wall myocardial infarction.

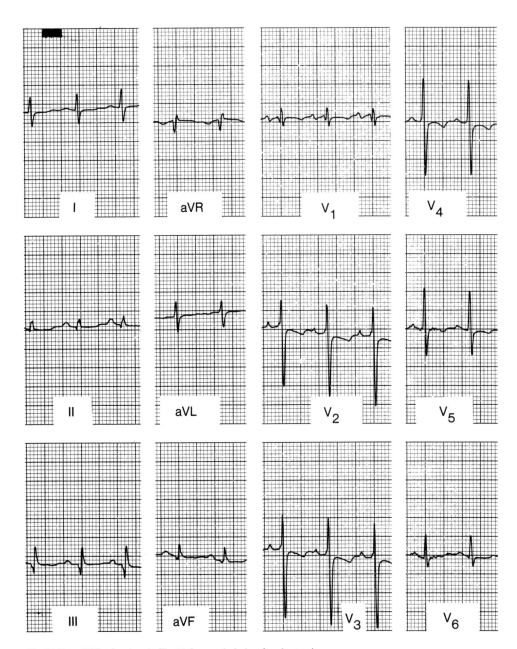

Fig 11-8b.—ECG of patient in Fig 11-8a on admission for chest pain.

Figure 11-9 shows a tracing of a patient with cor pulmonale. The abnormalities consist of atrial fibrillation, an axis of + 90°, $S_1 Q_3 T_3$, and a prominent R wave in lead V_1. Unless previous tracings are available, it is impossible to say whether these signs of right ventricular failure are acute or chronic, although the relatively slow ventricular response to atrial fibrillation suggests that this is not an acute problem.

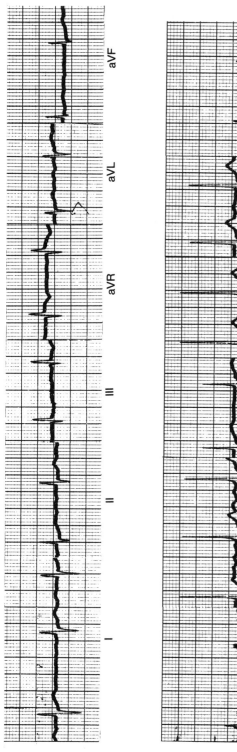
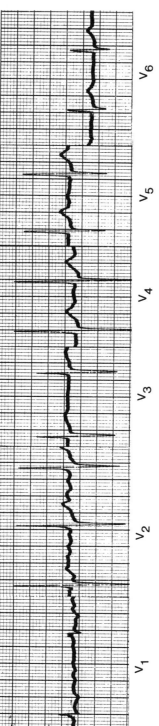

Fig 11-9.—ECG of patient with cor pulmonale.

A 39-year-old marathon runner was admitted to the hospital with chest pain. He was in excellent physical condition from training and had no significant history. The initial tracing (Fig 11-10a) is very unrevealing. There is sinus tachycardia, and leads II, III, and aVF show some nonspecific S-T and T wave abnormalities.

An ECG taken the next day (Fig 11-10b) shows a spread of the T wave inversions to the right precordial leads, suggesting a right ventricular problem.

The patient had a "shower" of pulmonary emboli, documented by lung scan. The nonspecific findings of sinus tachycardia and relatively minor abnormalities of T waves shown in Figure 11-10a are the only indications in most cases of this disorder.

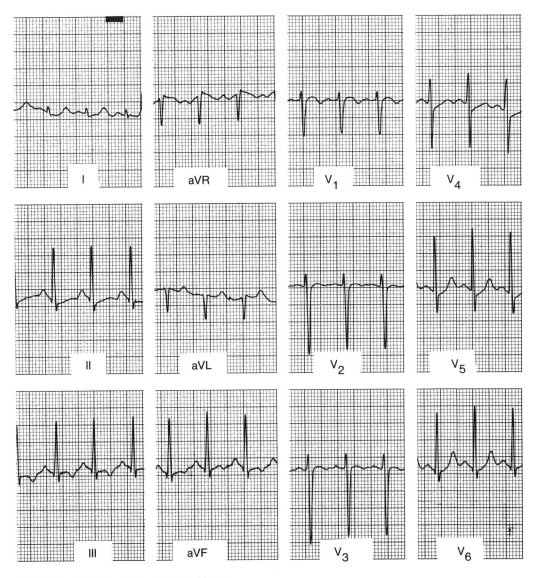

Fig 11-10a.—Admission ECG of 39-year-old man.

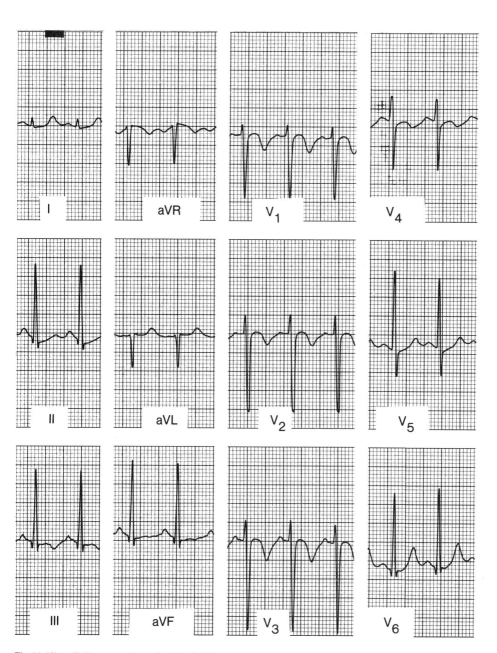

Fig 11-10b.—Follow-up tracing of patient in Fig 11-10a.

Low Voltage

Low voltage, per se, is a very nonspecific finding and is seen in anemia, diffuse myocardial damage, myxedema, obesity, hypothermia, malnutrition, and emphysema.[8] Voltages also decrease whenever fluid or air is interposed between the heart and the recording electrode, as may occur with such conditions as pneumothorax, pleural effusion, and pericardial effusion. The latter instances are of particular importance to the critical care nurse, since they may occur suddenly as a sign of a serious, previously unsuspected complication.

Criteria for low voltage

- QRS complexes 5 mm or less in leads I, II, and III
- QRS complexes 7½ mm or less in leads aVR, aVL, and aVF
- QRS complexes 10 mm or less in precordial leads

These criteria are taken from a personal communication from D. J. Scott, MD.

Voltage changes are difficult to assess from monitoring records, since most devices used for continuous ECG monitoring permit adjustments in gain, that is, they are not set to the standard of 10 mm = 1 mV. Therefore, if a change in voltage is suspected, a 12-lead ECG must be obtained to confirm the diagnosis.

Three tracings illustrate the usefulness of this procedure. Figure 11-11a, which was obtained at the time of admission, is within normal limits.

The patient required mechanical ventilation because of severe pneumonia. The second tracing (Fig 11-11b) was taken after treatment with a volume ventilator for 24 hours. There was a change in rhythm to multifocal atrial tachycardia and a shift in the frontal plane axis toward the right. These changes may have been due to pulmonary disease. The most dramatic change, however, was the sudden decrease in voltage. Even with severe lung disease, such a sudden decrease is not common. This patient had a pneumomediastinum due to barotrauma.

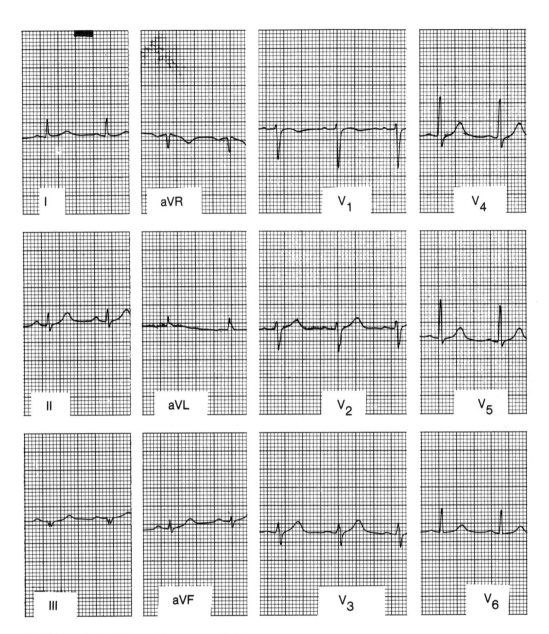

Fig 11-11a.—ECG of 60-year-old woman on admission.

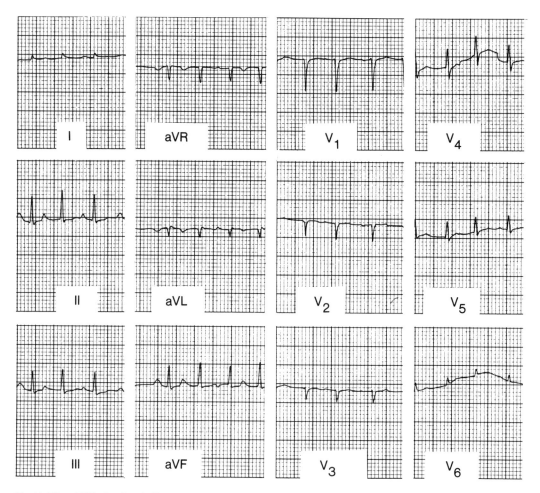

Fig 11-11b.—ECG of patient in Fig 11-11a, 2 days later.

The first ECG of a 55-year-old man is normal (Fig 11-12a). A second ECG, obtained 6 months later, shows a considerable loss of voltage, especially in the limb leads, as well as nonspecific flattening of the T waves throughout (Fig 11-12b). This man had a large pleural effusion.

In pleural effusion, the left precordial leads may show more of a voltage loss than the right precordial leads. This phenomenon (Fig 11-12b) is due to the fact that the right precordial leads are attached one intercostal space higher than the left leads and may be above the fluid level of the effusion.

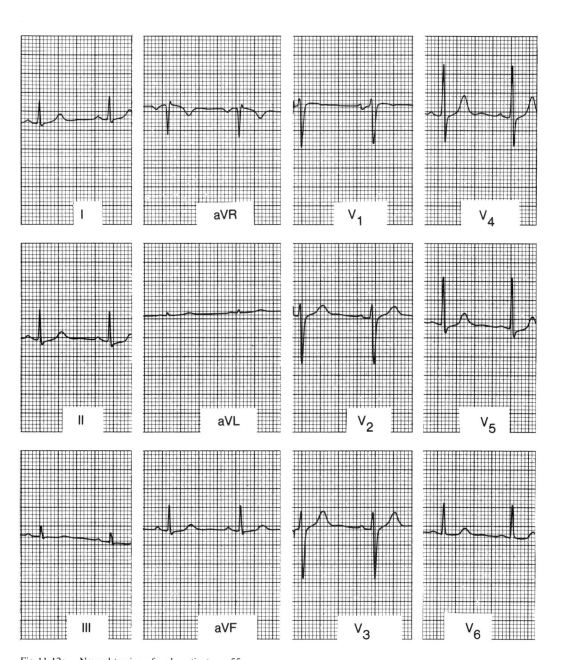

Fig 11-12a.—Normal tracing of male patient age 55.

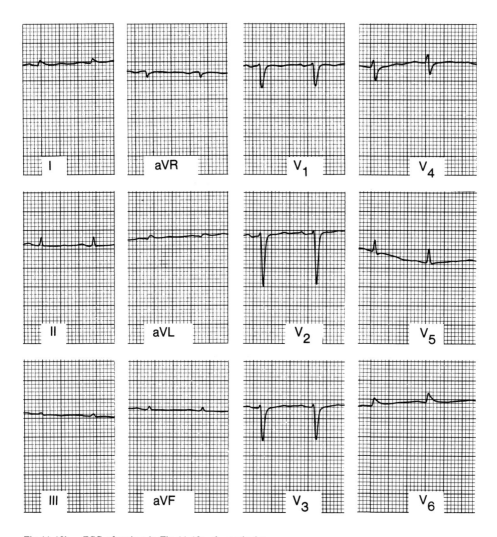

Fig 11-12b.—ECG of patient in Fig 11-12a, 6 months later.

The 20-year-old man, whose data appear in Figures 11-13a through c, was admitted unconscious in diabetic ketoacidosis (DKA). A subclavian catheter was inserted, since the peripheral veins proved unreliable. He responded well to the usual treatment and had begun to regain consciousness on the following morning, when the tracing in Figure 11-13a was obtained.

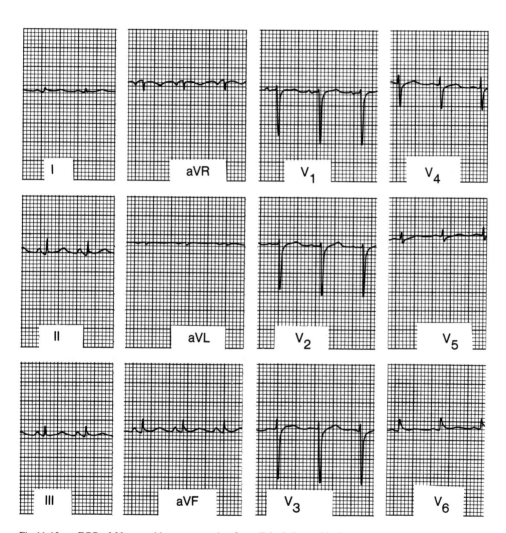

Fig 11-13a.—ECG of 20-year-old man recovering from diabetic ketoacidosis.

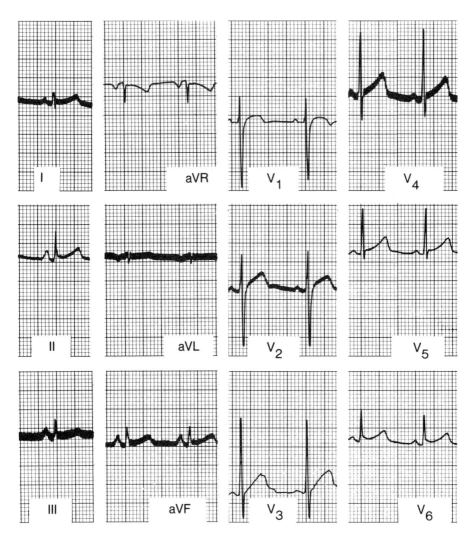

Fig 11-13b.—ECG of patient in Fig 11-13a obtained on previous admission.

Comparison with a tracing obtained on a previous admission revealed a considerable loss in voltage, especially in the left ventricular leads. A close examination of the chest X-ray (Fig 11-13c) reveals the cause of this problem; there is a 10% to 15% left-sided pneumothorax, probably produced by damage to the apex of the lung during insertion of the subclavian catheter. This did not pose a serious problem, and the patient made an excellent recovery. However, in a patient who requires mechanical ventilation, an unrecognized pneumothorax could lead to disaster.

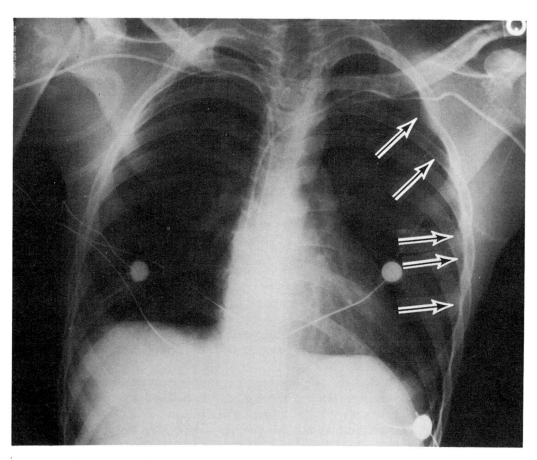

Fig 11-13c.—Chest X-ray of patient in Fig 11-13a; arrows indicate separation of visceral pleura from thoracic wall.

Drugs Used in Pulmonary Disease

The care of the patient with pulmonary disease is often complicated because the medications used to facilitate breathing have a tendency to produce cardiac arrhythmias or to make existing arrhythmias worse. The commonly used drugs include theophylline and β-adrenergic stimulants.[4,12]

The tachyarrhythmias, at worst, can be life-threatening; at best they greatly contribute to the patient's discomfort. They tend to increase oxygen consumption and often a vicious cycle is created in which more and more drugs are required, while the patient's condition worsens steadily. Careful management is required to ensure optimum pulmonary function while avoiding detrimental cardiac effects of drugs. The nurse plays a most important role in evaluating the impact of these medications on the patient's cardiopulmonary status.

Unfortunately, some of the drugs generally used to treat cardiac disorders may cause additional complications in patients with lung disease. Digitalis may be necessary to treat right-heart failure due to pulmonary disease or to coexisting heart disease. This drug must be used with great care, however, in patients who have chronic hypoxia, since this condition facilitates the development of digitalis toxicity.[4]

Many studies have shown that correction of hypoxia and metabolic disturbances is more effective in treating arrhythmias in this patient group than the customary antiarrhythmic agents.[1,2,4]

Most β-blockers, such as propranolol, which are very effective in the prevention and treatment of cardiac arrhythmias, may cause additional problems in the patient with pulmonary disease, by provoking bronchospasms. Some of the newer β_1-blockers, such as atenolol (Tenormin), offer some hope in this respect, as illustrated in the following case.

The ECG in Figure 11-14a was obtained in a 72-year-old woman who had emphysema. She was severely limited in her activities by constant shortness of breath and palpitations. The latter complaint was certainly justified: a rhythm strip (Fig 11-14b) taken at rest shows a heart rate averaging 150 beats/min.

Both tachycardias and complaints have persisted for years. Treatment with the customary drugs either had proven ineffective or, in the case of propranolol, had caused new complications.

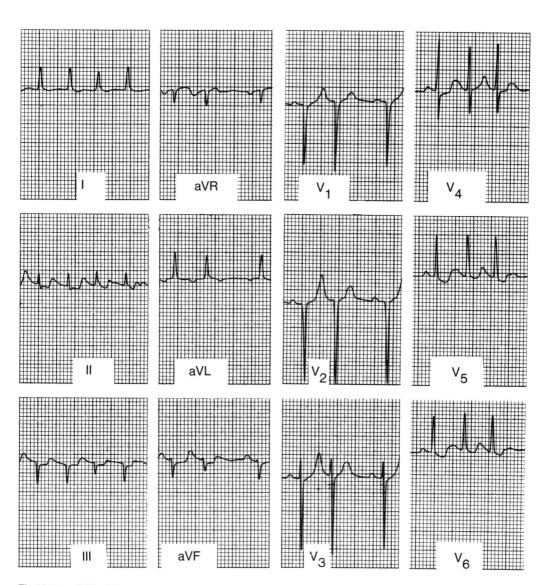

Fig 11-14a.—ECG of 72-year-old woman with emphysema.

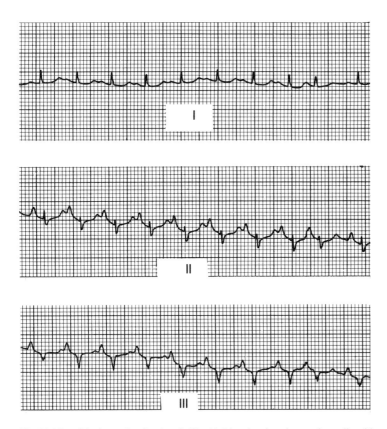

Fig 11-14b.—Rhythm strip of patient in Fig 11-14a, showing sinus tachycardia with premature atrial contractions.

The last tracing (Fig 11-14c) was obtained following treatment with atenolol. It shows normal sinus rhythm and is almost normal. This does not mean that she is cured; she still has emphysema. However, restoration of a regular rhythm at a normal rate has greatly improved her exercise tolerance, and she is once again able to enjoy moderate domestic and social activities.

Antiarrhythmic therapy in patients with chronic lung disease is generally best evaluated through Holter monitoring, while the patient carries out his accustomed activities.[4] It is usually impossible to maintain a patient who has chronic hypoxia and acid-base abnormalities in normal sinus rhythm. It would be futile and probably dangerous to increase antiarrhythmic drug dosages in an effort to achieve this goal. The most that can usually be accomplished is the suppression of life-threatening arrhythmias and a reasonable absence of symptoms in the patient.

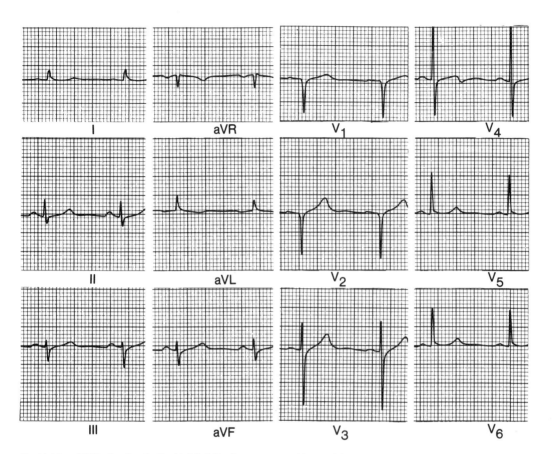

Fig 11-14c.—ECG of patient in Fig 11-14b following treatment with atenolol.

REFERENCES

1. Ayers SM, Grace WJ: Inappropriate ventilation and hypoxemia as a cause of cardiac arrhythmias. *Am J Med* 1969;46:495.

2. Ayers SM, Mueller H: Hypoxemia, hypercapnea and cardiac arrhythmias: The importance of regional abnormalities of vascular distensibility. *Chest* 1973;63:981.

3. Sweetwood HM: Oxygen administration in the coronary care unit. *Heart Lung* 1974;3:102.

4. Biggs FD, Lefrak SS, Kleiger RE, et al: Disturbances of rhythm in chronic lung disease. *Heart Lung* 1977;6:256.

5. Phibbs BP, Marriott HJL: Computer ECG programs: A critical appraisal. *Primary Cardiol* 1981;7:49.

6. Schamroth, L: *Electrocardiographic Excursions*. Oxford, England, Blackwell Scientific Publications, 1975, p 1.

7. Mitchell RS: The right ventricle in chronic airway obstruction. *Am Rev Respir Dis* 1976;114:147.

8. Friedman HH: *Diagnostic Electrocardiography and Vectorcardiography,* ed 2. New York, McGraw-Hill Book Co, 1977, pp 336-338.

9. Goldman MJ: *Principles of Clinical Electrocardiography,* ed 7. Los Altos, Calif, Lange Medical Publications, 1970, pp 111-116.

10. Dexter L, Dalen JE: Pulmonary embolism and acute cor pulmonale, in Hurst JW (ed): *The Heart.* New York, McGraw-Hill Book Co, 1978, p 1478.

11. Fitzmaurice JB, Sasahara AA: Current concepts of pulmonary embolism: Implications for nursing practice. *Heart Lung* 1974;3:209.

12. Greenbaum DM: Secondary cardiac dysrhythmias. *Heart Lung* 1977;6:308.

## Chapter 12

Electrolyte and Acid-Base Abnormalities

Electrolyte and acid-base disturbances are frequently reflected in the ECG. The most distinct and specific changes are seen with abnormal potassium levels. Since the ECG reflects intracellular and extracellular concentrations of some electrolytes, it is frequently more sensitive to changes in total body electrolyte stores than laboratory studies that record only serum levels.[1] This is of special importance when relative electrolyte concentrations shift rapidly and/or transiently, as is the case in acidosis and alkalosis.

Q-T Interval

The diagnosis of many of the abnormalities discussed in this and the following chapter is dependent on the length of the Q-T interval: the distance from the beginning of the ventricular complex to the end of the T wave. This interval varies directly with the heart rate. The slower the rate is, the longer the interval becomes. Generally, when the rate is 60 to 90 beats/min, the Q-T interval measures less than one half of the R-R interval. With faster rates, it may become slightly longer than half of the R-R interval.[2] This rule of thumb is sufficient for most purposes, but sometimes a more precise measurement is needed. Q-T intervals adjusted for heart rate and sex of the patient are listed in Table 7-2.

Abnormal Potassium Levels

Potassium plays a major role in the generation and conduction of electrical impulses, and abnormally high or low concentrations of this electrolyte have a distinct and sometimes fatal effect on myocardial depolarization and repolarization, as well as on automaticity.

415

Hyperkalemia

Hyperkalemia is most frequently seen in patients with renal failure, but it may occur following extensive burns or crushing injuries and during severe metabolic acidosis. It has also been observed following massive, rapid transfusion with bank blood.

The ECG changes seen with hyperkalemia relate to the serum potassium level but are more specific and sensitive to the actual clinical status than the laboratory studies.

Moderate

Moderate hyperkalemia (serum potassium level above 5.5 mEq/L) is reflected in a change in T wave configuration and is most readily recognized in the precordial leads. The T wave becomes tall and asymmetrical with a narrow base and is often peaked or "tented" (Fig 12-1).

Very tall T waves may also be seen in patients with bradycardia[3] and may be a sign of other disorders such as ischemia, so their appearance must be evaluated in light of the patient's clinical status.

The tracing in Figure 12-2 was obtained in a 20-year-old man who had had contusion of a kidney. His serum potassium level was within normal limits at 4 mEq/L, and he showed no signs of renal failure. Although the T waves are tall, they are not symmetrical or narrow at the base.

We have noted an interesting phenomenon in several of our renal patients who had LVH with inverted T waves: the T waves remained inverted as the serum potassium level rose, but assumed the other characteristics of the hyperkalemic T wave: they became symmetrical, pointed, and narrow at the base. The tracing in Figure 12-3 shows this T wave inversion. Combined hyperkalemia and hypocalcemia is a frequent finding in patients with chronic renal failure.

As the serum *potassium level rises* (serum potassium above 6.5 mEq/L), the amplitude of the R wave may decrease and there may be an increase in the depth of the S wave. At the same time, there may be prolongation of the QRS interval, the P-R interval lengthens, and the P waves become flat. Supraventricular as well as ventricular arrhythmias may occur, and the appearance of RBBB and hemiblocks has been reported.

In the tracing shown in Figure 12-4, the precordial leads show the characteristic T wave configuration of hyperkalemia. The P waves are flattened and cannot be seen at all in a number of leads. The QRS complexes are wide, and there are disturbances of cardiac rhythm.

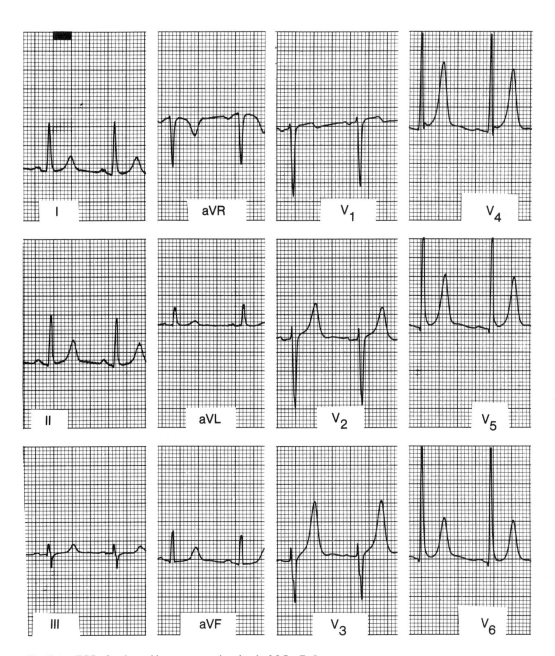

Fig 12-1.—ECG of patient with serum potassium level of 5.7 mEq/L.

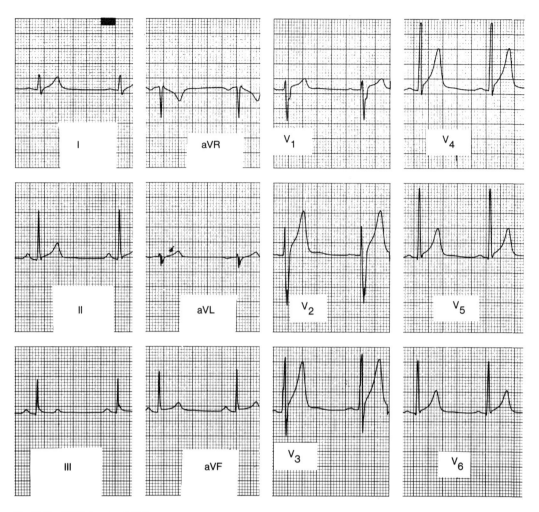

Fig 12-2.—ECG showing tall T waves.

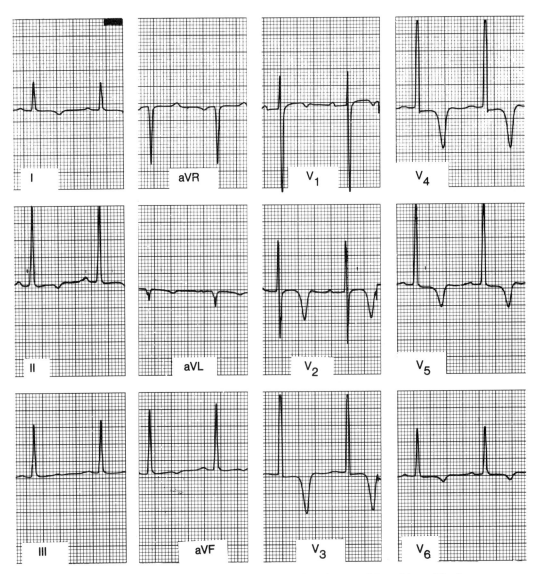

Fig 12-3.—ECG of patient with serum potassium level of 7.1 mEq/L and serum calcium of 8 mg/100 ml.

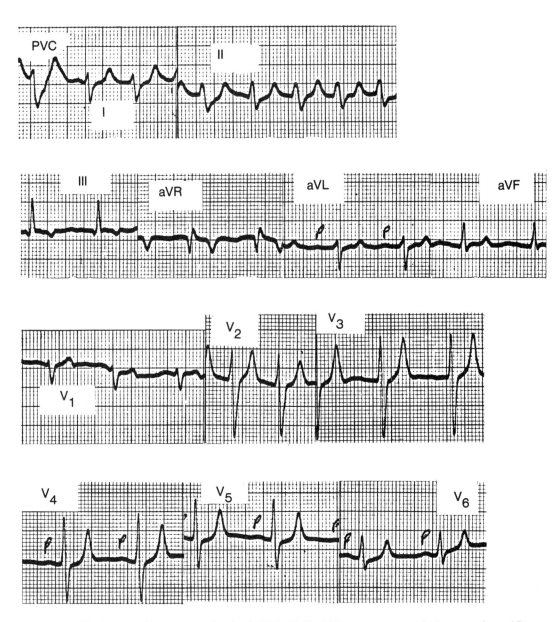

Fig 12-4.—ECG of patient with serum potassium level of 6.9 mEq/L. PVC = premature ventricular contraction and P = P wave.

Severe

In severe hyperkalemia (serum potassium level above 8 mEq/L), atrial activity usually can no longer be seen, although conduction of sinus impulses to the ventricles may continue through the internodal tracts, producing a sinoventricular rhythm. This phenomenon occurs because the cells of the atrial myocardium are more sensitive to potassium than those of the internodal tracts. At the same time, the QRS complexes widen markedly, and the characteristic peaked T waves may disappear or become inverted. It is usually impossible to determine from the surface ECG whether the resulting tracing reflects the sinoventricular rhythm described or represents sinus arrest with an idioventricular rhythm (Fig 12-5).

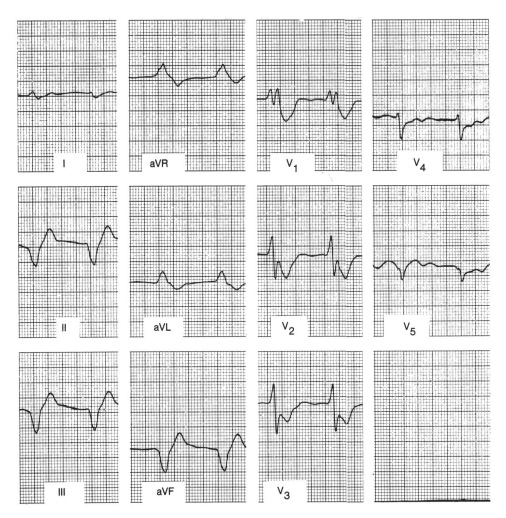

Fig 12-5.—ECG of patient with serum potassium level of 8 mEq/L.

The ECG shown in Figure 12-6a was obtained in a 61-year-old man with hypertension. The tracing shows LVH and a digitalis effect.

The tracing in Figure 12-6b was obtained in the same patient on emergency admission, when his serum potassium was 8.6 mEq/L. The QRS complexes have become extremely wide, and there are deep S-T segment depressions in many leads. Because the P wave cannot be seen in most leads, the rhythm cannot be determined unless the P waves in lead V_1 are recognized.

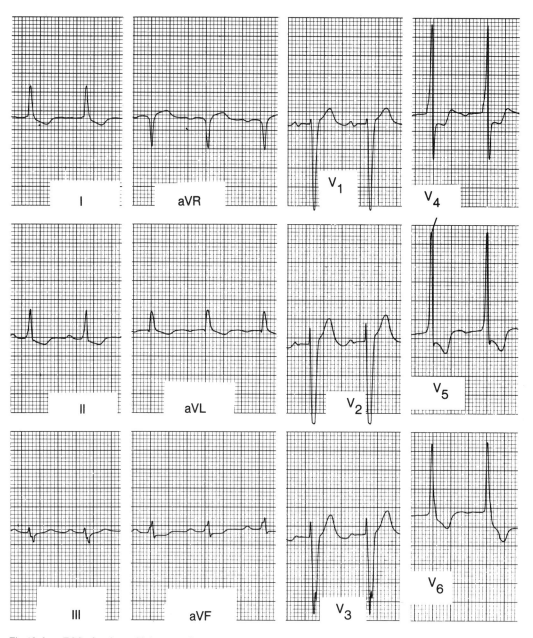

Fig 12-6a.—ECG of patient with hypertension.

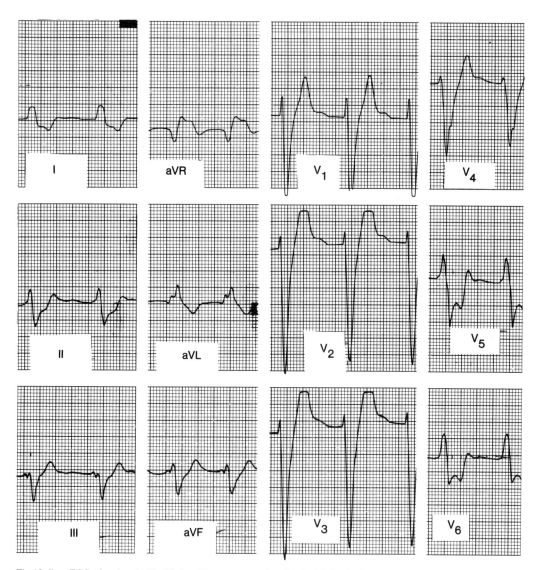

Fig 12-6b.—ECG of patient in Fig 12-6a with serum potassium level of 8.6 mEq/L.

The ventricular rhythm may become irregular due to underlying atrial fibrillation or because of a disturbance of the sinus mechanism. An instance of this disturbance is shown in Figure 12-6b. Because flat P waves with a prolonged P-R interval can be detected in lead V_1, the irregularity of the rhythm must be due to sinus arrhythmia.

The ECG changes often suggest a more serious problem than the laboratory studies do; this is revealed by the tracings in Figures 12-7a through c. They were obtained over a period of three days in a 55-year-old man with aortic stenosis, hypertension, and end-stage congestive heart failure.

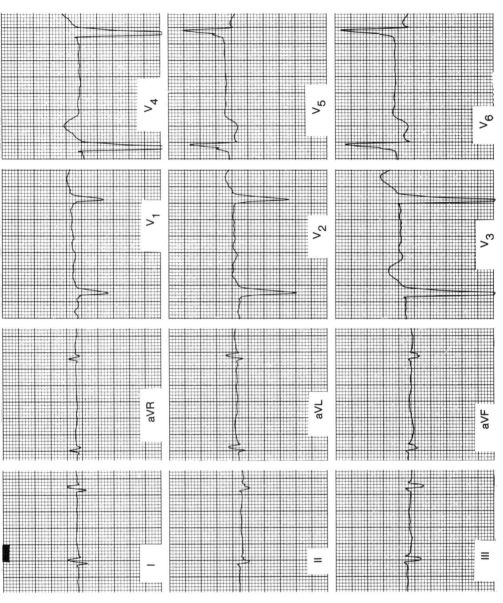

Fig 12-7a.—Serum potassium level of 4 mEq/L.

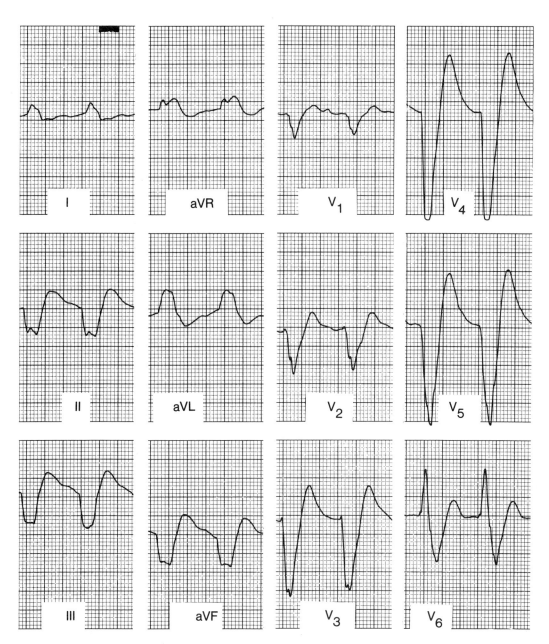

Fig 12-7b.—Serum potassium level of 4.9 mEq/L.

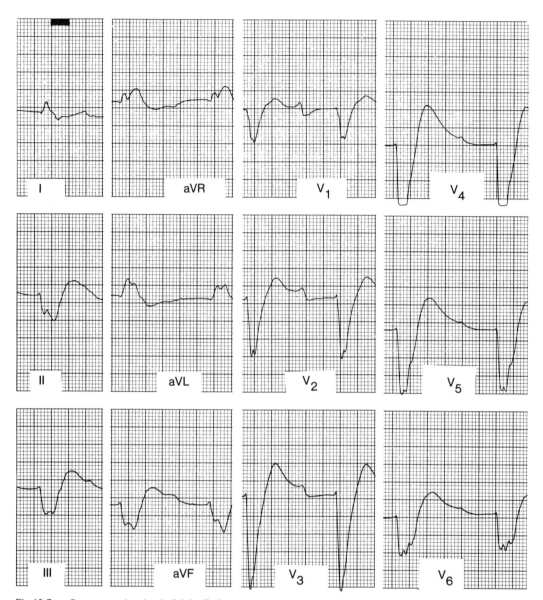

Fig 12-7c.—Serum potassium level of 6.6 mEq/L.

Very Severe

With very severe hyperkalemia there is progressive widening of the QRS complex, which merges smoothly with the inverted T wave, producing a sine-shaped configuration that resembles a "dying heart" complex. This is, in fact, a dying heart, unless therapy is promptly instituted.

At serum potassium levels of 10 to 14 mEq/L, deadly arrhythmias (ventricular fibrillation or standstill) invariably occur.[3] We have frequently observed immediately life-threatening arrhythmias (complete heart block and ventricular tachycardia) at serum potassium levels of 7 to 9 mEq/L (Fig 12-8a and b).

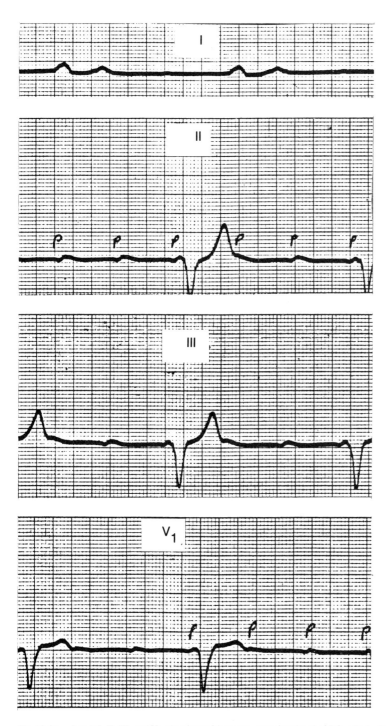

Fig 12-8a.—Leads I, II, III, and V_1 of patient with serum potassium level of 7.3 mEq/L. P = P wave.

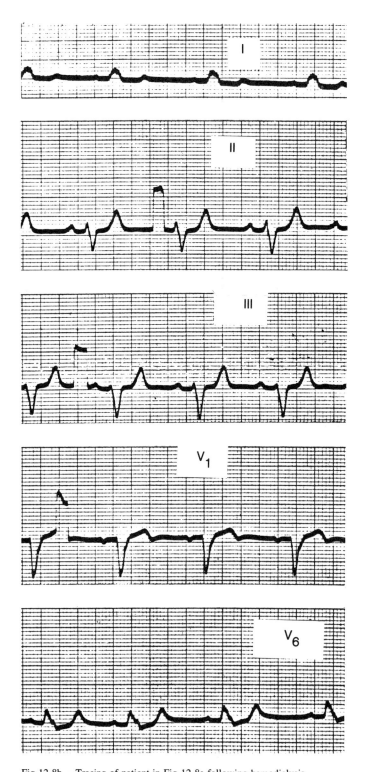

Fig 12-8b.—Tracing of patient in Fig 12-8a following hemodialysis.

The ECG shown in Figure 12-9 was taken in a young woman with chronic renal failure. She had not kept an appointment for hemodialysis and arrived in the emergency department two days later in a state of collapse, with ventricular tachycardia. The serum potassium level was 8.6 mEq/L. The arrhythmia failed to respond to all methods of treatment customarily used in this situation: lidocaine, sodium bicarbonate, calcium gluconate, glucose and insulin, and electric cardioversion.

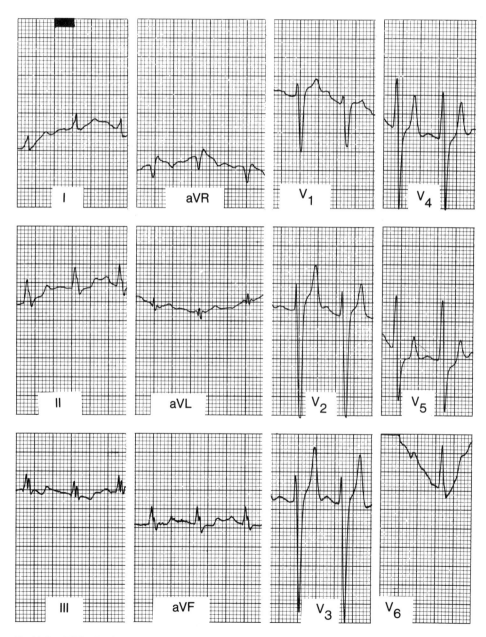

Fig 12-9.—ECG of patient with hyperkalemia.

The tracing in Figure 12-9 was obtained following hemodialysis. The QRS complexes are still wide, and the T waves show the characteristic configuration due to hyperkalemia, but sinus rhythm has been restored.

Significant hyperkalemia represents a serious threat to life. For example, the patients whose tracings are shown in Figures 12-5 and 12-6a and b died within an hour after admission. Critical care nurses should be alert for these characteristic changes, so therapeutic measures can be instituted in a timely manner.

Hypokalemia

Hypokalemia probably occurs most frequently as a result of vigorous or prolonged diuretic therapy. It can also be due to prolonged vomiting and diarrhea, or it can appear as a complication of steroid therapy or treatment of diabetic keto-acidosis. Alkalosis, too, can be the cause of low serum potassium levels.

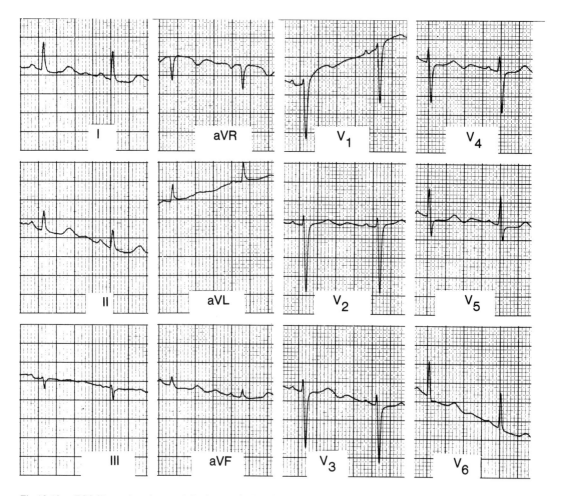

Fig 12-10.—ECG illustrating characteristic changes in T and U waves due to hypokalemia.

The first sign of hypokalemia is usually flattening of the T wave and an increase in the size of the U wave (Fig 12-10). Pronounced U waves may occasionally be seen in normal persons with slow heart rates and in patients with LVH. In these cases, however, the height of the T wave is not usually diminished.

The Q-T interval prolongation occasionally mentioned as a sign of hypokalemia is generally more apparent than real and is due to the difficulty in determining where the T wave ends and the U wave starts. This is true, for example, in leads V_4 to V_6 in Figure 12-11. In leads V_2 and V_3 of the same tracing, where the end of the T wave can be clearly seen, the Q-T interval measures 0.41 second, well within the normal limits for a heart rate of 57 beats/min. This ECG also shows another characteristic of hypokalemia, a notched T wave (arrow).

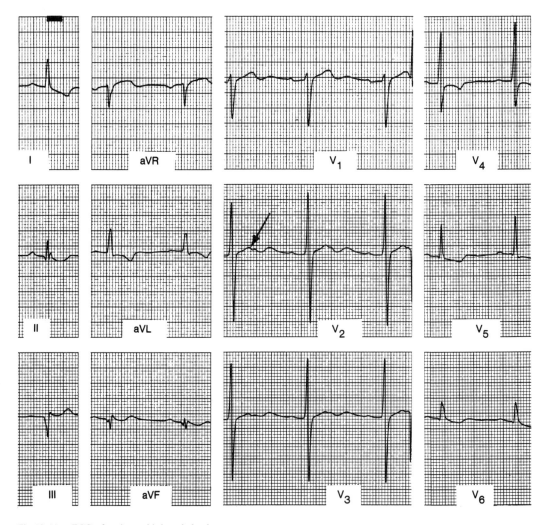

Fig 12-11.—ECG of patient with hypokalemia.

The S-T segment may be depressed and exhibit a trough-like appearance (Figure 12-12), and the T wave may also be inverted, as shown in Figures 12-11 and 12-12.

The relatively tall, upright wave following the QRS complex in Figure 12-13 is a U wave, not a T wave. The T wave is completely flat in most leads and slightly inverted in leads II, aVF, and V_6.

The QRS complex may widen slightly, in a nonspecific manner. This can be seen in several leads of Figure 12-11.

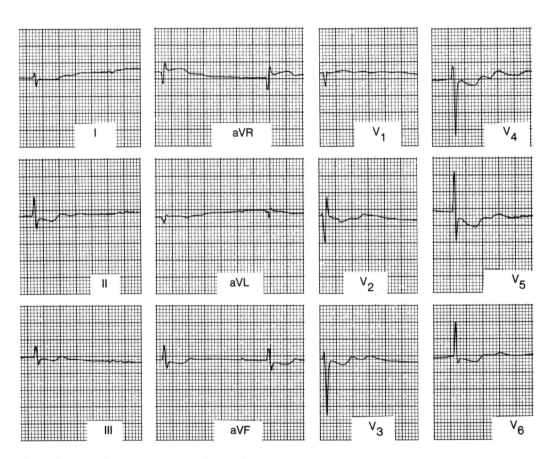

Fig 12-12.—ECG of patient with pronounced hypokalemia.

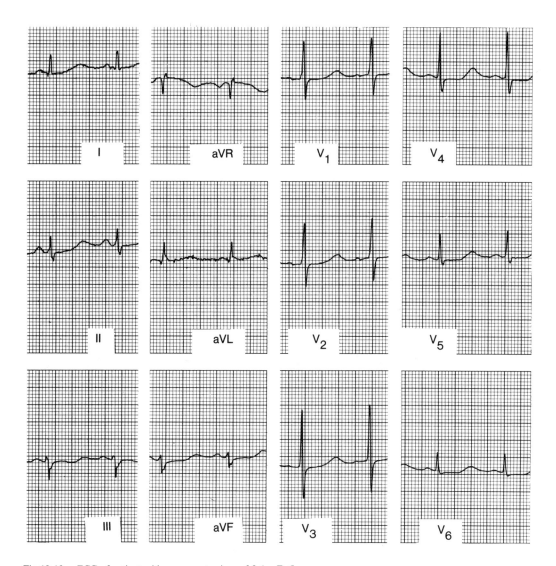

Fig 12-13.—ECG of patient with serum potassium of 2.1 mEq/L.

Hypokalemia frequently causes cardiac arrhythmias, such as 1° AV block, junctional rhythms (Fig 12-14), and supraventricular as well as ventricular arrhythmias. These occur in most individuals with serum potassium levels below 2.6 mEq/L, even in the absence of heart disease or digitalization.[3]

Hypokalemia is especially dangerous in the digitalized patient because it leads to the arrhythmias commonly associated with digitalis toxicity, in spite of normal serum levels of the drug.

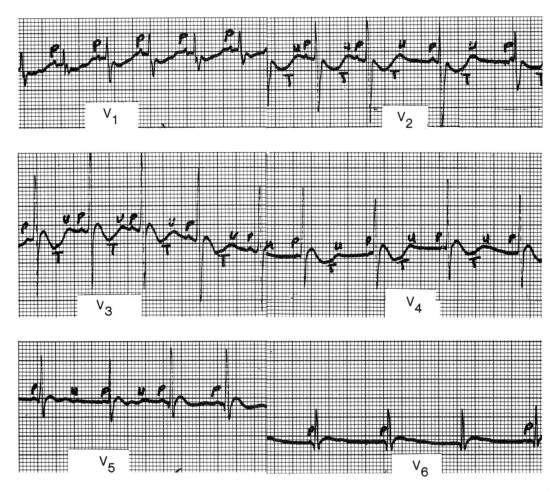

Fig 12-14.—ECG of 1-year-old child, showing sinus rhythm, junctional rhythm, and signs of hypokalemia. P = P wave, U = U wave, and T = T wave.

There are times when vigorous therapy can produce "overcorrection" of potassium imbalance. The ECG is an excellent means of observing the results of therapy and can be used to prevent dangerous overtreatment (Figures 12-15a through c).

The tracing in Figure 12-15a was obtained in a 31-year-old man with known renal failure and diabetes. At the time of emergency admission, the blood glucose level was 1,500 mg/100 ml and the serum potassium was 8.6 mEq/L. Treatment with insulin and peritoneal dialysis was begun immediately.

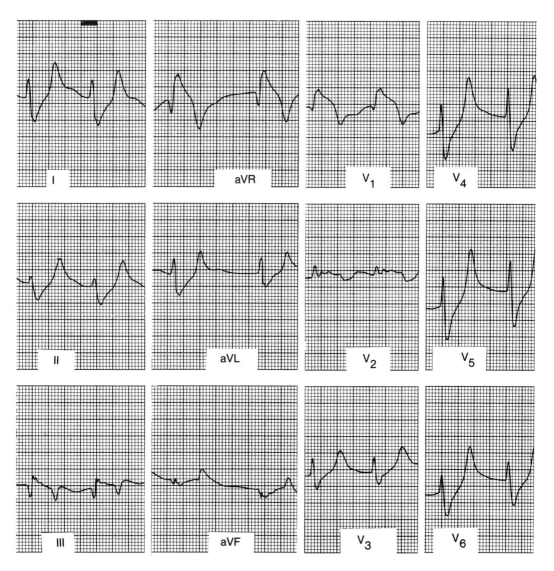

Fig 12-15a.—ECG showing severe hyperkalemia in patient with renal failure and diabetes.

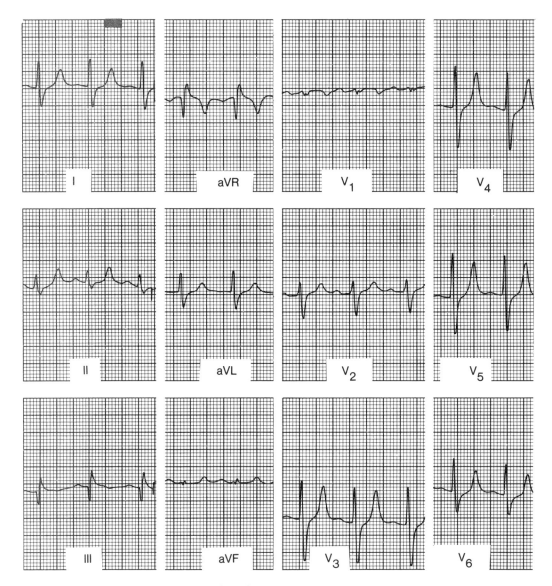

Fig 12-15b.—ECG of patient in Fig 12-15a, 4 hours later.

Although the ECG in Figure 12-15b still shows signs of hyperkalemia in the form of tented T waves, the condition is much improved, as reflected in the more normal QRS configuration and the reappearance of P waves.

An ECG obtained on the following morning, after continued treatment (Fig 12-15c), shows the beginning signs of hypokalemia: the T waves appear slightly flattened, and a U wave can be seen in several leads. The serum potassium level was 3.2 mEq/L at this time, and the composition of the dialysate was changed to prevent further extraction of potassium.

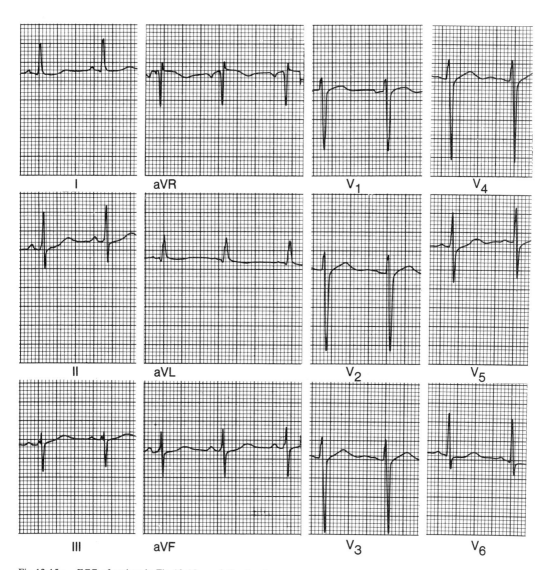

Fig 12-15c.—ECG of patient in Fig 12-15a on following day.

Abnormal Calcium Levels

Abnormal serum calcium levels are not seen as frequently as disturbances of potassium concentration, and they are not commonly found as isolated abnormalities.

Hypercalcemia

Hypercalcemia occurs in patients with hyperparathyroidism, malignancies involving bones, excessive intake of vitamin D, and a number of other conditions.[4]

The ECG characteristics of hypercalcemia consist of shortening of the Q-T interval and, in severe cases, upward rounding and widening of the T wave. Cardiac arrhythmias, as well as AV conduction disturbances, may occur, and shortening of the P-R interval and prolongation of QRS complexes have also been reported.[3]

The ECG manifestations of hypercalcemia are similar to those seen with administration of digitalis, and hypercalcemia may cause arrhythmias similar to those caused by digitalis toxicity. However, these changes are not necessarily diagnostic.

Dembin[5] and others recently reported finding no ECG changes in patients with significant hypercalcemia that was documented by laboratory studies. On the other hand, short Q-T intervals are seen not only after administration of digitalis but may also be observed in ECGs of healthy subjects who are receiving no medications. In my experience, the Q-T intervals in healthy young subjects are frequently shorter than those listed in commonly used tables (Fig 12-16).

Hypocalcemia

Hypocalcemia is seen in patients with several different conditions, including hypoparathyroidism, severe hypoperfusion, and massive burns.[6] Ionization of calcium is diminished in alkalosis, resulting in apparent hypocalcemia. Disturbances in calcium metabolism are frequently seen in combination with other electrolyte abnormalities, for example, with hyperkalemia in chronic renal failure.

The ECG characteristic of hypocalcemia is a flat, prolonged, S-T segment (Fig 12-17). Although the Q-T interval is prolonged, the T wave itself looks normal; the lengthening of the Q-T interval is due to the prolonged (0.18-second) S-T segment.

The P-R interval and QRS width may be shortened, and symmetrical inversion of the T wave has been seen. Hypocalcemia does not usually cause cardiac arrhythmias, but AV block has been reported.[3]

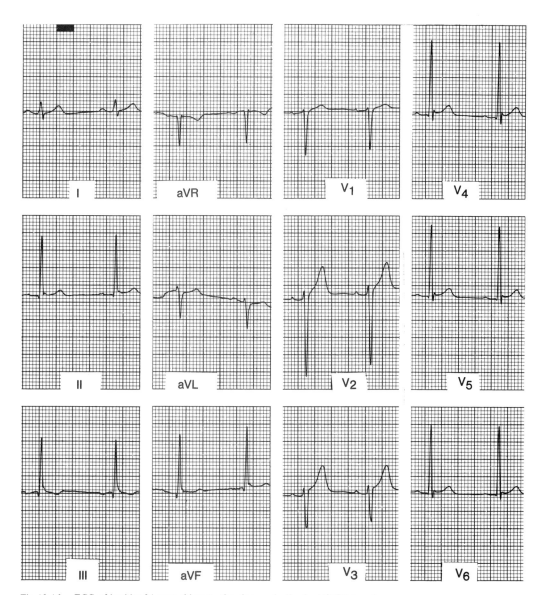

Fig 12-16.—ECG of healthy 24-year-old man, showing markedly short Q-T interval.

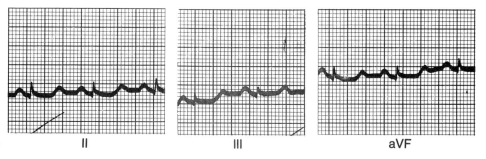

Fig 12-17.—Leads II, III, and aVF showing characteristic flattening and prolongation of S-T segment.

Abnormal Magnesium Levels

There is some question of whether abnormal magnesium levels cause specific, reproducible ECG findings.[7] This is probably due to the fact that changes in magnesium concentration are usually accompanied by other electrolyte abnormalities[8] that are reflected in the ECG. Since magnesium plays an important role in cardiac function, however, some of the changes described by various authors will be briefly discussed.

Hypermagnesemia

Increased serum magnesium concentrations may be found in patients with renal failure and in those who have had injections of magnesium sulfate.

The ECG characteristics have been described as: prolonged P-R interval, increased width of QRS complex, and elevation of the T wave.[6] Sinus blocks and AV blocks have reportedly been caused by this electrolyte abnormality.[9]

Hypomagnesemia

A deficiency in magnesium may be caused by severe malnutrition, chronic alcoholism, malabsorption, and several other conditions.[6]

The ECG characteristics include prominent U waves and diminished voltage of P waves and QRS complexes. Peaked, asymmetrical T waves, as well as flat or inverted T waves, have been reported.[8] Some of these findings may be attributable to accompanying abnormalities of serum potassium levels.

Hypomagnesemia may cause serious cardiac arrhythmias, especially in patients who are also digitalized or hypokalemic. For this reason it may be useful to check serum magnesium levels in patients whose arrhythmias fail to respond to conventional therapy.

Combined Abnormalities

Many diseases and conditions cause several electrolyte abnormalities to occur at the same time. The most frequently seen combination, hyperkalemia with hypocalcemia, is illustrated in Figure 12-18. Figure 12-19 shows the ECG of a patient with renal failure.

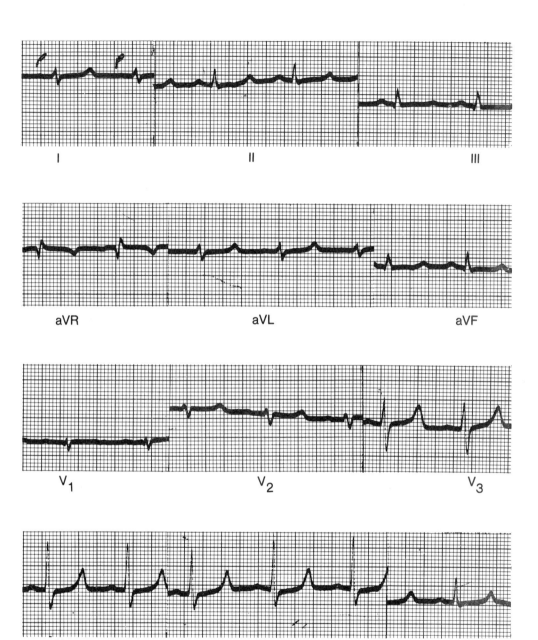

Fig 12-18.—ECG of patient with chronic renal failure, serum potassium level of 6.3 mEq/L, and serum calcium of 7.8 mg/100 ml.

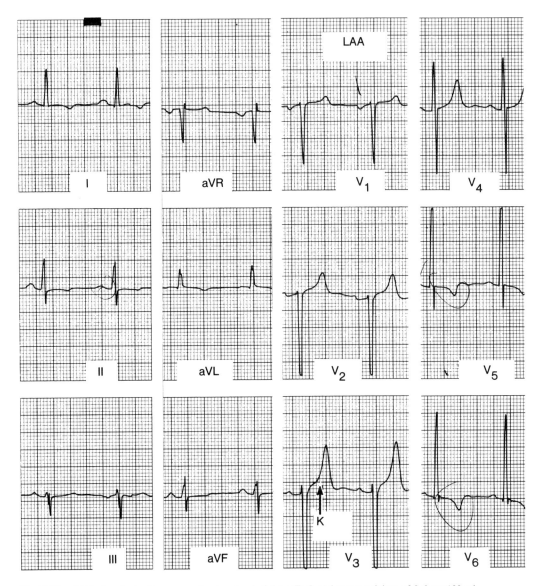

Fig 12-19.—ECG of patient with serum potassium level of 6.1 mEq/L and serum calcium of 8.6 mg/100 ml.

The cause of the hyperkalemia with hypocalcemia shown in Figure 12-20 is less common. The patient had a massive gastrointestinal hemorrhage and received 22 units of blood within a short period of time. When this ECG was taken, the serum calcium level had fallen to 6.5 mg/100 ml, and the potassium level was well above normal. This problem resulted from the administration of large amounts of stored, citrated blood. The case once again points out the importance of careful ECG monitoring in all critically ill patients.

A combination of hypokalemia and hypocalcemia is shown in Figure 12-21.

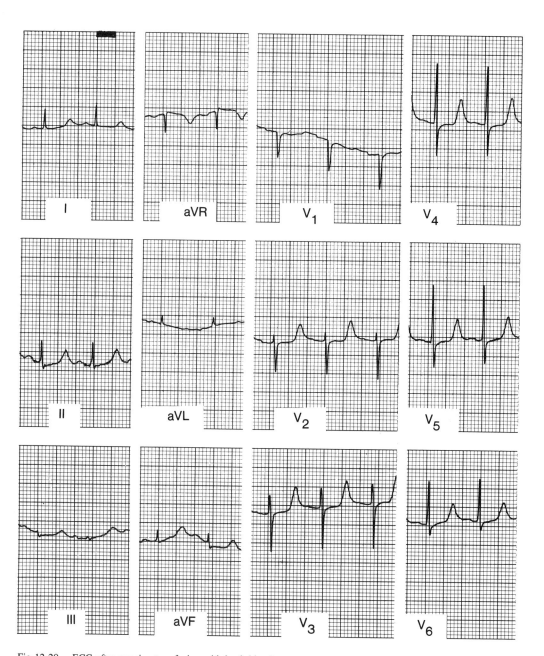

Fig 12-20.—ECG after massive transfusion with bank blood.

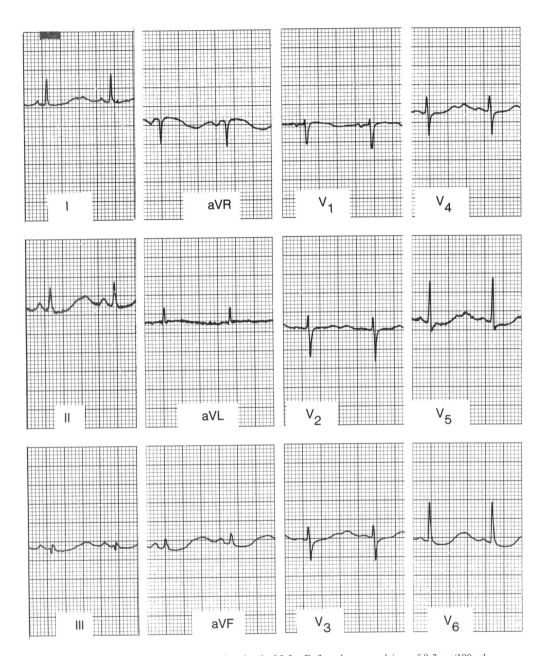

Fig 12-21.—ECG of patient with serum potassium level of 3.3 mEq/L and serum calcium of 8.3 mg/100 ml.

Acid-Base Disturbances

The ECG changes seen in acid-base imbalances are thought to be caused by changes in the concentration of potassium ions and, to a lesser extent, calcium ions.[3]

Alkalosis

In alkalosis, potassium ions enter the cells in exchange for hydrogen ions, creating a relative hypokalemia.

The ECG findings in patients with alkalosis are identical to those in patients with hypokalemia (Fig 12-22). An additional finding may be the "T-P phenomenon,"[3] a sinus tachycardia in which the P wave is superimposed on the delayed T wave.

Alkalosis may also cause a decrease in ionized calcium, as shown in Figure 12-23. This tracing illustrates the prolonged, flat S-T segment of hypocalcemia, especially in lead aVL. This patient also has fairly frequent PVCs, a common finding in alkalosis.

Acidosis

In acidosis, hydrogen ions enter the cells in exchange for potassium ions, producing a relative hyperkalemia. This can readily be seen in the patient with DKA as shown in Figures 12-24a and b. This tracing also shows slight S-T segment elevation in some of the precordial leads, especially lead V_3. The pattern, which is called "pseudomyocardial infarction," has recently been described in the literature.[10,11]

Great care must be taken in the correction of DKA, to avoid a sudden shift from hyperkalemia to hypokalemia. The latter condition can be caused during treatment because of two factors: correction of the acidosis allows potassium to move back into the cells, and the administration of glucose and insulin facilitates the transport of additional potassium into the cells. Careful attention to the ECG helps to prevent this problem and serves as a guide for the administration of supplementary potassium that is frequently required in this situation.

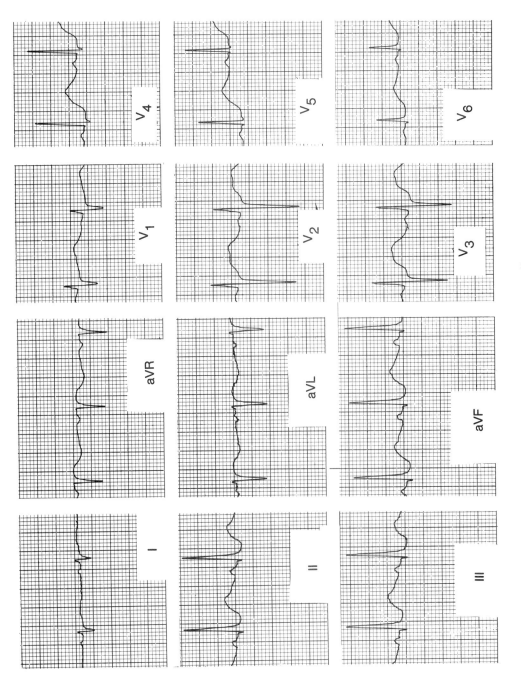

Fig 12-22.—ECG of patient in respiratory alkalosis, with $PaCO_2$ of 14 mm Hg and pH 7.67.

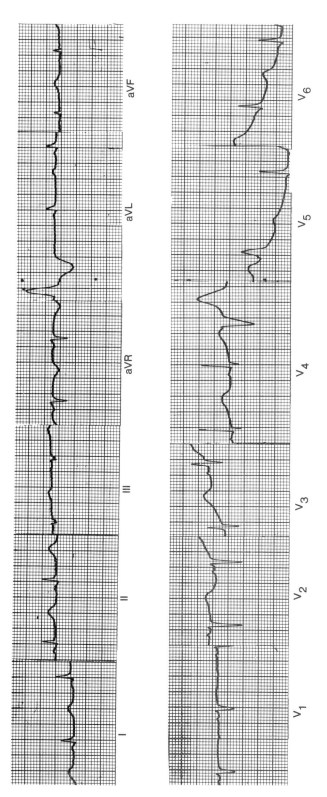

Fig 12-23.—ECG of patient in respiratory alkalosis, with pH 7.57, serum potassium level of 3.3 mEq/L, and serum calcium of 7 mg/100 ml.

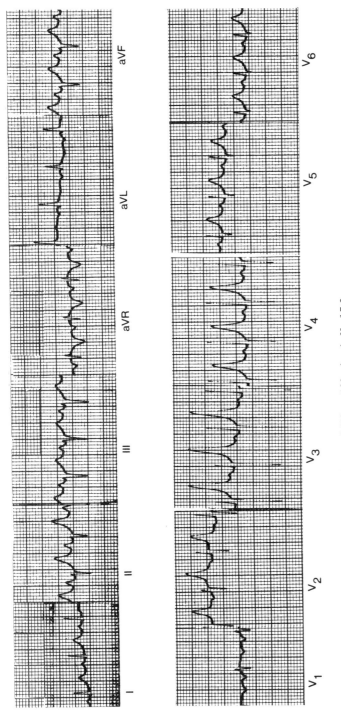

Fig 12-24a.—ECG of 20-year-old man with serum glucose of 600 mg/100 ml and pH of 7.2.

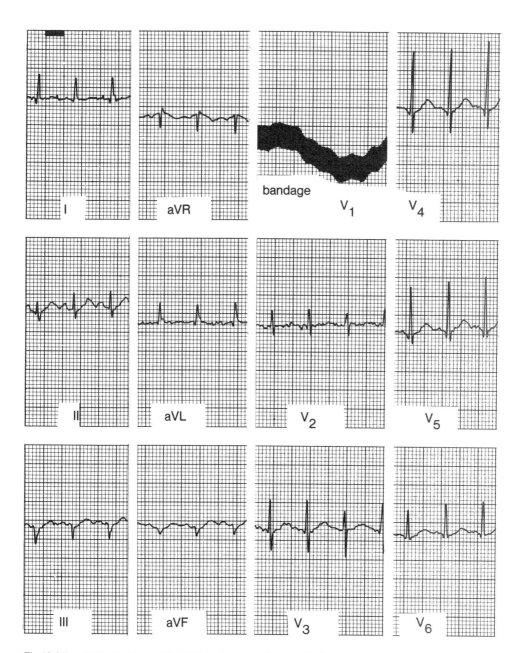

Fig 12-24b.—ECG of patient in Fig 12-24a, after correction of acidosis.

REFERENCES

1. Friedman, HH: *Diagnostic Electrocardiography and Vectorcardiography,* ed. 2. New York, McGraw-Hill Book Co, 1977, p 324.

2. Marriott HJL: *Workshop in Electrocardiography.* Tarpon Springs, Fla, Tampa Tracings, 1972, p 350.

3. Christy JH, Clements SD: Endocrine and metabolic disorders, in Hurst JW (ed): *The Heart,* ed 4. New York, McGraw-Hill Book Co, 1978, pp 1734-1753.

4. Zeluff GW, Suki WN, Jackson D: Hypercalcemia—etiology, manifestations, and management. *Heart Lung* 1980;9:146.

5. Dembin H: The rarity of Q-T interval shortening in significant hypercalcemia. *Crit Care Med* 1981;9:231.

6. Trunkey DD: Review of current concepts of fluid and electrolyte management. *Heart Lung* 1975;4:115.

7. Rothfeld EL: The itinerant S-T segment. *Heart Lung* 1977;6:857.

8. Burch GE, Giles TD: The importance of magnesium deficiency in cardiovascular disease. *Am Heart J* 1977;94:649.

9. Fish C: Electrolytes and the heart, in Hurst JW (ed): *The Heart,* ed 5. New York, McGraw-Hill Book Co, 1982, p 1609.

10. Burris AC, Chung EK: Pseudomyocardial infarction associated with acute bifascicular block due to hyperkalemia. *Cardiology* 1980;65:115.

11. Chawla KK, Cruz J, Kramer NE, et al: Electrocardiographic changes simulating acute myocardial infarction caused by hyperkalemia. Report of patient with normal coronary arteriograms. *Am Heart J* 1978;95:637.

## Chapter 13

Effect of Drugs on the Electrocardiogram

In discussing the effect of drugs on the ECG, it is necessary to define precisely what is meant by "effect." Some drugs produce characteristic changes in the configuration of ECG complexes, notably the S-T segment and the T wave, when they are administered in therapeutic doses. Others cause no changes in the appearance of the ECG, but their effect can be inferred from the disappearance of arrhythmias. Still other medications cause changes in metabolism that are seen as secondary effects on the ECG, and finally, a great variety of medications produce changes in the ECG when they are taken in toxic doses.

Unfortunately, too many physicians and nurses are not meeting their responsibility for patient education, so many patients are totally unaware of the name or purpose of the medications they are taking. This causes great problems when an emergency occurs and the patient's physician is not immediately available. In addition, inadequate instruction frequently leads to errors in taking medications, which may result in dangerous toxic effects.

Cardiac Drugs

Many of the medications used in the treatment of cardiovascular disease cause characteristic changes in the ECG when given in therapeutic doses. Their effectiveness can often be judged by the disappearance of arrhythmias and other untoward signs from the ECG. When toxicity occurs, distinct ECG abnormalities are produced that should be readily recognized by the nurse.

Digitalis

Digitalis, first described by Withering in 1785,[1] is still the most effective and widely used drug in the treatment of congestive heart failure.

ECG Changes

Therapeutic levels of digitalis can cause the S-T segment and the beginning portion of the T wave to sag in an upward concave configuration "as though you hooked your finger over it and pulled it down."[2] In leads in which the QRS is negative, the S-T segment may be slightly elevated and rounded upward. The *Q-T interval* is shortened.

The tracing in Figure 13-1 shows atrial fibrillation and the presence of LVH. In addition, the configuration of the S-T segment and the short Q-T interval strongly suggest a digitalis effect, that is, the ECG shows the characteristic changes normally seen in individuals who are taking digitalis.

The ECG in Figure 13-2 again shows the short Q-T interval and concave S-T segment depression characteristic of a digitalis effect. In this case, however, there is also a Wenckebach block, with brief periods of 2:1 conduction. This phenomenon, in a digitalized patient, should arouse suspicion of digitalis toxicity.

Digitalis Toxicity

Digitalis toxicity has been observed in as many as 35% of hospitalized patients who receive digitalis.[3]

Causes of digitalis toxicity

This "epidemic of digitalis toxicity," as Spann and Hurst[3] justly call it, appears to be due to a number of factors.

Excessive doses of digitalis are not usually the cause of the problem. When overdoses occur, they are generally accidental, as when the patient does not understand the instructions given.

Another circumstance that facilitates accidental overdose occurs when an out-of-town patient who has supraventricular tachyarrhythmias and congestive heart failure strongly denies having received digitalis previously. The patient is then digitalized in an effort to correct the problem. Two days later, when the physician is finally located, it is found that the patient had been taking digitalis and has now had a toxic dose. The urgent need for appropriate education is obvious if this type of problem is to be avoided.

The *increasing age* of the patient population poses a serious hazard, since pharmacokinetic and pharmacodynamic studies are usually performed on young, healthy subjects.[4,5] Doses that have been found to be safe and effective in these test subjects are generally too high for the patients in their 80s and 90s whom we tend to see in increasing numbers.

Hypokalemia is known to precipitate signs of digitalis toxicity, even in the presence of normal serum digitalis levels. The classic treatment of chronic as well as acute heart failure is a combination of digitalis and diuretics. Since the commonly used diuretics furosemide and thiazides cause a loss of potassium, there is always a danger of digitalis toxicity in these cases. Precautions used to prevent this problem include the administration of "balanced" diuretics and/or potassium supplements. However, many patients forget to take the potassium supplement and consequently have hypokalemia and digitalis toxicity.

Inadequate excretion of the drug is a frequent problem in the elderly, who tend to have reduced renal function[5] and are often dehydrated for a variety of reasons. This is a major concern in the management of patients with renal failure.

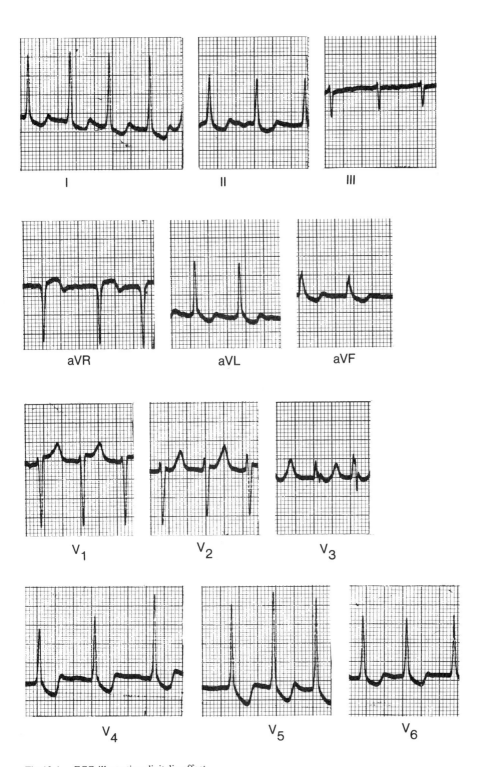

Fig 13-1.—ECG illustrating digitalis effect.

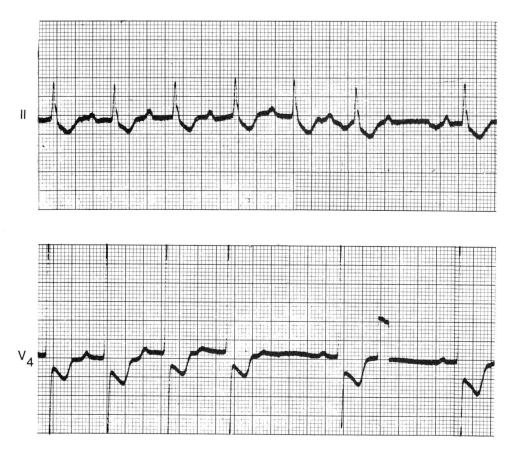

Fig 13-2.—Rhythm strip showing Mobitz I block and digitalis effect.

Recognition of digitalis toxicity

Because of the prevalence and potential lethal outcome of digitalis toxicity, nurses must be able to recognize the problem immediately. The time-honored practice of ''holding'' digitalis when the apical heart rate drops below 60 beats/min is simply not adequate. It does not even make much sense, considering that the immediately life-threatening arrhythmias caused by digitalis toxicity are frequently tachyarrhythmias.

Gastrointestinal symptoms of digitalis toxicity described by Withering[1] are not as likely to be the first signs of the problem today because of the refined products used and the frequency of intravenous (IV) administration.

Serum digitalis levels cannot be used as the sole guide to administration because there is variation in tolerance and need for the drug, as well as the various factors already described.

The ECG is generally the most reliable means of detecting signs of digitalis toxicity, which may produce almost any kind of arrhythmia, including atrial tachycardia with varying degrees of block, all types of AV block, junctional rhythms, and all forms of ventricular arrhythmias.

The tracing in Figure 13-3 shows a classic sign of digitalis toxicity: a completely regular ventricular rhythm in the presence of atrial fibrillation. This is only possible if there is complete AV block and if the focus for ventricular depolarization is in the junctional area or the ventricles. This ECG also illustrates a common cause of digitalis toxicity: hypokalemia.

Figure 13-4 shows another example of atrial fibrillation and complete AV block. In addition, the ECG shows ventricular bigeminy, a common result of digitalis toxicity.

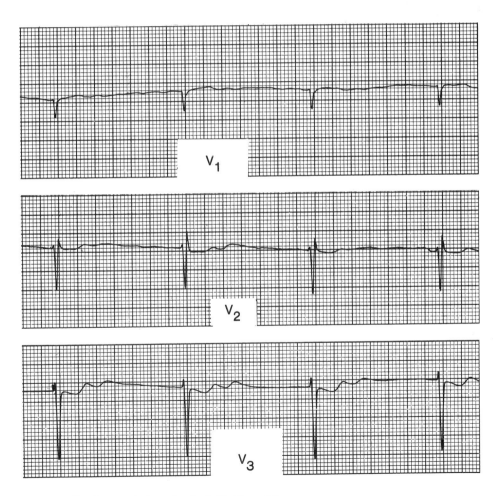

Fig 13-3.—Simultaneous rhythm strips: leads V_1, V_2, and V_3.

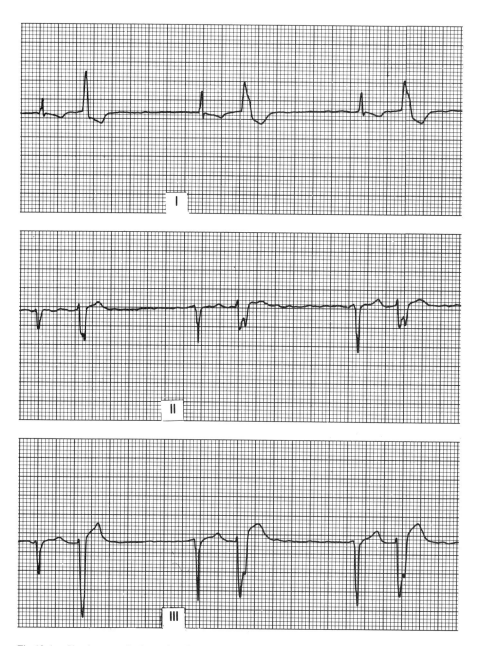

Fig 13-4.—Simultaneous rhythm strips: leads I, II, and III.

The tracings shown in Figures 13-5a through c illustrate a number of signs of digitalis toxicity. The first tracing was obtained on admission, when the 79-year-old man's serum digitalis level was 4.6 ng/ml. It shows an atrial tachycardia with an atrial rate of 170 beats/min, complete AV block with a ventricular rate of 36 beats/min, and ventricular bigeminy.

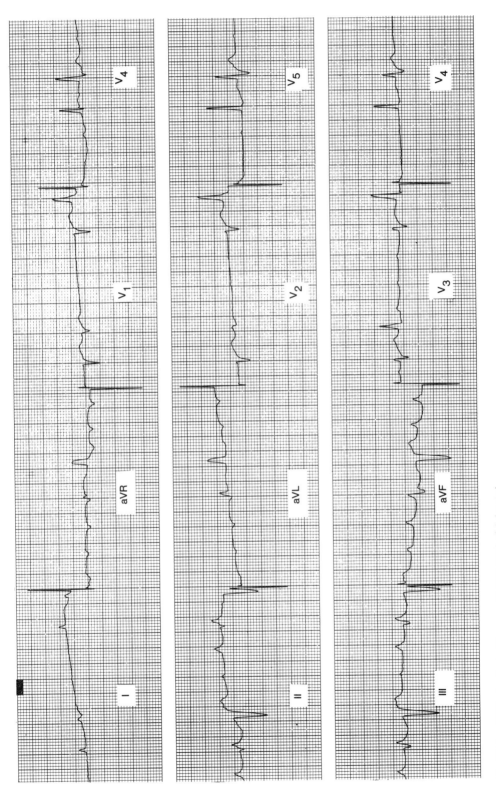

Fig 13-5a.—ECG of patient with serum digitalis level of 4.6 ng/ml.

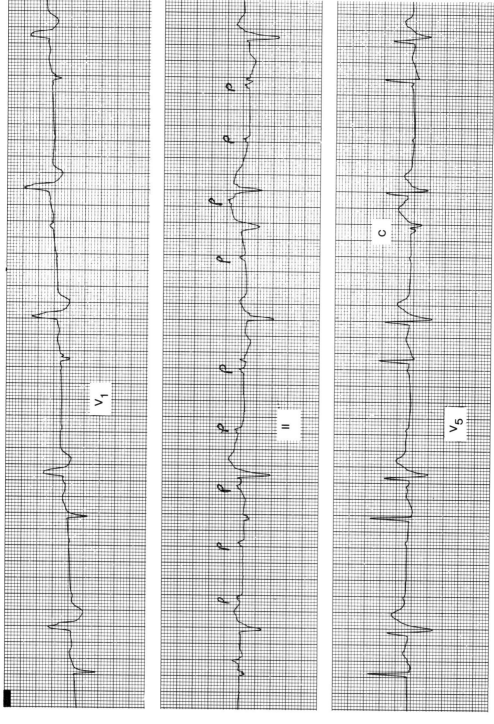

Fig 13-5b.—Simultaneous leads V$_1$, II, and V$_5$ of patient in Fig 13-5a on following day. C probably represents a beat conducted through atrioventricular node. P = P wave.

An ECG (Fig 13-5b), obtained on the following day, shows that the atrial rate slowed to 85 beats/min. There is again a high degree of AV block, with a junctional pacemaker at a rate of 31 beats/min, and ventricular bigeminy is still present. The QRS complex marked C appears to represent a beat conducted through the AV node, since it occurs somewhat earlier in the cycle.

An ECG (Fig 13-5c) taken two days after admission shows that there is still some delay in AV conduction, but an appropriate sinus rhythm has been restored. The short Q-T interval and configuration of the S-T segment clearly indicate the continued presence of a significant amount of digitalis in the bloodstream, even three days after the last dose was taken.

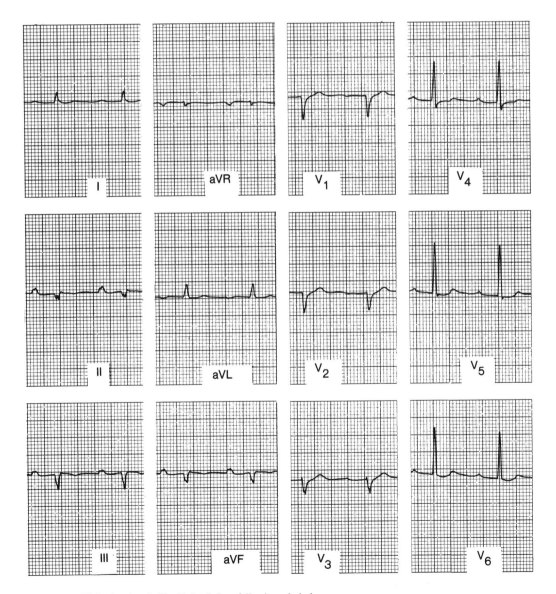

Fig 13-5c.—ECG of patient in Fig 13-5a, 2 days following admission.

The ECG in Figure 13-6 was obtained in a 75-year-old woman with renal failure, when her serum potassium was 8.6 mEq/L and her digitalis level was 5 ng/ml. It is interesting to speculate that the high serum potassium level may have prevented the arrhythmias that would be expected when the digitalis level is this high.

It is not possible to determine the rhythm, although the irregularity of the ventricular rhythm suggests the presence of underlying atrial fibrillation. The QRS complexes are very wide, probably the result of hyperkalemia, and the short Q-T interval reflects the presence of digitalis.

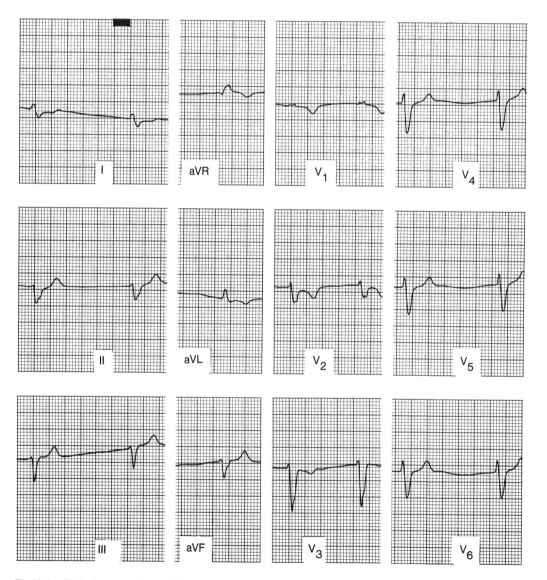

Fig 13-6.—ECG of patient with renal failure.

Antiarrhythmic Drugs

Class I

All class I antiarrhythmic drugs will hopefully produce an indirect effect on the ECG by abolishing arrhythmias. A number of them, namely procainamide (Pronestyl), quinidine, and disopyramide (Norpace), also cause characteristic ECG changes consisting of widening of the QRS complex and prolongation of the Q-T interval, when given in therapeutic doses.[6] In addition, procainamide and quinidine may also cause flattening and inversion of T waves and the appearance of prominent U waves.[7]

The patient whose ECG is shown in Figure 13-7 was treated with quinidine for frequent supraventricular and ventricular premature beats. The QRS complexes are widened to 0.10 second, and the Q-T interval is prolonged.

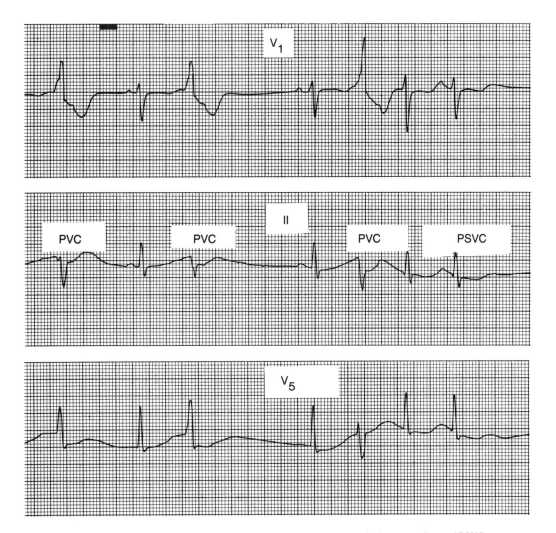

Fig 13-7.—Rhythm strip of patient treated with quinidine. PVC = premature ventricular contraction, and PSVC = premature supraventricular contraction.

The effects of procainamide (Fig 13-8) cannot be distinguished from those of quinidine. This tracing also shows a widening of the QRS complex and considerable prolongation of the Q-T interval.

Cardiotoxicity caused by procainamide and quinidine causes a delay in intraventricular conduction, expressed as a widening of the QRS complex. Therefore, as a general rule, therapy with either drug must be discontinued when the QRS complex widens by 25%. Frequent, careful measurements must be taken when procainamide is given IV, and when quinidine is administered in large oral doses.

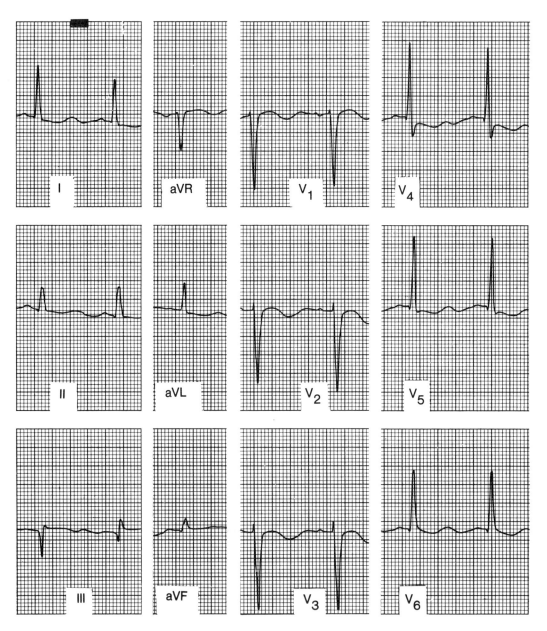

Fig 13-8.—ECG of patient treated with procainamide.

It has recently been suggested that administration of disopyramide be carefully monitored as well, since it, too, causes prolongation of the Q-T interval. This phenomenon increases the possibility that a PVC will be superimposed on the vulnerable portion of the T wave, with resultant ventricular tachycardia. The likelihood of such an event is greatly increased by concurrent administration of other class I antiarrhythmic agents.[8]

Lidocaine, one of the most frequently used class I antiarrhythmic agents, generally has no effect on the ECG other than abolishing ventricular arrhythmias.[6]

Diphenylhydantoin (Dilantin) either has no noticeable effect or may slightly decrease the P-R interval, QRS width, and/or Q-T interval.

Class II

In this country, the most commonly used class II antiarrhythmic drug is propranolol (Inderal), a β-blocker. In common with other β-blocking agents—metoprolol tartrate (Lopressor), and nadolol (Corgard)—it may increase the P-R interval, cause slight shortening of the Q-T interval, and produce slight, nonspecific changes in the T wave. All of these drugs cause slowing of the sinus rhythm; a mild sinus bradycardia is the expected effect, rather than a cause for discontinuation of the drug.

Class III

Bretylium tosylate (Bretylol), a class III antiarrhythmic agent, is not reported to cause any changes in the ECG, with the possible exception of prolongation of the P-R interval.[9]

Class IV

Verapamil (Calan, Isoptin), a class IV antiarrhythmic drug, has recently been released in the United States for use in the treatment of supraventricular tachyarrhythmias. Administration of this medication may cause prolongation of the Q-T interval. Toxic effects may include various degrees of AV block, bradycardia, or asystole. The drug should be used with caution in patients who are also receiving digitalis; concurrent administration of β-blockers and verapamil is contraindicated.[10,11]

Other Cardiac Drugs

Medications such as atropine or isoproterenol (Isuprel) that are used to increase the heart rate and/or to improve AV conduction produce no appreciable effect on the ECG, other than the desired response. This is illustrated in the rhythm strip in Figure 13-9.

Following the administration of atropine, there is a slight increase in the sinus rate and a reduction of the P-R interval to normal. This tracing also shows a slight decrease in the Q-T interval.

Isoproterenol increases ventricular automaticity and must be administered very carefully, especially in bolus form, to avoid serious ventricular arrhythmias (Fig 3-26b).

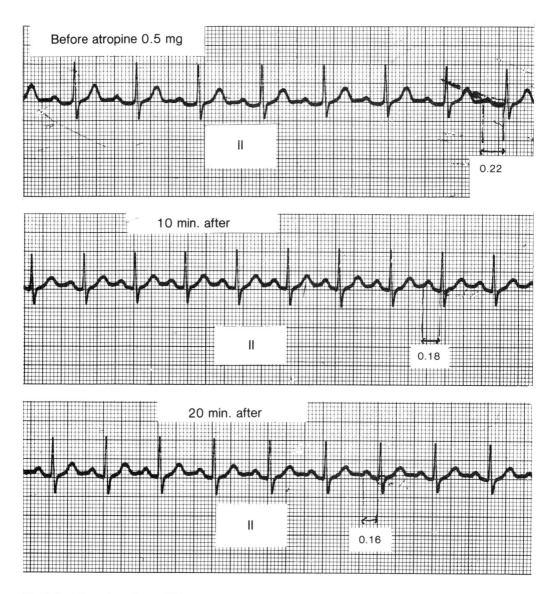

Fig 13-9.—Effect of atropine on ECG.

Antihypertensive Agents

Many of the antihypertensive agents contain a thiazide diuretic[12] and may, therefore, cause hypokalemia. Knowledge of the specific drug taken by the patient is essential to permit accurate evaluation of the ECG.

A number of these medications affect the heart rate. For example, bradycardia may be produced by guanethidine sulfate, methyldopa, *Rauwolfia serpentina,* and many other drugs, whereas tachycardia may be due to hydralazine HCl, nitroprusside, prazosin, and similar agents. In each instance the patient's medications must be known to permit evaluation of the arrhythmia.

Psychotherapeutic Agents

Many of the psychotherapeutic agents cause ECG changes when taken in therapeutic doses and result in serious, often lethal, arrhythmias when taken as an overdose.

The ECG in Figure 13-10 shows sinus tachycardia and "nonspecific" abnormalities of the S-T segments and T waves. The manufacturer of thioridazine HCl (Mellaril), one of the phenothiazines, lists the following ECG changes: prolongation of the Q-T interval, changes in the height of the T wave, and appearance of a bifid T or U wave.[13(p1575)]

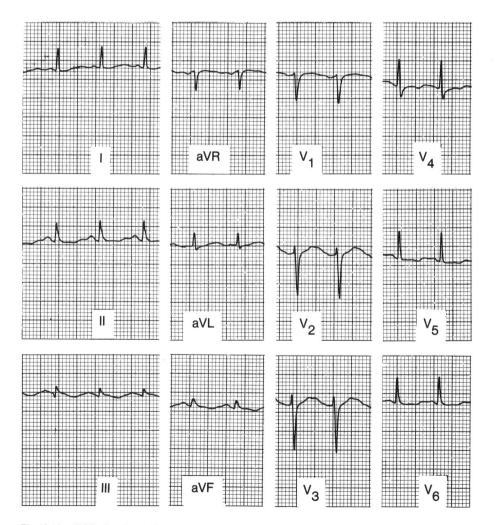

Fig 13-10.—ECG of patient taking therapeutic doses of thioridazine.

The ECG in Figure 13-11a was obtained in a 22-year-old woman who had taken an unspecified overdose of thioridazine. The tracing shows RBBB with LPH, an unusual finding in this age group, which may have been due to the tachycardia, since it disappeared on the following day, when the sinus rate had slowed (Fig 13-11b).

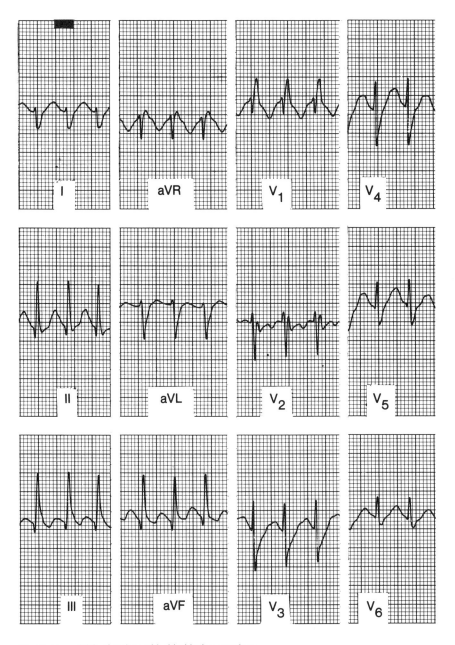

Fig 13-11a.—ECG of patient with thioridazine overdose.

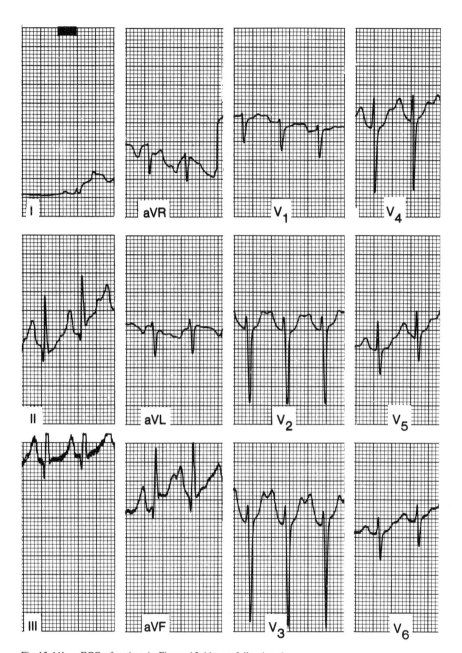

Fig 13-11b.—ECG of patient in Figure 13-11a on following day.

Tricyclic antidepressants (TCA) are known to cause ECG changes at therapeutic doses. These include lengthening of the P-R interval, QRS complex, and Q-T interval.[6]

Unfortunately, nurses see many patients who have ingested overdoses of these drugs. Cardiac arrhythmias ranging from sinus tachycardia to PVCs and standstill[14,15] have been reported as the result of overdoses. One study reports that the most reliable indicator of the seriousness of the problem is the width of the QRS complex.[14] It states that, in the absence of available plasma TCA levels, a QRS complex measuring 0.10 second or more is the best sign that the patient has taken an overdose.

A 52-year-old woman, who had ingested an unknown amount of TCA, was unconscious and required mechanical ventilation during the first 24 hours of hospitalization. The ECG (Fig 13-12) shows a nonspecific intraventricular conduction defect, with a QRS width of 0.11 second.

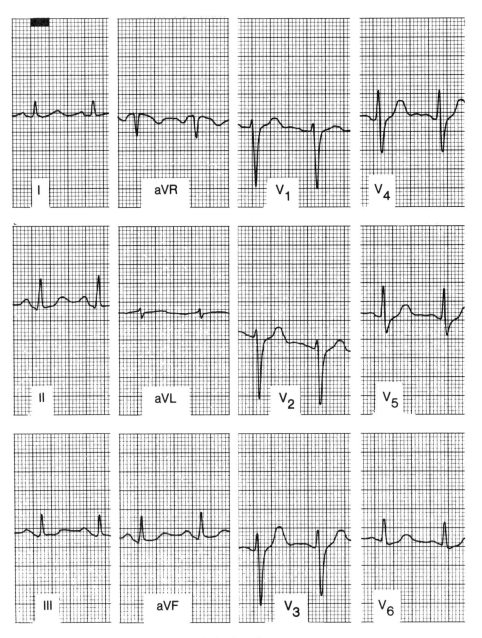

Fig 13-12.—ECG of patient with overdose of tricyclic antidepressant.

Social Drugs

Social "drugs" such as caffeine and nicotine are known to cause ectopic activity in sensitive individuals. Marijuana may cause supraventricular tachycardia, and amphetamines may cause severe arrhythmias as well as hypertension. It is often difficult to determine the cause of these arrhythmias when the patient is first examined, since there may be reluctance to admit the use of drugs.

Figures 13-13a and b illustrate a case in point. An alarming tracing (Fig 13-13a) was obtained in a 26-year-old man who came to the emergency department because of chest pain, palpitations, and shortness of breath. The ECG shows a supraventricular tachycardia at a rate of 220 beats/min. There is abnormal RAD, incomplete RBBB, and evidence of significant myocardial ischemia, especially in the left precordial leads. On questioning, he admitted the use of a large quantity of

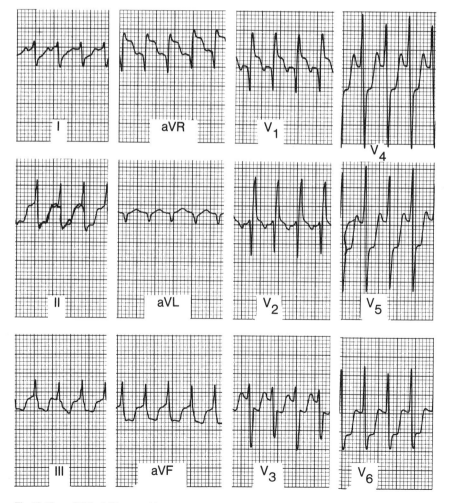

Fig 13-13a.—ECG of 26-year-old man.

cocaine during the preceding night. The arrhythmia was terminated by IV administration of edrophonium chloride (Tensilon), combined with carotid sinus pressure. A second bout of tachycardia occurred several hours later and was terminated by IV administration of verapamil.

An ECG obtained 24 hours later (Fig 13-13b) was within the broad normal limits for his age group. The electrical axis of $+90°$ is not unusual for a young person, and the incomplete RBBB may be a normal variant. Careful physical examination and diagnostic studies revealed no cardiac disease.

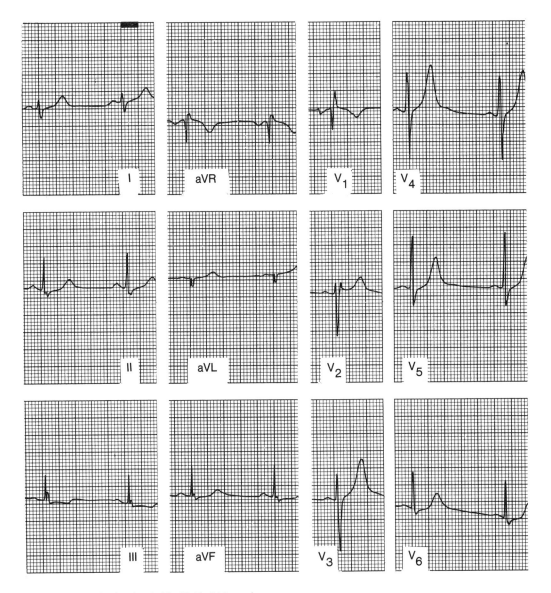

Fig 13-13b.—ECG of patient in Fig 13-13a 24 hours later.

Other Drugs

Numerous other drugs affect the ECG, and many of these changes will only become known as new drugs are used in the treatment of a large group of individuals and their results are reported.

Ritodrine HCl (Yutopar), a drug recently introduced in the practice of obstetrics, may serve as an example. Yutopar, which includes a β-sympathomimetic amine, is used to stop premature labor. It has been found that this medication may unmask previously unsuspected heart disease.[13(p1259)] For this reason, ECGs are normally obtained before and after start of therapy with this drug. Administration of ritodrine may cause the appearance of nonspecific changes in the S-T segments and T waves, as shown in Figure 13-14. Further trials and reports in the literature are needed to confirm this opinion.

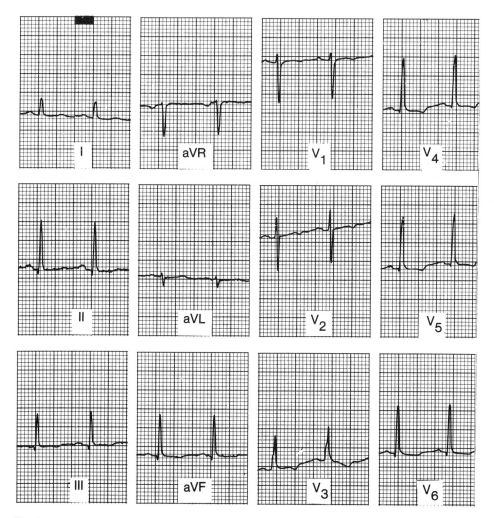

Fig 13-14.—ECG of healthy young woman, following administration of ritodrine HCl.

REFERENCES

1. Withering W: *An Account of the Foxglove, and Some of Its Medical Uses: With Practical Remarks on Dropsy and Other Diseases*. London, England, CGJ Robinson and J Robinson, 1785.

2. Marriott HJL: *Workshop in Electrocardiography*. Tarpon Springs, Fla, Tampa Tracings, 1972, p 351.

3. Spann JF, Hurst, JW: Treatment of heart failure, in Hurst JW (ed): *The Heart*. New York, McGraw-Hill Book Co, 1978, p 587.

4. Thompson WL: Dosage optimization in critical care: Use and abuse of drug analysis and computers, in *Critical Care*. Fullerton, Calif, Society of Critical Care Medicine, 1981, vol 2, p II(G):8.

5. Mullen EM, Granholm M: Drugs and the elderly patient. *J Gerontol Nurse* 1981;7:108.

6. Duke M: The effects of drugs on the electrocardiogram: A reference chart. *Heart Lung* 1981;10:698.

7. Friedman, HH: *Diagnostic Electrocardiography and Vectorcardiography,* ed 2. New York, McGraw-Hill Book Co, 1977, p 318.

8. Ellrodt G, Singh BN: Adverse effects of disopyramide (Norpace): Toxic interactions with other antiarrhythmic agents. *Heart Lung* 1980;9:469.

9. Lown B, Podrid PJ, De Silva RA, et al: Sudden cardiac death—management of the patient at risk. *Curr Probl Cardiol* 1980;4:1.

10. *The New Wave in Cardiology*. Searle Pharmaceuticals, 1981.

11. *Isoptin, Notes for the Physician*. Whippany, NJ, Knoll Pharmaceutical Co, 1981.

12. Gever LN (ed): *Nurse's Guide to Drugs*. Horsham, Pa, Nursing '80 Books, 1980, pp 192-209.

13. *Physicians' Desk Reference*. Oradell, NJ, Litton Industries, 1981, p 1575.

14. Briggs JT, Spiker DG, Petit JM, et al: Tricyclic antidepressant overdose. *JAMA* 1977;238:135.

15. Greenbaum DM: Secondary cardiac dysrhythmias. *Heart Lung* 1977;6:308.

## Chapter 14

Some Ill-Assorted Problems

In this last chapter, we will examine a variety of unusual problems. Some of these are normal, others are due to cardiac or systemic disorders, and a few are caused by human error.

Pediatric Electrocardiograms

The interpretation of abnormal ECGs of infants and children requires highly specialized study. The normal ECG[1(pp361-366),2-5] of the young child, and especially the infant, differs so radically from that of the adult that one could easily be misled into assuming the presence of disease in a normal, healthy baby.

ECG Criteria for Infants and Children

1. Heart rate
   - At birth, a sinus tachycardia rate of 125 to 165 beats/min is normal.
   - The rate slows gradually and reaches the normal adult rate by age 10.
   - Teenaged athletes may have sinus bradycardia at rest.
2. P wave
   - The duration of the P wave is < 0.07 s, and the height is < 2.5 mm.
   - The P wave axis is about +60° and changes little throughout life.
3. P-R interval
   - In the newborn, the P-R interval is 0.07 to 0.12 s.
   - By age 5, it is normally < 0.16 s.
4. QRS duration in the term infant is 0.04 to 0.06 s.
5. QRS axis

- In the newborn, the axis is generally about $+137°$, with a permissible range of $+75°$ to $+190°$.
- By the age of 6 months, the axis is usually $+70°$, with a permissible range of $+30°$ to $+135°$.
- At age 12, the axis is usually about $+60°$, with a permissible range of $-15°$ to $+110°$.

6. QRS voltage
   - QRS voltage may be low during the 1st day of life, but it is generally greater in young children than in adults.
   - The voltage criteria for LVH in infants and young children are: R wave in lead $V_5 > 50$ mm; R wave in $V_6 > 30$ mm; or R wave in leads III or aVF > 30 mm.

7. Q wave
   - A small Q wave is usually present in leads II, III, and V_6.
   - A Q wave in lead V_1 is usually a sign of severe RVH, especially if the Q wave is absent in lead V_6.[2]

8. R wave
   - There is often a monophasic R wave in leads V_{4R} and V_1 and the R/S ratio is > 1.
   - By the age of 3 months, the QRS complex tends to become equiphasic in lead V_1.
   - At 6 months of age, the R waves may be the same height in V_1 and V_6.
   - By the age of 5, the precordial leads tend to show the same type of R wave progression that is seen in the adult.

9. The T waves undergo rapid and remarkable changes after birth.

T Wave Changes after Birth

1. Initially, the T wave is upright in the limb leads and the precordial leads.
2. Within 1 to 6 hours after birth, the T wave becomes inverted in leads I, aVL, and V_6.
3. Within a period of 3 to 7 days after birth, the T waves become upright in these leads but inverted in lead V_1.
4. Persistence of a positive T wave in lead V_1 beyond 7 days after birth is a sign of an abnormality such as respiratory distress, corrected transposition of the great vessels, or RVH.
5. The T waves then become inverted successively across the precordium from right to left.
6. During childhood, the T waves generally become upright in reverse order (from left to right), and by age 10 they usually show an adult pattern.
7. Inverted T waves may persist in leads V_1 and V_2 into young adulthood and are referred to as a juvenile pattern.

In an adult the tracing in Figure 14-1a would represent severe RVH. Figure 14-1b shows how the QRS axis "normalizes" with age.

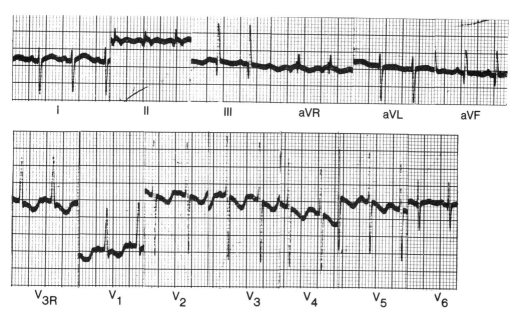

Fig 14-1a.—ECG of baby boy, 4 days old.

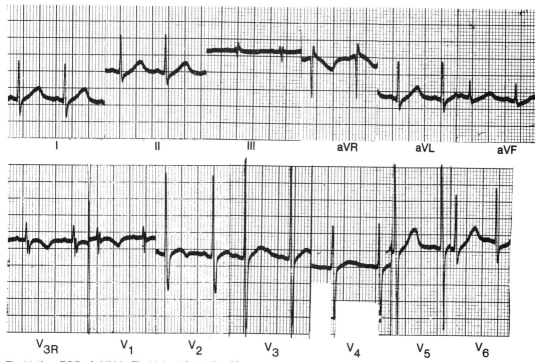

Fig 14-1b.—ECG of child in Fig 14-1a, 16 months old.

The main QRS axis is now $+40°$, and the R waves in leads V_{3R} and V_1 have become biphasic. The voltages in the midprecordial leads are much greater than would be appropriate in the adult, but there is much less muscle and fat between the heart and the recording electrode than there would be in the adult.

In the tracing of a 5-year-old child in Figure 14-2, the juvenile T wave inversion in the right precordial leads can be seen, but the R wave progression across the precordium resembles that of the adult.

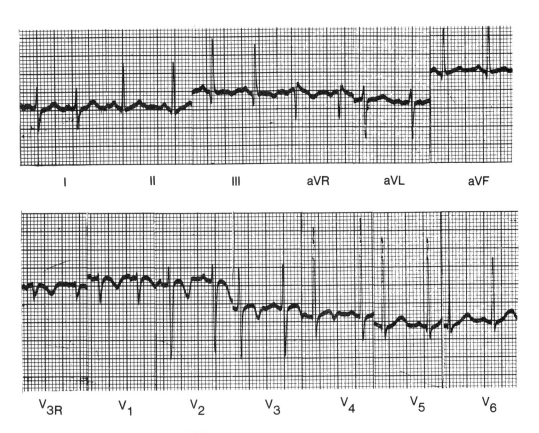

I   II   III   aVR   aVL   aVF

V_{3R} V_1 V_2 V_3 V_4 V_5 V_6

Fig 14-2.—ECG of healthy 5-year-old child.

Congenital Problems

The following tracings illustrate a few congenital abnormalities that may be encountered in adult patients.

Negative P Wave in Lead I

The normal P wave is upright in lead I, with three exceptions. The first is a junctional rhythm, in which there may be a negative P wave immediately before the QRS complex.

In Figure 14-3, the P-R interval is normal, so this is not a junctional rhythm. The tracing shows pronounced RAD in the frontal plane, but the precordial leads look fairly normal. The problem is that someone has reversed the arm electrodes. This phenomenon appears with amazing regularity, especially when ECGs are taken hurriedly.

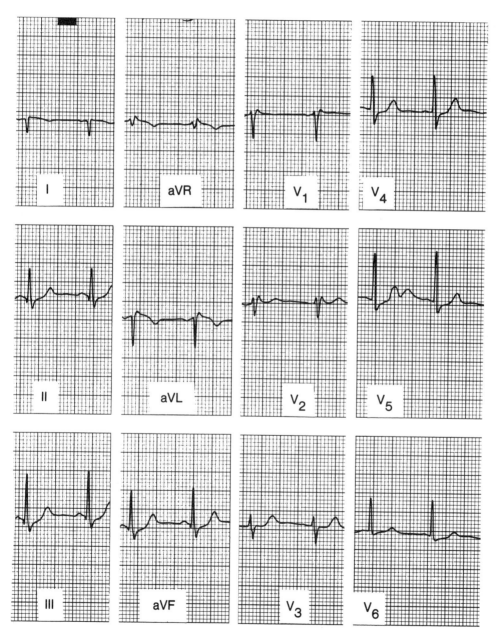

Fig 14-3.—Unknown tracing for identification.

The frontal plane leads look peculiar in Figure 14-4a, with an axis of +150°, but the complexes in the precordial leads grow smaller and smaller from the right toward the left of the tracing, and they remain negative.

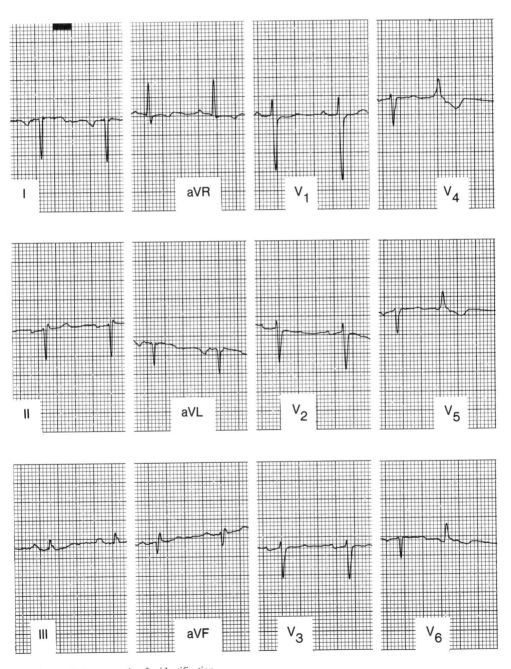

Fig 14-4a.—Unknown tracing for identification.

The tracing in Figure 14-4b is the mirror image of the one shown in Figure 14-4a and appears to be normal. This tracing was obtained by deliberately reversing the arm electrodes, and the precordial electrodes were placed, as marked, mainly across the right chest. This is a true case of dextrocardia with situs inversus. The subject is completely healthy, but all of his organs are on the "wrong" side.

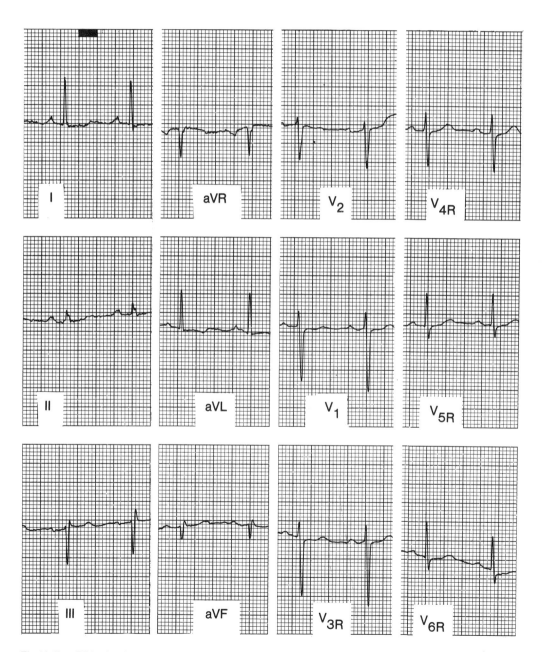

Fig 14-4b.—ECG of patient in Fig 14-4a.

Prolonged Q-T Interval

Some persons are born with a greatly prolonged Q-T interval (Fig 14-5a) and maintain this configuration through life. This is not a disease, but if the person should have PVCs, they are very likely to be superimposed on the vulnerable portion of the T wave and to precipitate ventricular arrhythmias. This is illustrated in Figure 14-5b, in which PVCs superimposed on the T wave produce coupling in two instances. These two short strips were obtained in a 21-year-old woman who came to our emergency department with ventricular tachycardia.

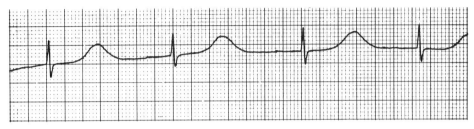

Fig 14-5a.—Rhythm strip of young woman with prolonged Q-T interval.

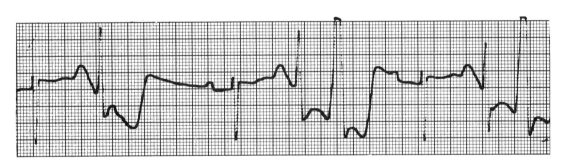

Fig 14-5b.—Rhythm strip of patient in Fig 14-5a with frequent PVCs.

A congenitally prolonged Q-T interval, found in persons who are also deaf-mute from birth, has been named Jervell and Lange-Nielsen syndrome. In those with normal hearing, it is called the Romano-Ward syndrome.[6] Both syndromes are characterized by ventricular dysrhythmias, syncope, and sudden death, often in childhood. The problem, although rare, must be looked for in children and young people with a history of arrhythmias or syncope, since a mortality of 73% has been reported in untreated persons with a history of syncope.[6] Treatment with β-blockers reduces mortality to a considerable extent.

S-T Segment Elevation

Elevation of S-T segments in one or more leads (Fig 14-6) is frequently seen in young, healthy athletes. It is usually found in males, and is common in blacks.[7]

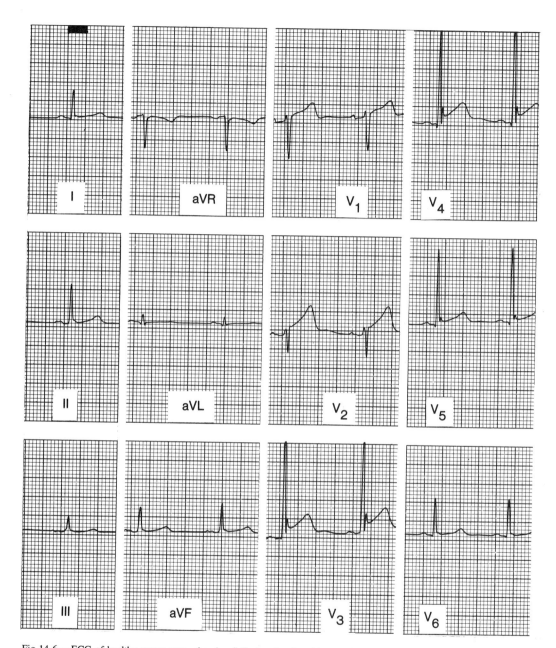

Fig 14-6.—ECG of healthy young man, showing S-T elevation in midprecordial leads.

This condition, often referred to as "early repolarization," is thought to be due to vagotonia and generally disappears when the heart rate is increased by exercise. The S-T elevation is most frequently observed in the left ventricular leads and is associated with normal QRS complexes and T waves.[8] This is not a disease, but it is occasionally mistaken for a sign of myocardial injury.

Myocarditis

The ECG signs of myocarditis may also be mistaken for evidence of CAD. They reflect myocardial injury, but the cause is inflammation of muscle, rather than the more common ischemic process.

Almost every known bacterial, viral, rickettsial, mycotic, and fungal disorder can attack the myocardium and start an inflammatory process.[9]

ECG characteristics [9,10]

- prolongation of P-R interval (rheumatic myocarditis)
- prolongation of Q-T interval
- S-T segment depression
- inversion of T waves (often widespread)
- voltages may be low

The tracing in Figure 14-7 shows widespread inversion of the T waves that could be easily interpreted as a sign of ischemia. This points out, once again, that the ECG is only one diagnostic tool. To arrive at the diagnosis, a detailed history and physical examination of the patient are essential.

Thyroid Disorders

Both hypothyroidism and hyperthyroidism have an effect on cardiac function and produce characteristic ECG findings.

Thyrotoxicosis

Thyrotoxicosis places a great strain on the heart, causing tachyarrhythmias and congestive heart failure.

ECG characteristics [10,11]

- tachycardia and supraventricular arrhythmias, mainly atrial fibrillation in adults
- prolongation of P-R interval and complete heart block reported
- prominent T waves and T wave inversion
- voltage criteria for LVH
- changes reflecting LVH usually disappear when thyroid disease is corrected

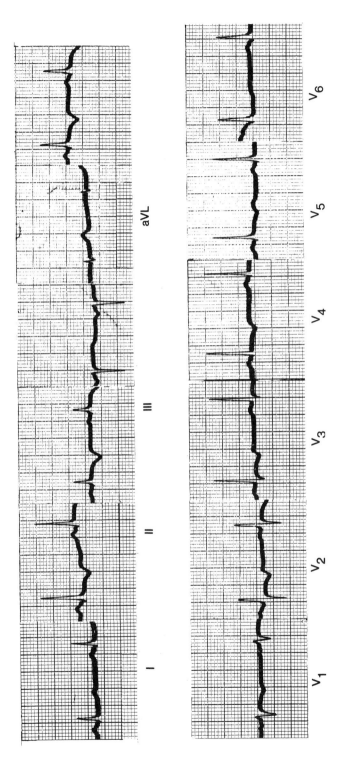

Fig 14-7.—ECG of patient with myocarditis.

The tracing in Figure 14-8 shows atrial fibrillation with a rapid ventricular response and S-T segment depression and T wave inversion, suggesting left ventricular "strain." The arrhythmia failed to respond to electric countershock, but the tracing returned to normal when the thyroid disorder was corrected.

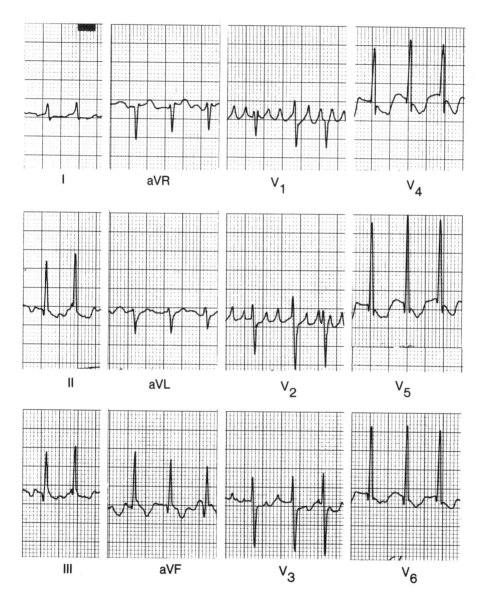

Fig 14-8.—ECG of patient with thyrotoxicosis.

Hypothyroidism

The most commonly seen changes in hypothyroidism are sinus bradycardia, low voltage, and nonspecific T wave changes.[11]

The rhythm strip of a patient with myxedema (Fig 14-9) shows atrial fibrillation with an exceedingly slow ventricular response, very low voltage, and inversion of the T waves.

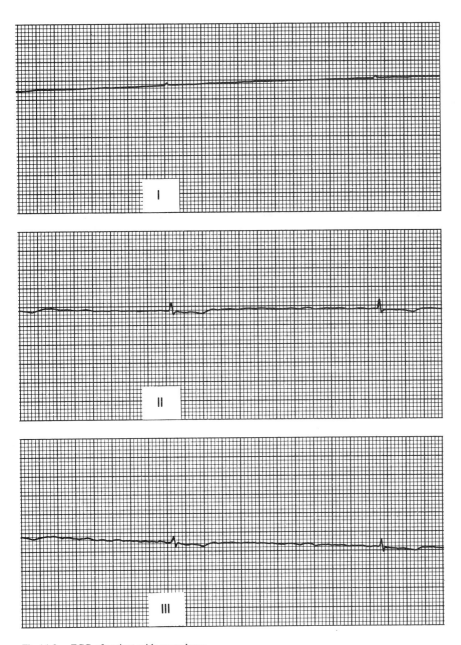

Fig 14-9.—ECG of patient with myxedema.

Intracranial Problems

Cerebrovascular accidents, neurosurgical procedures, and intracranial injuries may cause ECG changes. The mechanism producing these changes is not known.[1(p304)]

ECG characteristics of subarachnoid hemorrhage

- possibility of flat T waves
- T waves usually abnormally long and may be inverted, resembling those seen in myocardial ischemia
- large U waves and marked prolongation of the Q-T interval
- abnormal Q waves, occasionally
- abnormalities most frequently in left ventricular leads (I, aVL, and V_4 through V_6)
- sinus bradycardia may be present
- abnormalities tending to be reversible

The ECG in Figure 14-10 illustrates most of these abnormalities: sinus bradycardia, inversion of T waves, and prolongation of the Q-T interval.

In the tracing in Figure 14-11, the sinus mechanism is somewhat irregular, and not all of the P waves are conducted, so this rhythm represents a high degree of AV block. The most remarkable feature is the greatly prolonged T wave, which is especially noticeable in leads V_4 through V_6.

Brain Death

A recent study[12] describes ECG findings characteristically seen in brain death. This condition is defined as an irreversible state of unconsciousness, with complete cessation of cerebral activity. The ECG changes are not dependent on the patient's disease.

ECG characteristics

- a completely regular heart rate
- prolonged Q-T interval
- nonspecific S-T segment and T wave changes
- presence of an Osborn wave[12,13]

The Osborn wave consists of a deformation of the S-T segment close to the J point. This configuration has also been called a J wave, or hypothermic hump, and is well illustrated in Figures 14-12c and e.

The series of tracings in Figures 14-12a through e was obtained from an 80-year-old woman, who arrived in the emergency department as a "code" and died three days later without having regained consciousness. Her pulmonary and cardiac arrest were thought to be due to an intracranial event.

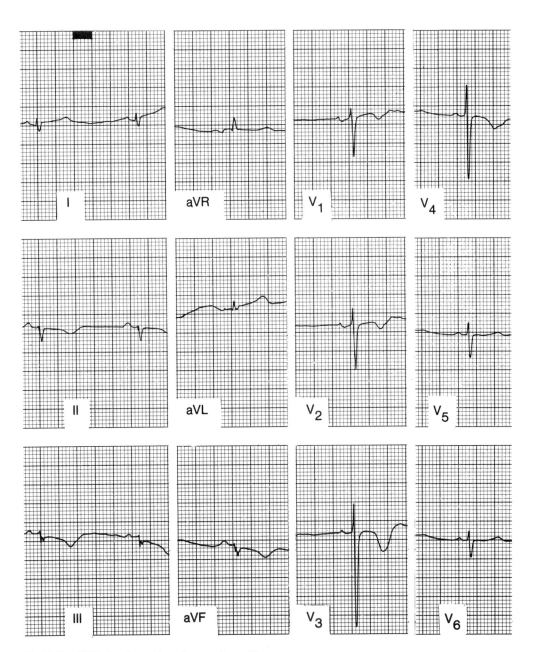

Fig 14-10.—ECG of patient with cerebrovascular accident.

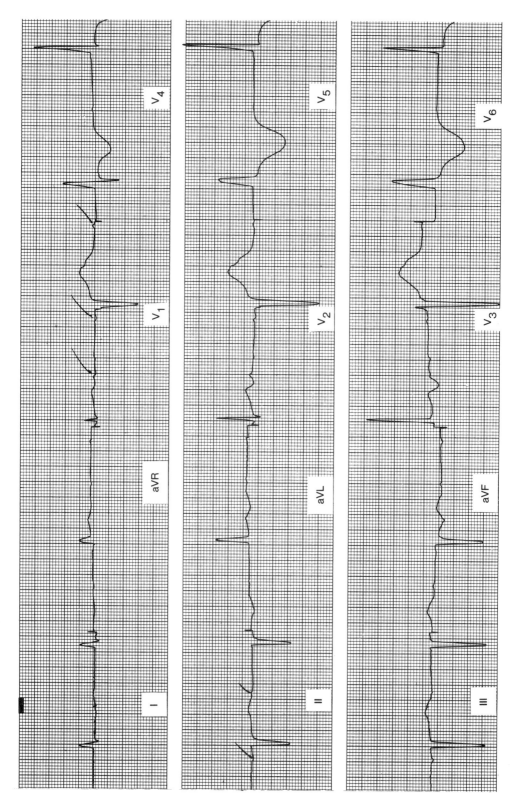

Fig 14-11.—ECG of 91-year-old woman with cerebrovascular accident.

The first tracing (Fig 14-12a) does not look especially abnormal, except that the Q-T interval is prolonged. The tracing taken several hours later (Fig 14-12b) shows sinus bradycardia, further prolongation of the Q-T interval, and inversion of the T waves in leads V_1 and V_2.

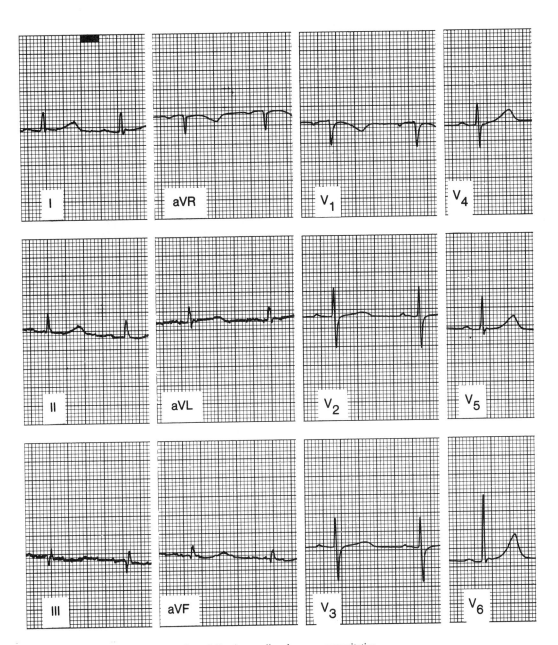

Fig 14-12a.—ECG of 80-year-old patient, following cardiopulmonary resuscitation.

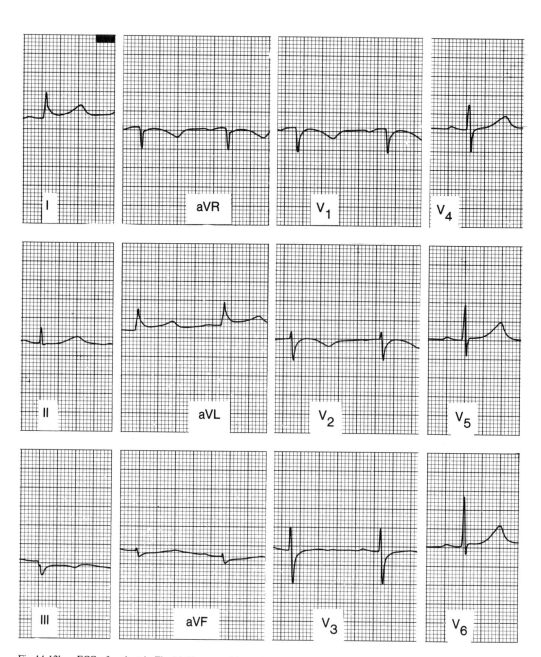

Fig 14-12b.—ECG of patient in Fig 14-12a several hours later.

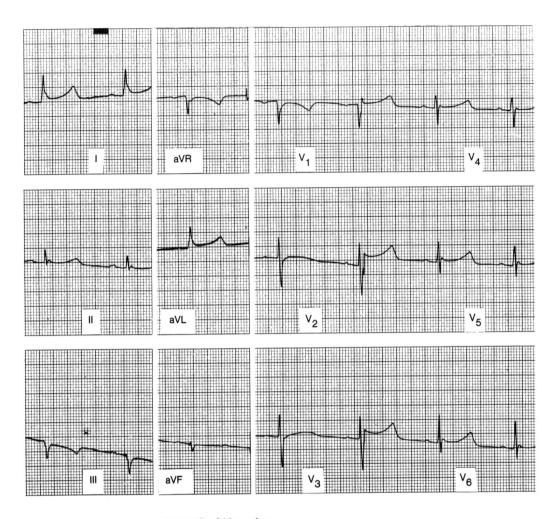

Fig 14-12c.—ECG of patient in Fig 14-12a, 24 hours later.

On the second day, there is sinus bradycardia with 1° AV block (Fig 14-12c). There is some S-T elevation, and the T waves are greatly prolonged.

The rhythm has changed to atrial fibrillation on the third day (Fig 14-12d). The most outstanding feature of this tracing is the appearance of Osborn waves. These are seen especially well in leads I, aVL, V_5, and V_6. Body temperature at this time had fallen to 30.6°C.

The final tracing (Fig 14-12e) shows a slow (37 beats/min) sinus mechanism, with Osborn waves and a greatly prolonged Q-T interval.

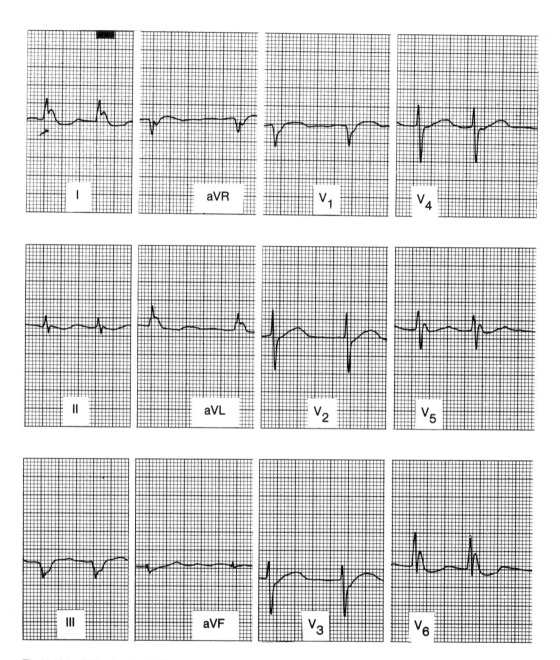

Fig 14-12d.—ECG of patient in Fig 14-12a on 3rd day.

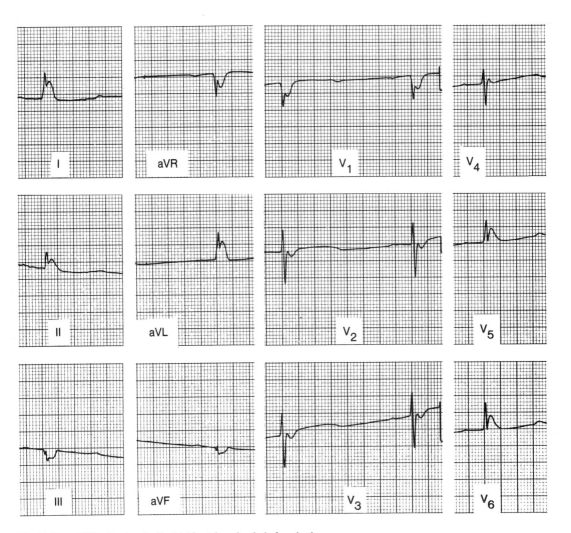

Fig 14-12e.—ECG of patient in Fig 14-12a, taken shortly before death.

Hypothermia

Not all patients whose ECGs show the characteristics described above have brain death. The same findings are seen in patients who have hypothermia;[13] the condition is readily reversible, as shown in Figures 14-13a and b.

The ECG in Figure 14-13a was taken on admission of a 21-year-old man with DKA. He had apparently lost consciousness, and had lain in an alley most of the night before he was discovered and brought to the hospital. The tracing shows sinus bradycardia and an Osborn wave. In several of the leads the J wave, or hypothermic hump, is taller than the R wave.

In the second tracing (Fig 14-13b), obtained following treatment of DKA and warming, the Osborn wave is still visible but has greatly decreased in size.

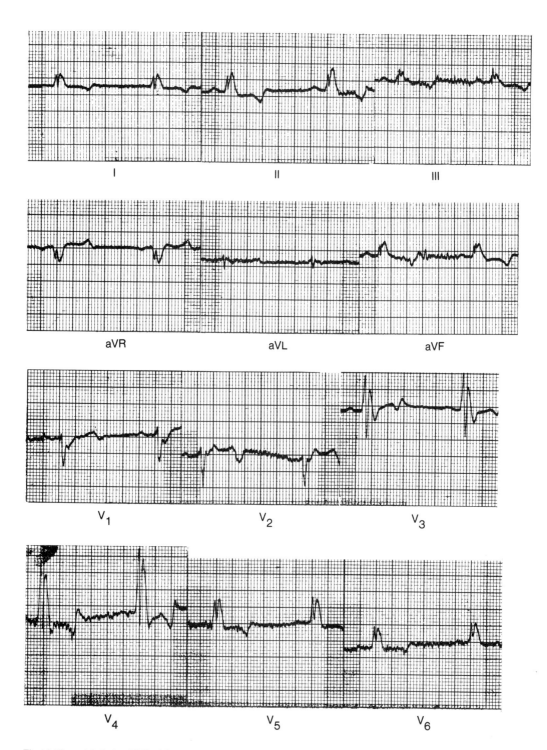

Fig 14-13a.—Admission ECG of 21-year-old man with diabetic ketoacidosis and hypothermia.

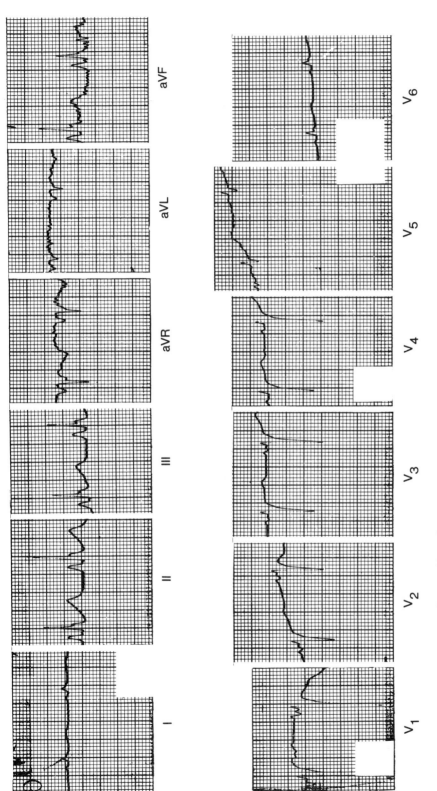

Fig 14-13b.—ECG of patient in Fig 14-13a several hours later.

A Final Word of Caution

The ECG in Figure 14-14 suggests a number of abnormalities. The R/S ratio is greater than 1, suggesting RVH. There is no R wave in lead V_2 or V_3, indicating the possibility of anteroseptal infarction. The patient appears to be a perfectly healthy young man. There is no disease present; someone has placed the precordial electrodes incorrectly.

This illustrates two essential points in electrocardiology.

1. Before interpreting an ECG, make sure it was taken correctly.
2. All ECG diagnoses must be made in light of the total clinical picture.

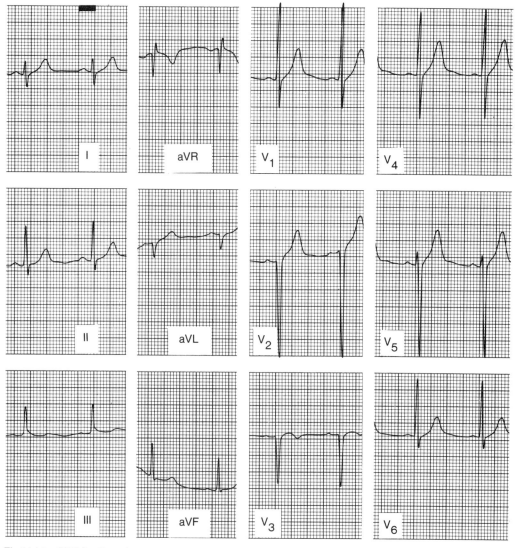

Fig 14-14.—ECG for discussion.

REFERENCES

1. Friedman HH: *Diagnostic Electrocardiography and Vectorcardiography,* ed 2. New York, McGraw-Hill Book Co, 1977.

2. Chandra N: *Handbook of Pediatric Electrocardiograms.* Medical Products Division, 3M Co, 1978.

3. Rowe RD, Mehrizi A: *The Neonate With Congenital Heart Disease.* New York, WB Saunders, 1968.

4. Engle MA: *Pediatric Cardiovascular Disease.* Philadelphia, FA Davis Co, 1981.

5. Nadas AS, Fyler DC: *Pediatric Cardiology,* ed 3. Philadelphia, WB Saunders, 1972, pp 36-76.

6. Denes P: Congenital and acquired syndrome of a long Q-T interval. *Chest* 1977;71:126.

7. St Mary E, Virgin H, Castillo C, et al: The "variant normal" electrocardiogram of the professional football player. *Phys Sports Med* 1978;6:85.

8. Schamroth L: *The Electrocardiology of Coronary Artery Disease.* Oxford, England, Blackwell Scientific Publications, 1975, p 30.

9. Wenger NK: Myocarditis, in Hurst JW (ed): *The Heart.* New York, McGraw-Hill Book Co, 1978, p 1529.

10. Goldman MJ: *Principles of Clinical Electrocardiography,* ed 7. Los Altos, Calif, Lange Medical Publications, 1970, p 282.

11. Christy JH, Clements SD: Endocrine and metabolic disorders; in Hurst JW (ed): *The Heart.* New York, McGraw-Hill Book Co, 1978, p 1735.

12. Drory Y, Quaknine G, Kosary IZ, et al: Electrocardiographic findings in brain death: description and presumed mechanism. *Chest* 1975;67:435.

13. Gilbert CA: Temperature and humidity, radiation, underwater environment, hyperbaric oxygen and the cardiovascular system; in Hurst JW (ed): *The Heart.* New York, McGraw-Hill Book Co, 1978, p 1830.

Bibliography

Antman E, et al: Nifedipine therapy for coronary artery spasm. *N Engl J Med* 1980;302:1269.

Aranda JM, Befeler B, Castellanos A, et al: His bundle recordings: Their contribution to the understanding of human electrophysiology. *Heart Lung* 1976;5:907.

Arcebal AG, Lemberg L: Angina pectoris in the absence of coronary artery disease. *Heart Lung* 1980;9:728.

Arcebal AG, Lemberg L: Acute myocardial infarction and left bundle branch block. *Heart Lung* 1981;10:532.

Arcebal AG, Lemberg L: Acute myocardial infarction and fascicular block. *Heart Lung* 1981;10:717.

Arcebal AG, Lemberg L: The diagnosis of myocardial infarction in patients with permanent pacemakers. *Heart Lung* 1981;10:1111.

Arcebal AG, Lemberg L: The diagnosis of myocardial infarction in patients with permanent pacemakers. Part II. *Heart Lung* 1982;11:99.

Aroesty JM, et al: Bradycardia-tachycardia syndrome. *Chest* 1974;66:257.

Ayers SM, Grace WJ: Inappropriate ventilation and hypoxemia as a cause of cardiac arrhythmias. *Am J Med* 1969;46:495.

Ayers SM, Mueller H: Hypoxemia, hypercapnea and cardiac arrhythmias; The importance of regional abnormalities of vascular distensibility. *Chest* 1973;63:981.

Bachman S, Sparrow D, Smith KL: Effect of aging on the electrocardiogram. *Am J Cardiol* 1981;48:513.

Bailey JC: The electrophysiologic basis for cardiac electrical activity: Normal and abnormal. *Heart Lung* 1981;10:455.

Barold SS, Falkott MD, Ong LS, et al: Interpretation of electrocardiograms produced by a new unipolar multiprogrammable ''committed'' AV sequential demand (DVI) pulse generator. *PACE* 1981;4:692.

Berman JL, Wynne J, Cohn PF: Multiple lead QRS changes with exercise testing, diagnostic value and hemodynamic implications. *Circulation* 1980;61:53.

Biggs FD, Lefrak SS, Kleiger RE, et al: Disturbances of rhythm in chronic lung disease. *Heart Lung* 1977;6:256.

Bognolo DA, Vigainagar R, Eckstein PF, et al: Two leads in one introducer technique for A-V sequential implantations. *PACE* 1982;5:217.

Boincey P, Zellinger A, Levine PA: *Pacesetter Puzzles*. Sylmar, Calif, Pacesetter Systems, Inc, 1981.

Boineau JP, Moore EN, Spear JF, et al: Basis of clinical ECG variation in right and left ventricular pre-excitation, in Dreifus LS, Watanabe Y (eds): *Cardiac Arrhythmias*. New York, Grune & Stratton, Inc, 1973, p 421.

Botvinick EH, et al: Thallium-201 myocardial perfusion scintigraphy for the clinical clarification of normal, abnormal, and equivocal electrocardiographic stress tests. *Am J Cardiol* 1978;41:43.

Braunwald E: Idiopathic hypertrophic subaortic stenosis, in Hurst JW (ed): *The Heart*. New York, McGraw-Hill Book Co, 1978, p 1560.

Braunwald E, Maroko PR: The reduction of infarct size—an idea whose time (for testing) has come. *Circulation* 1974;50:206.

Braunwald E, et al: *Cardiology Reference Book*. New York, Pfizer, Inc, 1980.

Briggs JT, Spiker DG, Petit JM, et al: Tricyclic antidepressant overdose. *JAMA* 1977;238:135.

Bruce RA, Irving JB: Special electrocardiographic examination of the heart, in Hurst JW (ed): *The Heart*. New York, McGraw-Hill Book Co, 1978, pp 336-348.

Burch GE, Giles TD: The importance of magnesium deficiency in cardiovascular disease. *Am Heart J* 1977;94:649.

Burris AC, Chung EK: Pseudomyocardial infarction associated with acute bifascicular block due to hyperkalemia. *Cardiology* 1980;65:115.

Cain RS, et al: Variant angina: A nursing approach. *Heart Lung* 1979;8:1122.

Calcium in Cardiac Metabolism. Whippany, NJ, Knoll Pharmaceutical Co, 1981.

Castellanos A, Agha AS, Castillo CA, et al: Ventricular activation in the presence of Wolff-Parkinson-White syndrome, in Dreifus LS, Watanabe Y (eds): *Cardiac Arrhythmias*. New York, Grune & Stratton, Inc, 1973.

Castellanos A, Myerburg RJ: The resting electrocardiogram, in Hurst JW (ed): *The Heart*. New York, McGraw-Hill Book Co, 1978, p 308.

Chandra N: *Handbook of Pediatric Electrocardiograms*. Medical Products Division, 3M Co, 1978.

Chawla KK, Cruz J, Kramer NE, et al: Electrocardiographic changes simulating acute myocardial infarction caused by hyperkalemia: Report of patient with normal coronary arteriograms. *Am Heart J* 1978;95:637.

Chernow B, Smith J, Rainey TG, et al: Hypomagnesemia: Implications for the critical care specialist. *Crit Care Med* 1982;10:193.

Chia BL: Alternating Wolff-Parkinson-White pattern. *Heart Lung* 1981;10:769.

Christy JH, Clements SD: Endocrine and metabolic disorders, in Hurst JW (ed): *The Heart*. New York, McGraw-Hill Book Co, 1978, pp 1734-1753.

Chung EK: Diagnosis and clinical significance of atrioventricular (AV) dissociation, in Sandoe E, et al (eds): *Cardiac Arrhythmias*. Södertälje, Sweden, AB Astra, 1970.

Chung EK: Reappraisal of parasystole. *Heart Lung* 1973;2:82.

Chung EK: Tachyarrhythmias related to the Wolff-Parkinson-White syndrome. *Heart Lung* 1977;6:262.

Chung EK: Sick sinus syndrome: Current views. *Mod Concepts Cardiovasc Dis* 1980;49:67.

Cohen FL, Fruehan CT, King RR: Carotid sinus syndrome. *J Neurosurg* 1976;45:78.

Cohn JN: Right ventricular infarction revisited. *Am J Cardiol* 1979;43:666.

Collins VJ: *Principles of Anesthesiology*. Philadelphia, Lea & Febiger, 1978.

Crawley IS, Morris DC, Silverman BD: Valvular heart disease, in Hurst JW (ed): *The Heart*. New York, McGraw-Hill Book Co, 1978, p 1015.

Curry PVL, Rowland E, Krikler DM: Dual-demand pacing for refractory atrioventricular re-entry tachycardia. *PACE* 1979;2:137.

Damato AN, Bonkle F: Definition of terms related to cardiac rhythm. *Am Heart J* 1978;95:796.

Damato AN, Caracta AR: Significance of His bundle electrocardiography, in Fowler N (ed): *Cardiac Diagnosis*, 1979.

DeJoseph RL: *Introduction to Electrocardiography: The Vectorial Approach*. Sandoz Pharmaceuticals, 1977.

Dembin H: The rarity of Q-T interval shortening in significant hypercalcemia. *Crit Care Med* 1981;9:231.

Denes P: Congenital and acquired syndrome of a long Q-T interval. *Chest* 1977;71:126.

Dexter L, Dalen JE: Pulmonary embolism and acute cor pulmonale, in Hurst JW (ed): *The Heart*. New York, McGraw-Hill Book Co, 1978, p 1478.

Dreifus LS, Watanabe Y: AV conduction block associated with Wolff-Parkinson-White syndrome, in Dreifus LS, Watanabe Y (eds): *Cardiac Arrhythmias*. New York, Grune & Stratton, Inc, 1973, p 467.

Drory Y, Quaknine G, Kosary IZ, et al: Electrocardiographic findings in brain death: Description and presumed mechanism. *Chest* 1975;67:435.

Duke M: The effects of drugs on the electrocardiogram: A reference chart. *Heart Lung* 1981;10:698.

Edwards WD, Tajik AJ, Seward JB: Standardized nomenclature and anatomic basis for regional tomographic analysis of the heart. *Mayo Clin Proc* 1981;56:479.

El Gamal M, Van Gelder B: Suppression of an external demand pacemaker by diaphragmatic myopotentials: A sign of electrode perforation? *PACE* 1979;2:191.

Ellrodt G, Singh BN: Adverse effects of disopyramide (Norpace): Toxic interactions with other antiarrhythmic agents. *Heart Lung* 1980;9:469.

Engel HJ, Lichtlein PR: Beneficial enhancement of coronary blood flow by nifedipine. *Am J Med* 1981;71:658.

Engle MA: *Pediatric Cardiovascular Disease*. Philadelphia, FA Davis Co, 1981.

Farshidi A, Josephson ME, Horowitz LN: Electrophysiologic characteristics of concealed bypass tracts: Clinical and electrocardiographic correlates. *Am J Cardiol* 1978;41:1052.

Favis JV, Morris SN: Detection, prevalence and significance of arrhythmias during exercise. *Heart Lung* 1981;10:644.

Fester A: Provocative testing for coronary arterial spasm with ergonovine malleate. *Am J Cardiol* 1980;46:338.

Fiol M, Ibañez J, DeLuna AR, et al: Significance of the prematurity index and sinus rate in warning arrhythmias of ventricular fibrillation. *Crit Care Med* 1981;9:229.

Fish C: Electrophysiologic basis of arrhythmias. *Heart Lung* 1974;3:51.

Fish C: Electrolytes and the heart, in Hurst JW (ed): *The Heart,* ed 5. New York, McGraw-Hill Book Co, 1982, p 1609.

Fitzmaurice JB, Sasahara AA: Current concepts of pulmonary embolism: Implications for nursing practice. *Heart Lung* 1974;3:209.

Fletcher RD: Complications of temporary transvenous cardiac pacing, in *A Clinical Update*. NSCI Cardiology and Radiology Division, 1981, p 20.

Freeman WR, Peter T, Mandel WJ: Verapamil therapy in variant angina pectoris refractory to nitrates. *Am Heart J* 1981;102:358.

Friedman HH: *Diagnostic Electrocardiography and Vectorcardiography,* ed 2. New York, McGraw-Hill Book Co, 1977.

Fuller CM, et al: Exercise-induced coronary arterial spasm: Angiographic demonstration, documentation of ischemia by myocardial scintigraphy and results of pharmacologic intervention. *Am J Cardiol* 1980;46:500.

Furman S: The present status of cardiac pacing. *Surg Gynecol Obstet* 1976;143:645.

Furman S: Recent developments in cardiac pacing. *Heart Lung* 1978;7:813.

Gallagher JJ, Gilbert M, Svenson RH, et al: The Wolff-Parkinson-White syndrome. *Circulation* 1975;51:767.

Gever LN (ed): *Nurse's Guide to Drugs*. Horsham, Pa, Nursing '80 Books, 1980, pp 192-209.

Goldman, MJ: *Principles of Clinical Electrocardiography,* ed 10. Los Altos, Calif, Lange Medical Publications, 1979.

Gozensky C, Thorne D: Rabbit ears: An aid in distinguishing ventricular ectopy from aberration. *Heart Lung* 1974;3:634.

Greenbaum DM: Secondary cardiac dysrhythmias. *Heart Lung* 1977;6:308.

Hamer HS, Lemberg L: Accelerated idioventricular rhythm masquerading as complete AV block. *Heart Lung* 1978;7:505.

Harrison DH (ed): *Cardiac Arrhythmias*. Boston, GK Hall, 1981.

Hartzler GO: Pathologic/electrophysiologic perspectives, in *A Clinical Update*. Billerica, NSCI Cardiology and Radiology Division, 1981.

Hecht HH, Kossman CE, Childers RW, et al: Atrioventricular and intraventricular conduction. *Am J Cardiol* 1973;31:232.

Heger J, Prystowsky EN, Zipes DP: New drugs for the treatment of ventricular arrhythmias. *Heart Lung* 1981;10:476.

Helfant RH: Coronary spasm. *Am J Cardiol* 1979;44:839.

Henriques HZ, Schamroth L: Sinus rhythm complicated by second-degree sino-atrial block. *Heart Lung* 1976;5:45.

Heupler FA: Provocative testing for coronary arterial spasm: Risk, method and rationale. *Am J Cardiol* 1980;46:335.

Hope RR, Scherlag BJ, Lazzara R: Excitation of the ischemic myocardium: Altered properties of conduction, refractoriness and excitability. *Am Heart J* 1980;99:753.

Hudson RB: The pathology of heart failure, in Hurst JW (ed): *The Heart*. New York, McGraw-Hill Book Co, 1978, p 536.

Hummelgard AB, Esrig BC: Calcium and calcium slow channel blockers: An overview. *Crit Care Quart* 1981;4:17.

Hurst JW, Logue RB, Rackley CE, et al: *The Heart,* ed 5. New York, McGraw-Hill Book Co, 1982.

Isoptin, Notes for the Physician, Whippany, NJ, Knoll Pharmaceutical Co, 1981.

James TN: Morphology of the human antrioventricular node, with remarks pertinent to its electrophysiology. *Am Heart J* 1961;62:756.

Kannel WB: Incidence, prevalence and mortality of cardiovascular disease, in Hurst JW (ed): *The Heart,* ed 5. New York, McGraw-Hill Book Co, 1982, p 627.

Kaplan BM: Tachycardia-bradycardia syndrome (so-called sick sinus syndrome). *Am J Cardiol* 1973;31:497.

Keith JD, Rowe RD, Vlad P: *Heart Disease in Infancy and Childhood*. New York, Macmillan Co, 1958.

Kennedy GT: Variant angina: Clinical spectrum, pathophysiology, and management. *Heart Lung* 1981;10:1073.

Kennedy HL, Underhill SJ: Electrocardiographic recognition of ventricular ectopic beats in lead V_1—a preliminary report. *Heart Lung* 1975;4:921.

Kent AFS: Researches on the structure and function of the mammalian heart. *J Physiol* 1893;14:233.

Khan MM, Logan KR, McComb JM, et al: Management of recurrent ventricular tachyarrhythmias associated with Q-T prolongation. *Am J Cardiol* 1981;47:1301.

Killip T, et al: *National Heart, Lung, and Blood Institute Coronary Artery Surgery Study*. Dallas, American Heart Association, 1981.

Kinney MR, Dear CB, Packa DR, et al. *AACN's Clinical Reference for Critical-Care Nursing*. New York, McGraw-Hill Book Co, 1981.

Lemberg L, Vinsant M: *Pacer Electrode Location*. Read before the National Teaching Institute, American Association of Critical Care Nurses, New Orleans, 1974.

Leppo J, et al: Thallium-201 myocardial scintigraphy in patients with triple-vessel disease and ischemic exercise stress tests. *Circulation* 1979;59:715.

Levine PA: *Pacemaker Puzzles*. Sylmar, Calif, Pacesetter Systems, Inc, 1978.

Levy S, et al: Long-term results of permanent atrioventricular sequential demand pacing. *PACE* 1979;2:175.

Lewis BS, Schamroth L: The hyperacute phase of true posterior infarction. *Heart Lung* 1977;6:331.

Lown B, De Silva RA: Roles of psychological stress and autonomic nervous system changes in provocation of ventricular premature complexes. *Am J Cardiol* 1978;41:979.

Lown B, Ganong WF, Levin SA: The syndrome of short P-R interval, normal QRS complex and paroxysmal rapid heart action. *Circulation* 1952;5:693.

Lown B, et al: Symposium on nifedipine and calcium flux inhibition in the treatment of coronary arterial spasm and myocardial ischemia. *Am J Cardiol* 1979;44:780.

Lown B, Podrid PJ, De Silva RA, et al: Sudden cardiac death—management of the patient at risk. *Curr Probl Cardiol* 1980;4:1.

Lyon AF: The hemiblocks and peri-infarction blocks. *ECG Self-Reviews,* No 4, Maxon Davis, Inc, 1980.

Lyon AF: Right ventricular hypertrophy. *ECG Self-Reviews,* No. 6. Maxon Davis, Inc, 1980.

Lyons CJ, Han G: Premature ventricular contractions: Which ones require treatment? *Heart Lung* 1981;10:691.

Mahaim A: Kent fibers and the paraspecific conduction through the upper connection of the bundle of His—Tawara. *Am Heart J* 1947;33:651.

Marriott HJL: *Workshop in Electrocardiography.* Tarpon Springs, Fla, Tampa Tracings, 1972.

Marriott HJL: Arrhythmias in coronary care: A renewed plea. *Heart Lung* 1982;11:33.

Marriott HJL. Fogg E: Constant monitoring for cardiac dysrhythmias and blocks. *Mod Concepts Cardiovasc Dis* 1979;6:103.

Marriott HJL, Myerburg RJ: Recognition and treatment of cardiac arrhythmias and conduction disturbances, in Hurst JW (ed): *The Heart.* New York, McGraw-Hill Book Co, 1978.

Marriott HJL, Sandler IA: Criteria old and new for differentiating between ectopic ventricular beats and aberrant ventricular conduction in the presence of atrial fibrillation. *Prog Cardiovasc Dis* 1966;9:18.

Martell RW, Schamroth L: A study of ventricular conduction vs ventricular ectopy. *Heart Lung* 1981;10:886.

Masters AM, et al: Coronary artery disease and the "two-step exercise test." *NY State J Med* 1957;57:1051.

McCarthy E: Hemodynamic effects and clinical assessment of dysrhythmias. *Crit Care Quart* 1981;4:9.

McKibbin J, Schamroth L: Phasic aberrant ventricular conduction manifesting as right bundle branch block with left anterior hemiblock. *Heart Lung* 1975;4:441.

Messineo FC, Al-Hani AJ, Katz AM: The relationship between frequent and complex ventricular ectopy during 24-hour ambulatory electrocardiographic monitoring. *Cardiology* 1981;68:91.

Millar S, et al: *Methods in Critical Care.* Philadelphia, WB Saunders, 1980.

Mitchell RS, et al: The right ventricle in chronic airway obstruction. *Am Rev Respir Dis* 1976;114:147.

Monroe MT, Chung EK: Pacemaker bigemini: pseudomalfunction. *Heart Lung* 1975;4:927.

Moss AJ, Rivers RJ: Termination and inhibition of recurrent tachycardias by implanted pervenous pacemaker. *Circulation* 1975;50:942.

Mullen EM, Granholm M: Drugs and the elderly patient. *J Gerontol Nurse* 1981;7:108.

Nadas AS, Fyler DC: *Pediatric Cardiology,* ed 3. Philadelphia, WB Saunders, 1972.

Narula OS: *Cardiac Arrhythmias: Electrophysiology, Diagnosis and Management.* Baltimore, Williams and Wilkins, 1979.

Page H: NIH study finds nitroglycerine beneficial in acute infarction. *Hospital Tribune,* April 1975, p 21.

Pantaleo N, Rozanski A, Maddahi J, et al: Diagnostic application of thallium-201 myocardial scintigraphy in patients with coronary artery disease. *Crit Care Quart* 1981;4:43.

Papa LA, Saia JA, Chung EK: Ventricular fibrillation in Wolff-Parkinson-White syndrome, type A. *Heart Lung* 1978;7:1015.

Parsonnett V: Routine implantation of permanent pacemaker electrodes in both chambers: A technique whose time has come. *PACE* 1981;4:109.

Parsonnett V: Temporary transvenous cardiac pacing, in *A Clinical Update.* Billerica: NSCI Cardiology and Radiology Division, 1981.

Parsonnett V, Furman S, Smyth NPD: A revised code for pacemaker identification. *PACE* 1981;4:400.

Parsonnett V, Manhardt M: Permanent pacing of the heart: 1952-1976. *Am J Cardiol* 1977;39:250.

Pelletier JB, Marriott HJL: Atrioventricular block: Incidence in acute myocardial infarction and determinants of its "degrees." *Heart Lung* 1977;6:327.

Pepine CJ, Conti CR: Calcium blockers in coronary heart disease. *Mod Concepts Cardiovasc Dis* 1981;50:61.

Perloff JK, Roberts NK, Cabeen WR: Left axis deviation. *Circulation* 1979;60:12.

Peter T: The electrocardiographic recognition of the Wenckebach phenomenon in sites other than the atrioventricular junction. *Heart Lung* 1976;5:747.

Petty T, Morganroth M: Respiratory failure and the heart—revisited. *Heart Lung* 1982;11:29.

Phibbs BP, Marriott HJL: Computer ECG programs: A critical appraisal. *Primary Cardiol* 1981;7:49.

Physicians' Desk Reference. Oradell, N.J., Litton Industries, 1981.

Preston TA: The use of pacemaking for the treatment of acute arrhythmias. *Heart Lung* 1977;6:249.

Prinzmetal M, et al: Angina pectoris I: A variant form of angina pectoris. *Am J Med* 1959;27:375.

Programmer III, Instructions for Use. Miami, Cordis Corp, 1981.

Racchini AP, Chunn PO, Dick M: Ventricular tachycardia in children. *Am J Cardiol* 1981;47:1091.

Rackley CE, et al: Mitral valve disease, in Hurst JW (ed): *The Heart,* ed 5. New York, McGraw-Hill Book Co, 1982, p 892.

Reicheck N, Devereux RB: Left ventricular hypertrophy: Relationship of anatomic, echocardiographic, and electrocardiographic findings. *Circulation* 1981;63:1391.

Reynolds SF: Cardiac trauma and tamponade. *Crit Care Quart* 1981;4:27.

Riccioni N, Bartolomei C: Treatment of bradycardia-tachycardia syndrome with low doses of amiodarone. *Cardiology* 1982;2:3.

Rosen KM, Arostegui FL, Pouget JM: Pre-excitation with normal P-R intervals. *Chest* 1972;62:581.

Rosen MR, Hoffman BF, Wit AL: Electrophysiology and pharmacology of cardiac arrhythmias. V. Cardiac antiarrhythmic effect of lidocaine. *Am Heart J* 1975;98:526.

Rosenbaum MB, Elizari MV, Lazzari JO: *The Hemiblocks.* Tarpon Springs, Fla, Tampa Tracings, 1970.

Rosenbaum M: Intraventricular trifascicular block. *Heart Lung* 1972;1:216.

Rothfeld EL: The itinerant ST-T segment. *Heart Lung* 1977;6:857.

Rowe MA: The use of electro-physiological mapping studies in treating recurrent sustained ventricular tachycardia. *Crit Care Quart* 1981;4:67.

Rowe RD, Mehrizi A: *The Neonate with Congenital Heart Disease.* New York, WB Saunders, 1968.

Sandler IA, Marriott HJL: The differential morphology of anomalous ventricular complexes of RBBB type in lead V_1. *Circulation* 1965;31:551.

Schamroth L: *The Disorders of Cardiac Rhythm.* Oxford, England, Blackwell Scientific Publications, 1971.

Schamroth L: *Electrocardiographic Excursions.* Oxford, England, Blackwell Scientific Publications, 1975.

Schamroth L: *The Electrocardiology of Coronary Artery Disease.* Oxford, England, Blackwell Scientific Publications, 1975, p 30.

Schamroth L, et al: Ventricular interpolation with prolonged effect. *Heart Lung* 1979;8:349.

Scheidt S, et al: *Cornell Postgraduate Course on Cardiac Arrhythmias: A Clinical Workbook.* New York, Medcom, Inc, 1980.

Schneider JF, et al: Newly acquired left bundle branch block: The Framingham study. *Ann Intern Med* 1979;5:303.

Schoenberger JA: Myocardial reinfarction: Mechanisms, incidence and prognosis. *Primary Cardiol* 1982;1(suppl):2.

Sclarovsky S, Strasberg B, Martonovich G, et al: Ventricular rhythms with intermediate rates in acute myocardial infarction. *Chest* 1978;74:180.

Severi S, et al: Long-term prognosis of "variant" angina with medical treatment. *Am J Cardiol* 1980;46:228.

Shand DG: Comparative pharmacology of the beta-adrenoreceptor blocking agents. *Primary Cardiology* 1982;1(suppl):6.

Sherf L, Neufeld H: *The Pre-excitation Syndromes: Facts and Theories.* New York, Yorke Medical Books, 1978.

Singh BN: The genesis of arrhythmias, in *Cornell Postgraduate Course in Cardiac Arrhythmias.* New York, Medcom, Inc, 1979.

Skapinker A, Schamroth L: "Postextrasystolic" change. *Heart Lung* 1977;6:343.

Slota MC: Cardiac pacemakers in children. *Crit Care Nurse* November-December 1981, p 35.

Slota MC, Beerman L, Sanchez G: Pediatric electrocardiography overview. *Heart Lung* 1982;11:69.

Smart R, Schamroth L: A case of idionodal (non-paroxysmal) tachycardia. *Heart Lung* 1978;7:1053.

Spann JF, Hurst JW: in Hurst JW (ed): *The Heart,* New York, McGraw-Hill Book Co, 1978, p 587.

Spence MI, Lemberg L: Cardiac pacemakers. III. Pacemakers in the management of reciprocating tachycardia. *Heart Lung* 1975;4:128.

Spence MI, Lemberg L: Glucose-insulin-potassium in acute myocardial infarction. *Heart Lung* 1980;9:905.

St Mary E, Virgin H, Castillo C, et al: The "variant normal" electrocardiogram of the professional football player. *Phys Sports Med* 1978;6:85.

Strumpfer G: History of the nuclear demand pacemaker. *Media Fact Sheet.* Minneapolis, Medtronic, Inc, 1973.

Sunquist JM, et al: Right ventricular infarction: Recognition, treatment, and nursing considerations. *Heart Lung* 1980;9:706.

Sweetwood HM: Oxygen administration in the coronary care unit. *Heart Lung* 1974;3:102.

Sweetwood HM: Evaluation of cardiac arrhythmias. *Nurse Pract* March-April, 1980, p 12.

Sweetwood HM, Boak JG: Aberrant conduction. *Heart Lung* 1977;6:73.

The Cordis Pacer Systems Analyzer. Miami, Cordis Corp, 1976.

The New Wave in Cardiology. Searle Pharmaceuticals, 1981.

Thompson WL: Dosage optimization in critical care: Use and abuse of drug analysis and computers, in *Critical Care,* Society of Critical Care Medicine. 1981, vol 2, p 11g:8.

Torres M, et al: Spectrum of myocardial contusion. *Crit Care Med* 1981;9:154.

Trunkey DD: Review of current concepts of fluid and electrolyte management. *Heart Lung* 1975;4:115.

Uhley HN: Comparison of A-V block due to acute myocardial infarction and chronic conduction system disease. *Heart Lung* 1975;4:430.

Underhill SL, Woods SL, Sivaragain ES, et al: *Cardiac Nursing.* Philadelphia, JB Lippincott Co, 1982.

Venkatesh A, Pauls DL, Crowe R, et al: Mitral valve prolapse in anxiety neurosis. *Am Heart J* 1980;100:302.

Vera Z, Awan NA, Amsterdam E: Cardiac pacemakers: Indications and complications. *Heart Lung* 1975;4:444.

Vera Z, et al: His bundle electrography for evaluating criteria in differentiating ventricular ectopy from aberrancy in atrial fibrillation. *Circulation* 1972;46(suppl II):90.

Villforth C: *Policy Statement: Cardiac Pacemaker Warning Signs Near Microwave Ovens.* US Food and Drug Administration, Washington, DC, September 1976.

Weidner NJ, Ganm WE, Chon TC: Hyperkalemia—electrocardiographic abnormalities. *J Pediatr* 1978;93:462.

Wenger NK: Myocarditis, in Hurst JW (ed): *The Heart.* New York, McGraw-Hill Book Co, 1978, p 1529.

White PD: Wolff-Parkinson-White syndrome, in Sandoe E, Jensen EF, Olesen KH (eds): *Cardiac Arrhythmias.* Södertälje, Sweden, AB Astra, 1970, p 368.

Widman WD, et al: Pitfalls in measuring R waves in pacemaker dependent patients. *PACE* 1979;2:186.

Williams ES: Supraventricular tachycardias. *Heart Lung* 1981;10:634.

Withering W: *An Account of the Foxglove, and Some of Its Medical Uses: With Practical Remarks on Dropsy, and Other Diseases.* London, England, CGJ Robinson and J Robinson, 1785.

Wolff G, Han J, Curran J: Wolff-Parkinson-White syndrome in the neonate. *Am J Cardiol* 1978;41:559.

Wolff L, Parkinson J, White PD: Bundle branch block with short P-R interval in healthy young people prone to paroxysmal tachycardia. *Am Heart J* 1930;5:685.

Zeluff GW, Suki WN, Jackson D: Hypercalcemia—etiology, manifestations, and management. *Heart Lung* 1980;9:146.

Zipes DP, Noble JD: Assessment of electrical abnormalities, in Hurst JW (ed): *The Heart,* ed 5. New York, McGraw-Hill Book Co, 1982, p 337.

Zohman LR, Kattus AA: Exercise testing in the diagnosis of coronary heart disease: A perspective. *Am J Cardiol* 1977;40:243.

Zoll PM: Resuscitation of the heart in ventricular standstill by external electrical stimulation. *N Engl J Med* 1952;247:768.

Self-Assessment

Tracings

The following representative ECG strips are provided to assess your comprehension of ECG interpretation skills discussed in the text. Interpretation of each strip can be found in the following section.

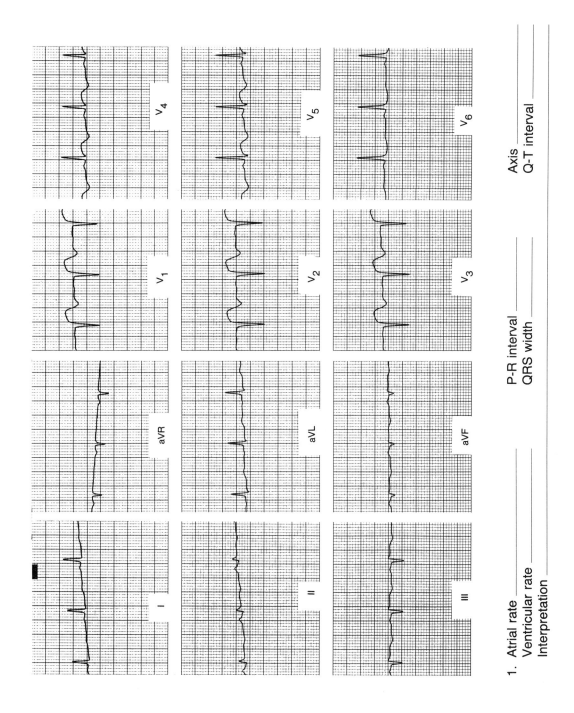

1. Atrial rate _____   P-R interval _____   Axis _____
   Ventricular rate _____   QRS width _____   Q-T interval _____
   Interpretation _____

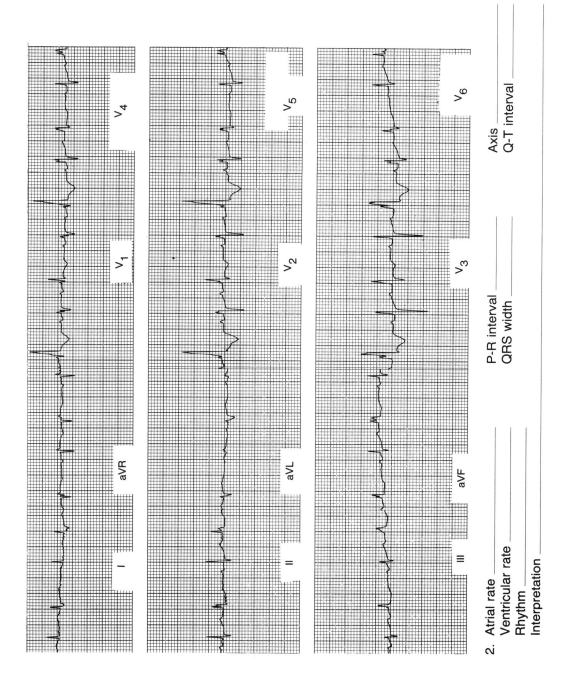

2. Atrial rate _____   P-R interval _____   Axis _____
   Ventricular rate _____   QRS width _____   Q-T interval _____
   Rhythm _____
   Interpretation _____

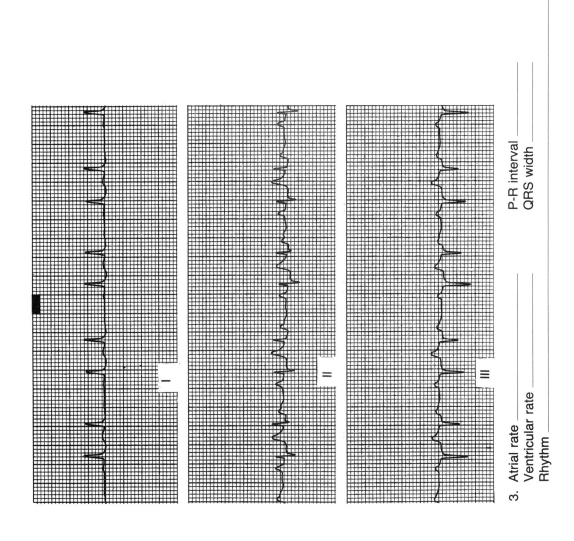

I

II

III

3. Atrial rate _____
   Ventricular rate _____
   Rhythm _____

P-R interval _____
QRS width _____

Axis _____

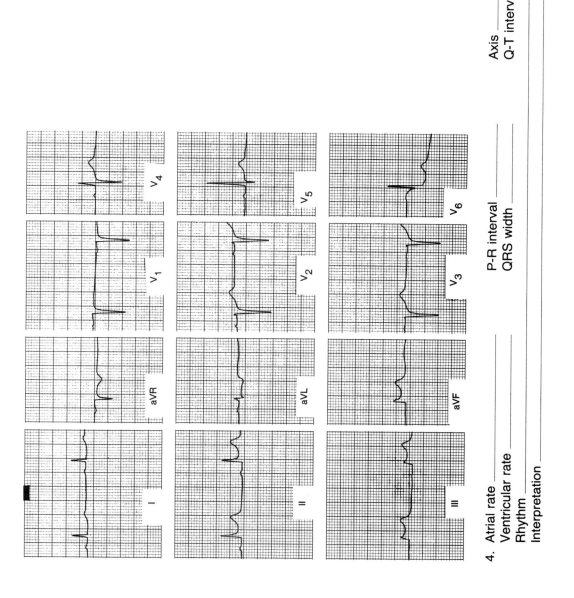

4. Atrial rate _____

Ventricular rate _____

Rhythm _____

Interpretation _____

P-R interval _____

QRS width _____

Axis _____

Q-T interval _____

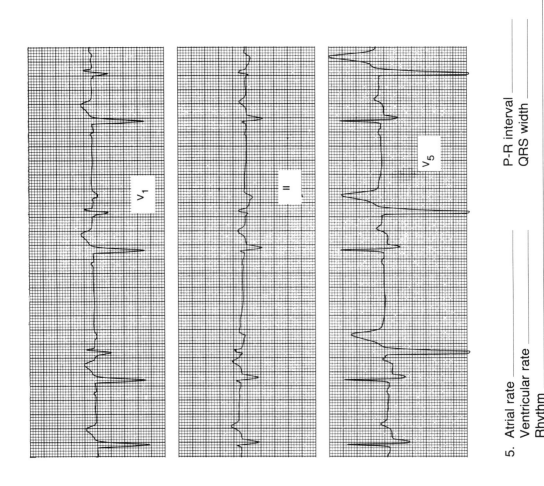

5. Atrial rate _____   P-R interval _____
    Ventricular rate _____   QRS width _____
    Rhythm _____

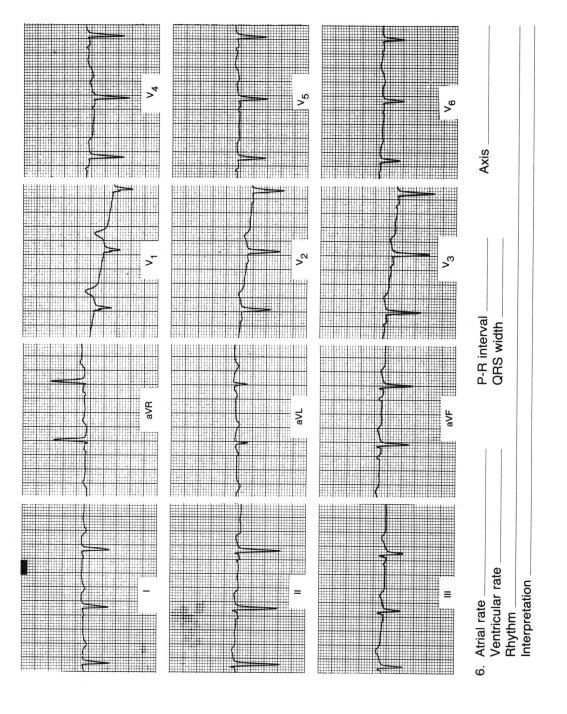

6. Atrial rate _____   P-R interval _____   Axis _____
   Ventricular rate _____   QRS width _____
   Rhythm _____
   Interpretation _____

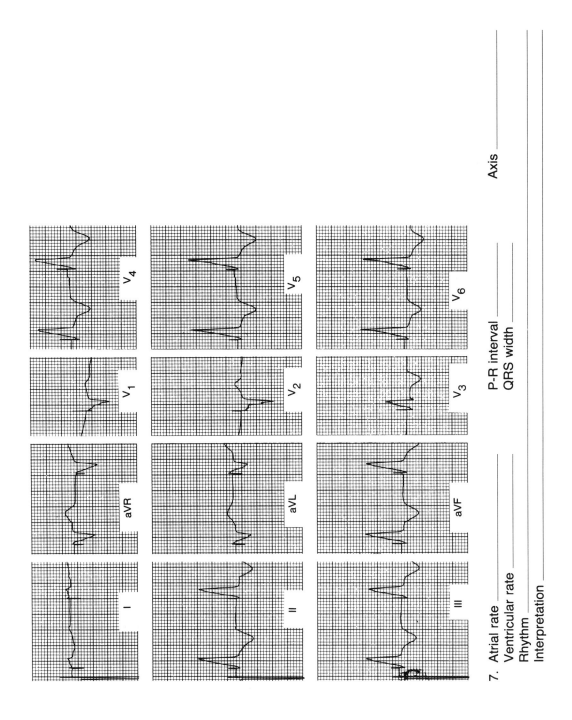

7. Atrial rate _____

Ventricular rate _____

Rhythm _____

Interpretation _____

P-R interval _____

QRS width _____

Axis _____

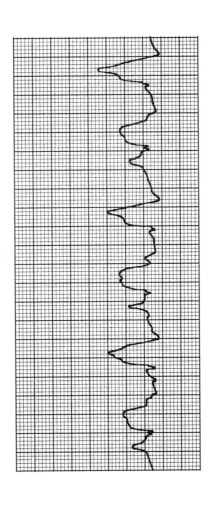

8. Atrial rate _____   P-R interval _____

Ventricular rate _____   QRS width _____

Rhythm _____

Interpretation _____

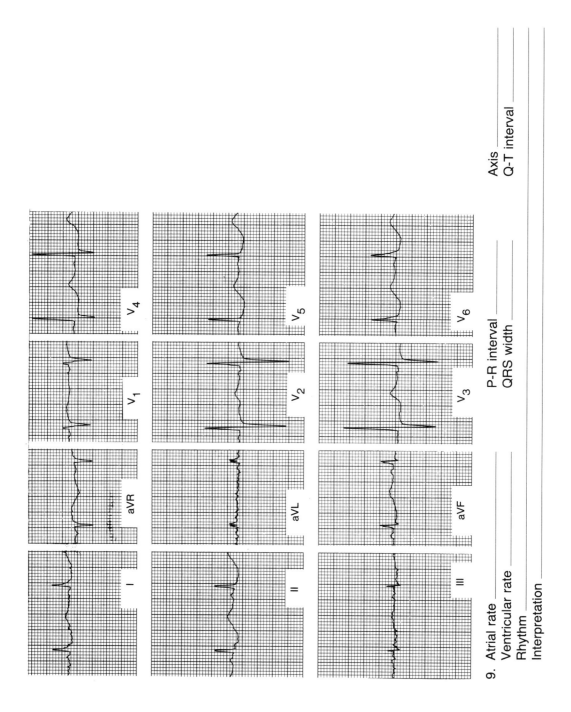

9. Atrial rate _____   Axis _____
   Ventricular rate _____   Q-T interval _____
   Rhythm _____
   Interpretation _____

P-R interval _____
QRS width _____

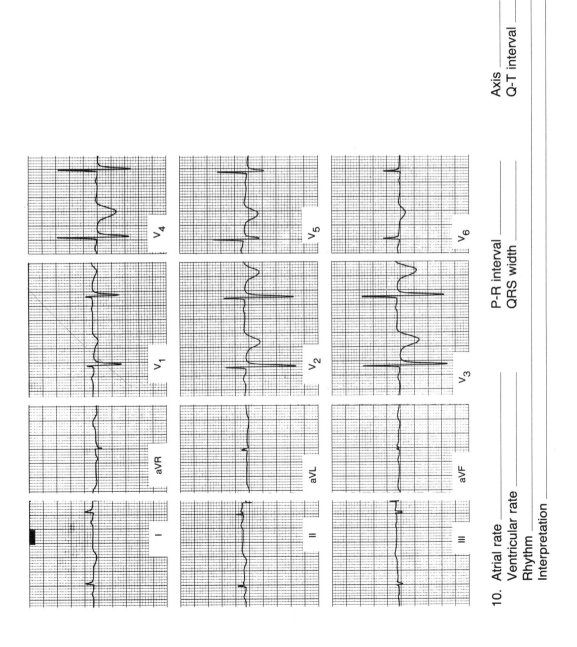

10. Atrial rate _____   Axis _____
    Ventricular rate _____   Q-T interval _____
    Rhythm _____
    Interpretation _____

P-R interval _____
QRS width _____

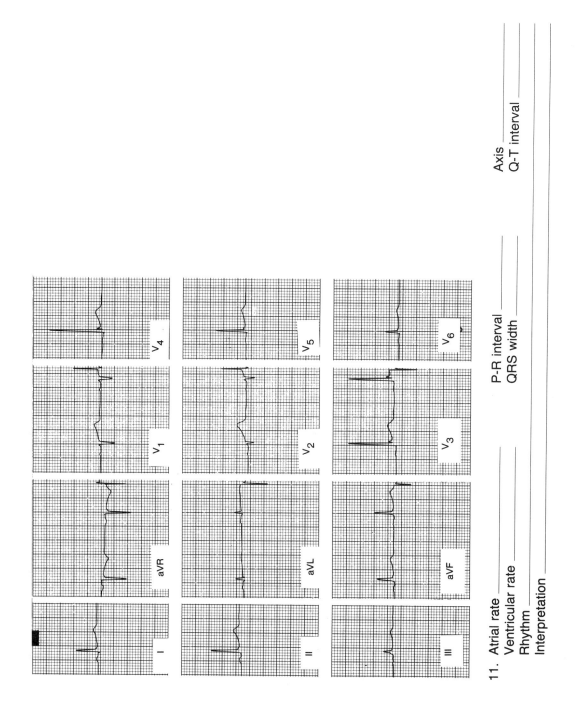

11. Atrial rate _____   Axis _____

Ventricular rate _____   P-R interval _____   Q-T interval _____

Rhythm _____   QRS width _____

Interpretation _____

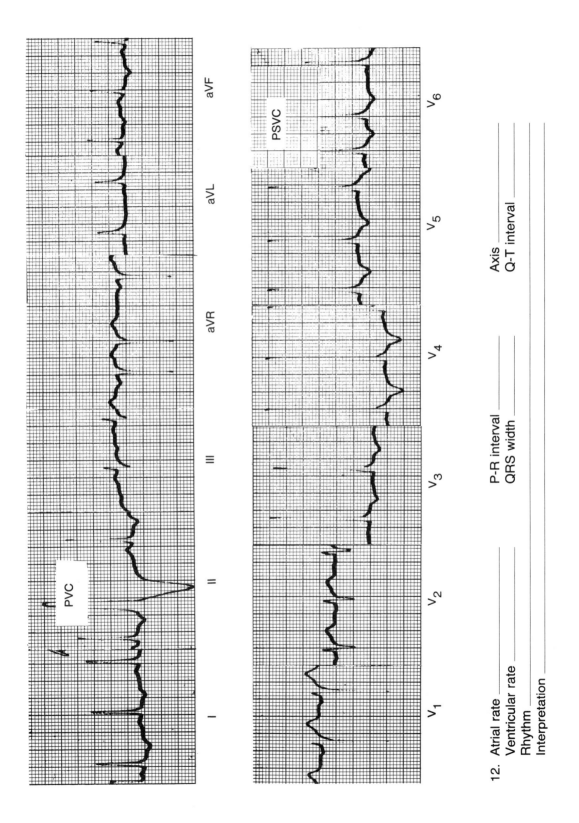

I   II   III   aVR   aVL   aVF

PVC

PSVC

V1   V2   V3   V4   V5   V6

12. Atrial rate _____   P-R interval _____   Axis _____

Ventricular rate _____   QRS width _____   Q-T interval _____

Rhythm _____

Interpretation _____

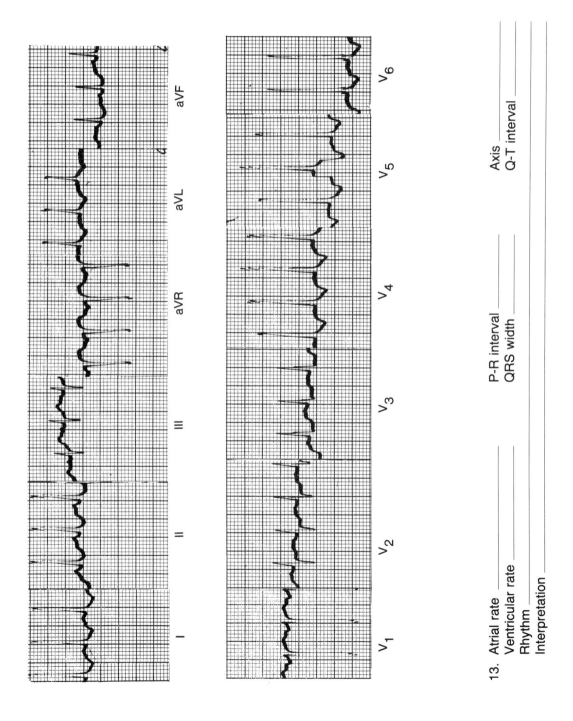

13. Atrial rate _____   Axis _____
    Ventricular rate _____   Q-T interval _____
    Rhythm _____   P-R interval _____
    Interpretation _____   QRS width _____

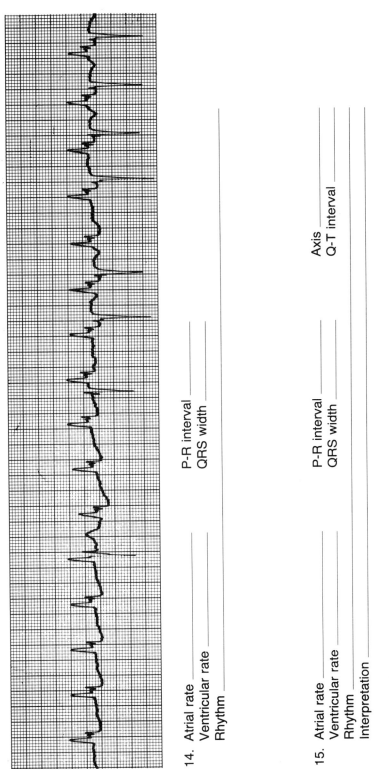

14. Atrial rate _____   P-R interval _____
    Ventricular rate _____   QRS width _____
    Rhythm _____

15. Atrial rate _____   P-R interval _____   Axis _____
    Ventricular rate _____   QRS width _____   Q-T interval _____
    Rhythm _____
    Interpretation _____

(Note: The ECG for question 15 is on the next page.)

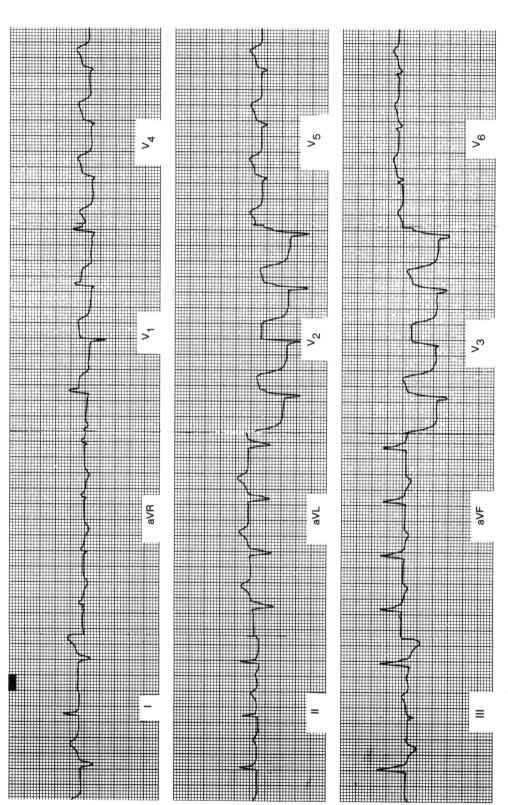

This ECG is to be used in answering question 15.

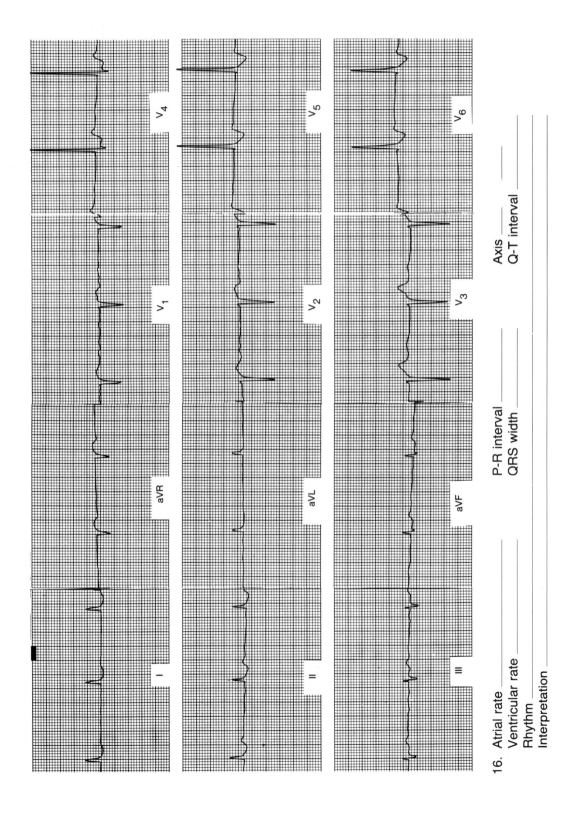

16. Atrial rate _____   Axis _____
    Ventricular rate _____   Q-T interval _____
    P-R interval _____
    QRS width _____
    Rhythm _____
    Interpretation _____

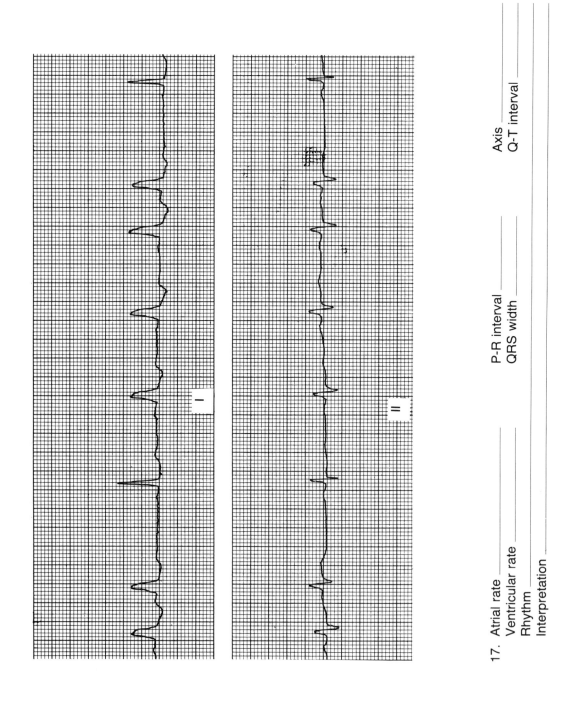

17. Atrial rate _____   P-R interval _____   Axis _____
    Ventricular rate _____   QRS width _____   Q-T interval _____
    Rhythm _____
    Interpretation _____

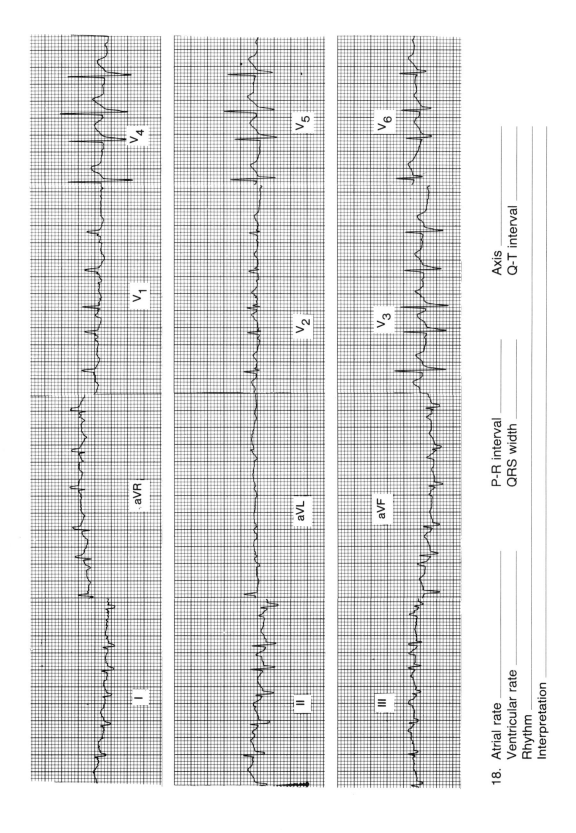

18. Atrial rate _____   Axis _____
    Ventricular rate _____   Q-T interval _____
    Rhythm _____   P-R interval _____
    Interpretation _____   QRS width _____

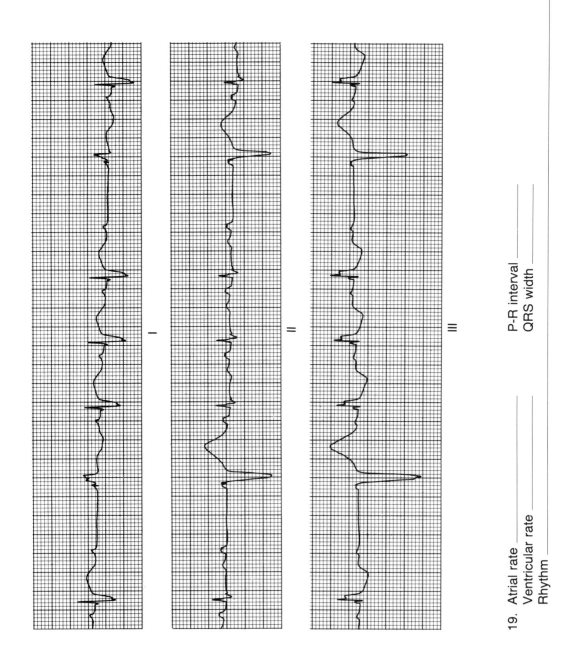

I

II

III

19. Atrial rate _____   P-R interval _____
     Ventricular rate _____   QRS width _____
     Rhythm _____

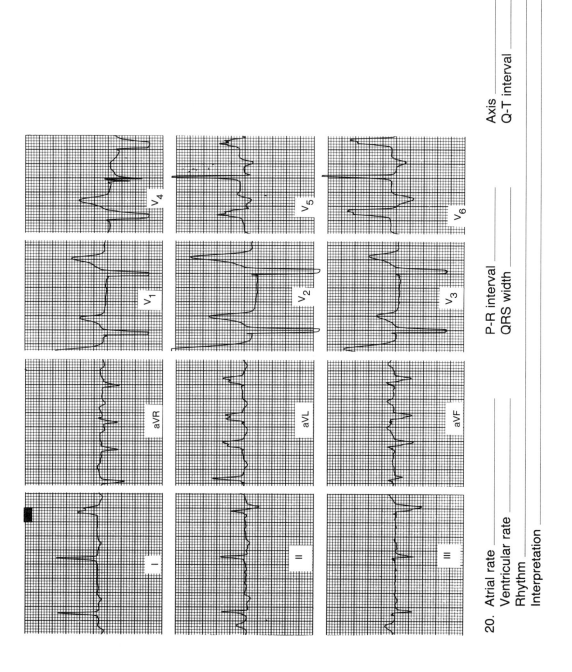

20. Atrial rate _____
    Ventricular rate _____
    Rhythm _____
    Interpretation _____

    P-R interval _____
    QRS width _____

    Axis _____
    Q-T interval _____

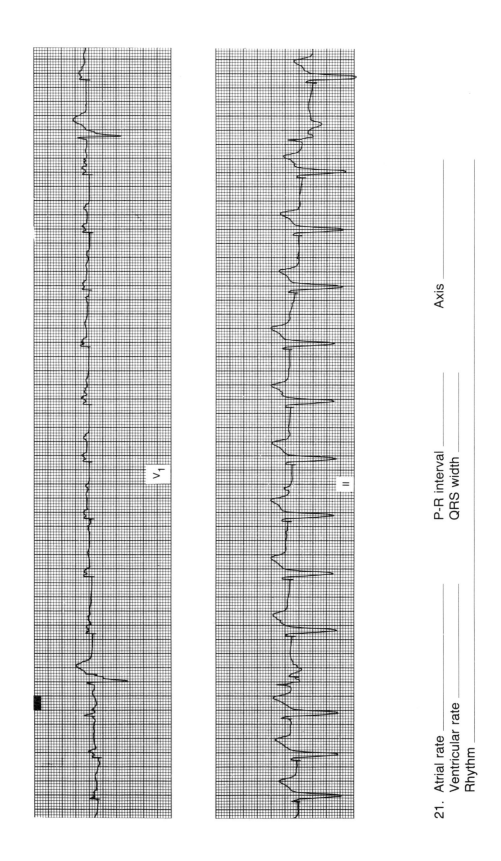

V₁

II

21.   Atrial rate _____   P-R interval _____   Axis _____
       Ventricular rate _____   QRS width _____
       Rhythm _____

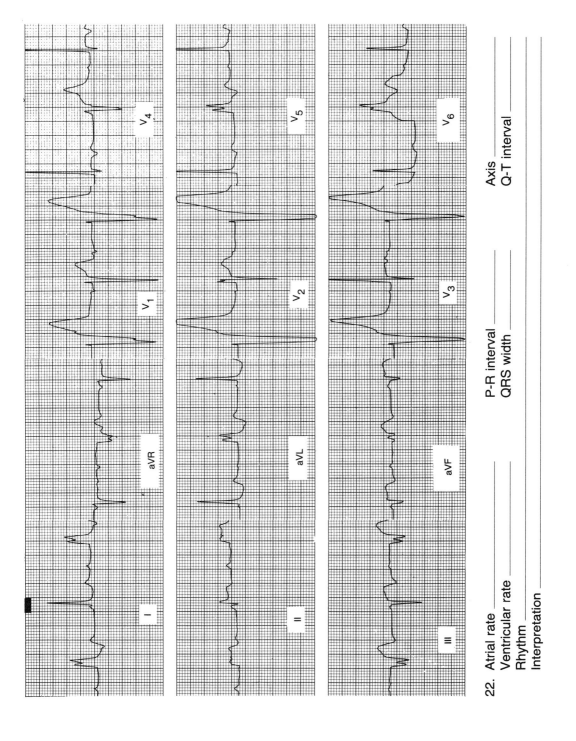

22. Atrial rate _____   Axis _____
    Ventricular rate _____   P-R interval _____   Q-T interval _____
    Rhythm _____   QRS width _____
    Interpretation _____

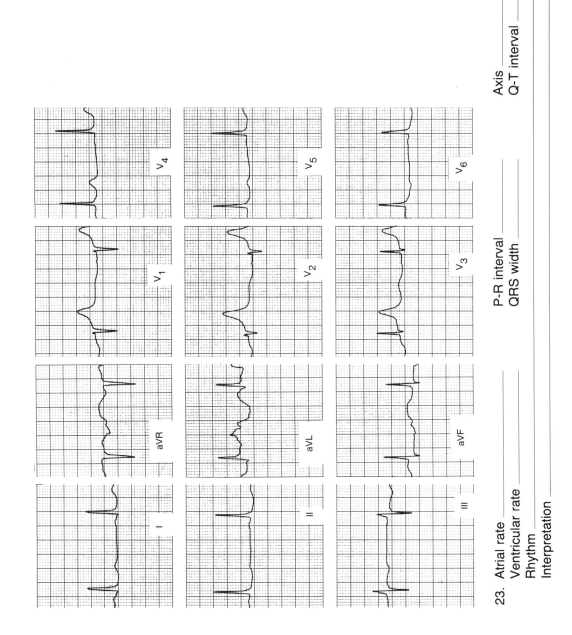

23. Atrial rate _____
Ventricular rate _____
Rhythm _____
Interpretation _____

P-R interval _____
QRS width _____

Axis _____
Q-T interval _____

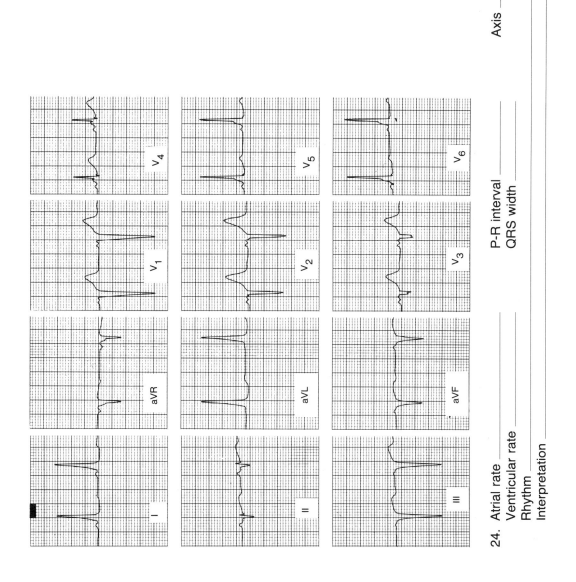

24. Atrial rate _____   Axis _____

Ventricular rate _____

Rhythm _____   P-R interval _____

Interpretation _____   QRS width _____

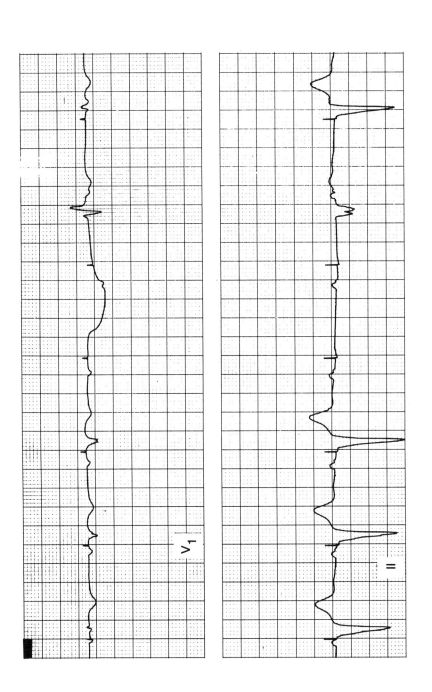

V₁

II

25. Atrial rate _____   P-R interval _____
    Ventricular rate _____   QRS width _____
    Rhythm _____

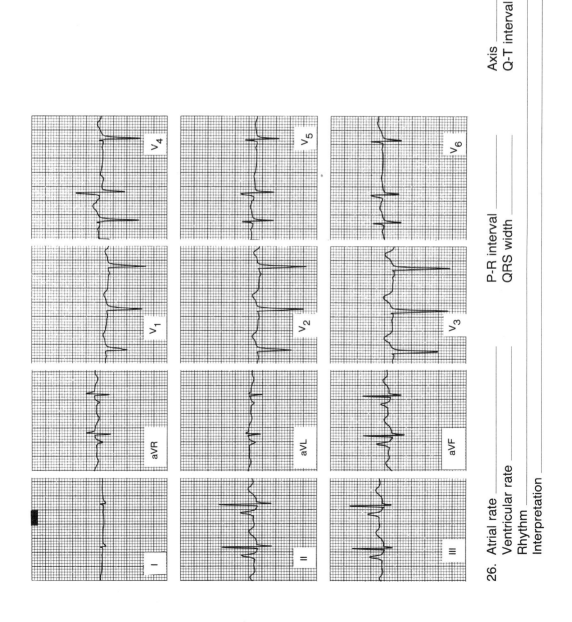

26. Atrial rate _____

Ventricular rate _____

Rhythm _____

Interpretation _____

P-R interval _____

QRS width _____

Axis _____

Q-T interval _____

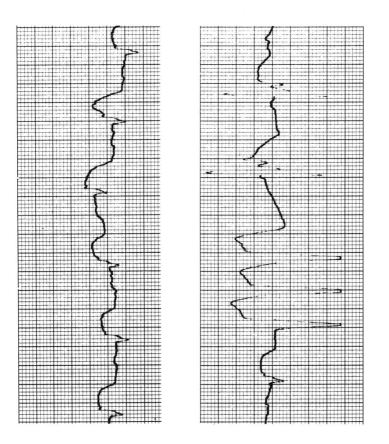

27. Atrial rate _____   P-R interval _____
    Ventricular rate _____   QRS width _____
    Rhythm _____
    Interpretation _____

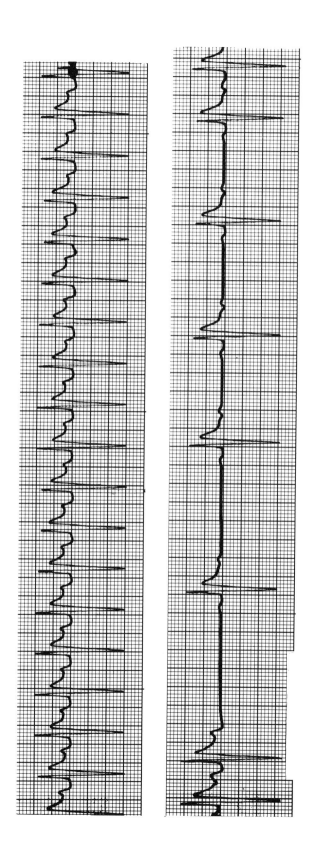

28. Atrial rate _____   P-R interval _____
     Ventricular rate _____   QRS width _____
     Rhythm _____

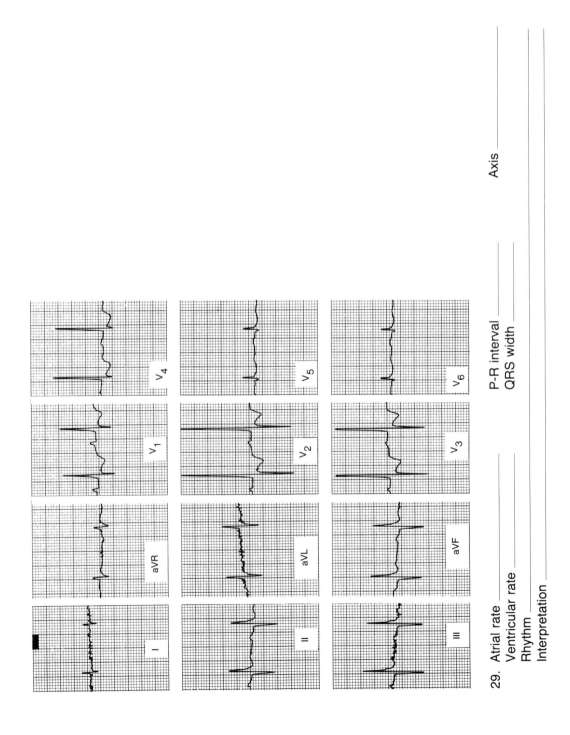

29. Atrial rate _____   P-R interval _____   Axis _____

Ventricular rate _____   QRS width _____

Rhythm _____

Interpretation _____

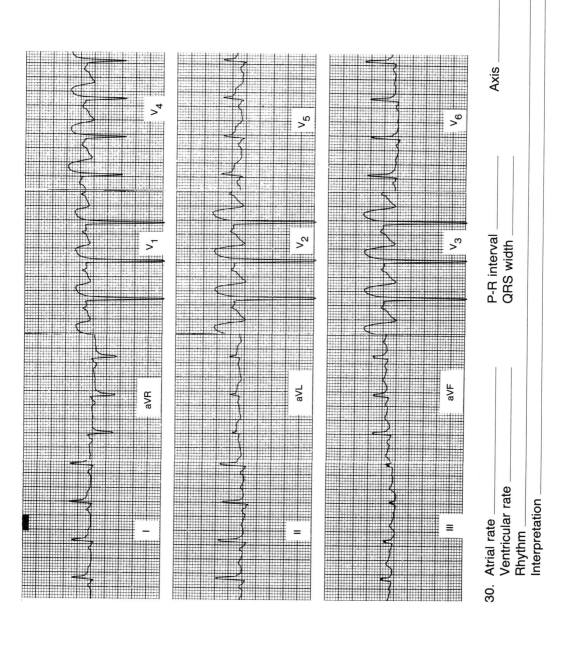

30. Atrial rate _____   P-R interval _____   Axis _____
     Ventricular rate _____   QRS width _____
     Rhythm _____
     Interpretation _____

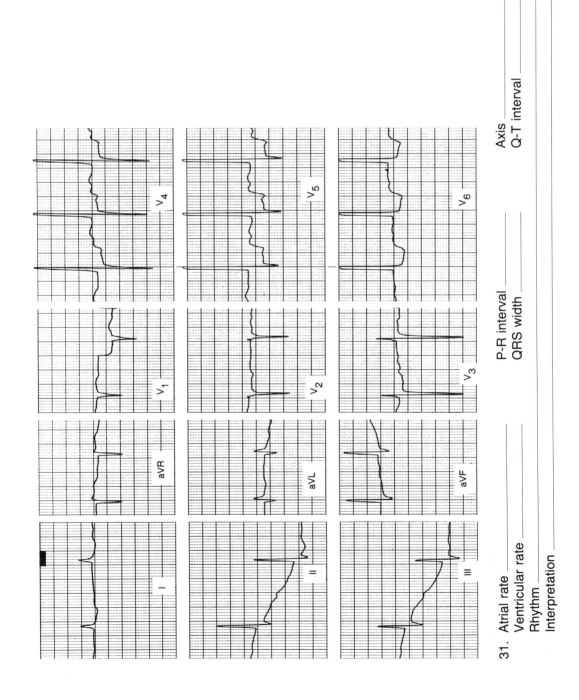

31.   Atrial rate _____   P-R interval _____   Axis _____
       Ventricular rate _____   QRS width _____   Q-T interval _____
       Rhythm _____
       Interpretation _____

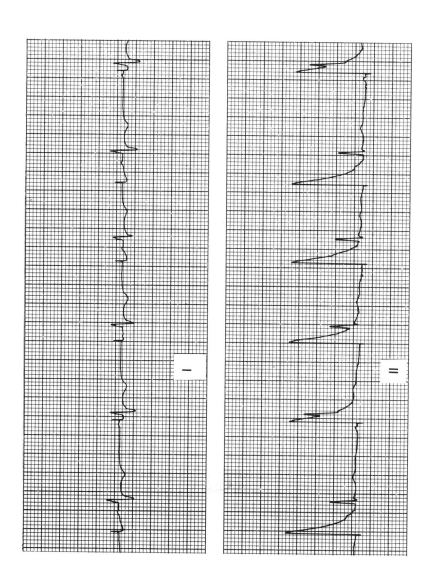

32. Atrial rate _____   P-R interval _____
    Ventricular rate _____   QRS width _____
    Rhythm _____

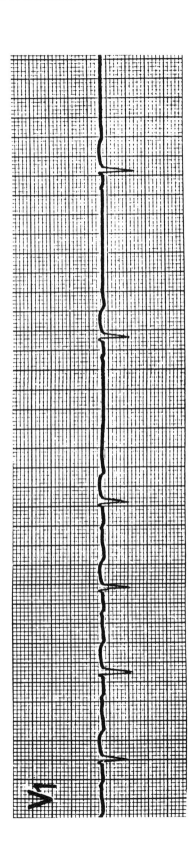

P-R interval _____
QRS width _____

33. Atrial rate _____
    Ventricular rate _____
    Interpretation _____

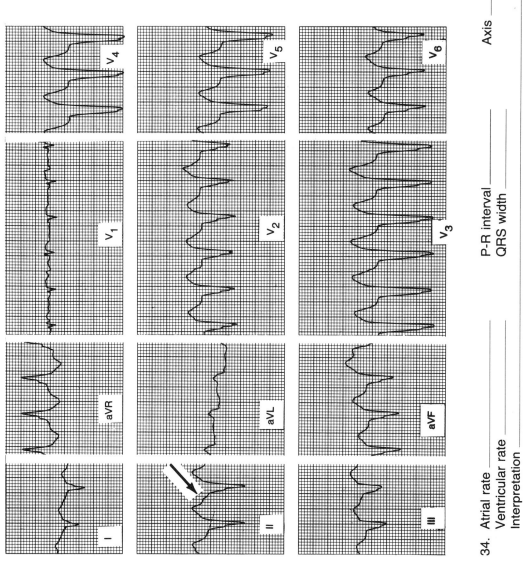

34. Atrial rate _____   P-R interval _____   Axis _____

Ventricular rate _____   QRS width _____

Interpretation _____

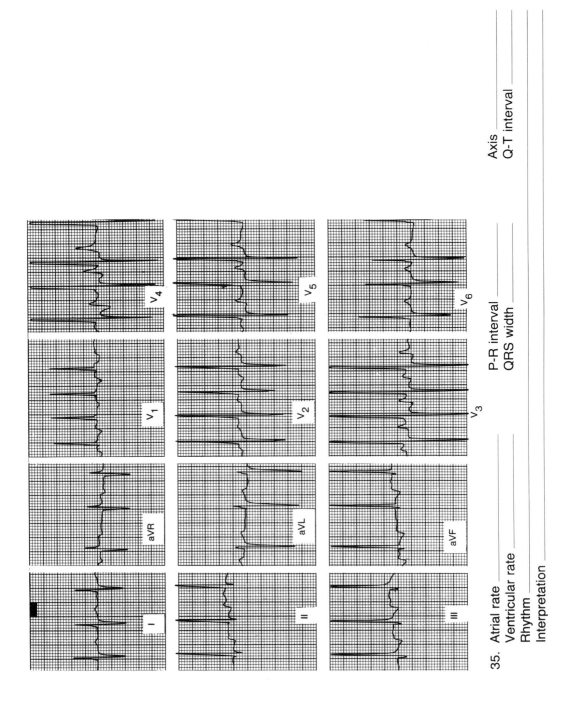

35. Atrial rate _____   P-R interval _____   Axis _____
    Ventricular rate _____   QRS width _____   Q-T interval _____
    Rhythm _____
    Interpretation _____

Interpretations

1. Atrial rate: *82 beats/min*   P-R interval: *0.16 s*   Axis: *−15°*
   Ventricular rate: *82 beats/min*   QRS width: *0.08 s*   Q-T interval: *0.40 s*
   Interpretation: *Acute anteroseptal MI and IWMI, probably recent.*

2. Atrial rate: *120 beats/min*   P-R interval: *0.14 s*   Axis: *+60°*
   Ventricular rate: *120 beats/min* QRS width: *0.08 s*   Q-T interval: *0.28 s*
   Rhythm: *Atrial bigeminy. The premature beats are conducted with a slightly longer P-R interval and an RBBB type of aberrancy.*
   Interpretation: *A number of features suggest the presence of a pulmonary problem. These include: arrhythmia, low voltage, clockwise rotation, and nonspecific ST-T abnormalities. Conditions likely to be present include: COPD, pleural effusion, and pneumothorax. Diagnosis would be facilitated by comparison with previous tracings and knowledge of the clinical findings.*

3. Atrial rate: *190 beats/min*   P-R interval: *Variable*   Axis: *−30°*
   Ventricular rate: *120 beats/min* QRS width: *0.06 s*
   Rhythm: *Atrial tachycardia with Wenckebach conduction. The first P wave in each instance is conducted normally. The P-R interval of the second P wave is slightly longer, the QRS complex is slightly aberrant, and the third P wave is not conducted at all.*

4. Atrial rate: *55 beats/min*   P-R interval: *0.20 s*   Axis: *+60°*
   Ventricular rate: *55 beats/min*   QRS width: *0.08*   Q-T interval: *0.40 s*
   Rhythm: *Sinus bradycardia*
   Interpretation: *Acute IWMI*

5. Atrial rate: *65 beats/min*   P-R interval: *0.18 s*
   Ventricular rate: *65 beats/min*   QRS width: *0.11 s*
   Rhythm: *Normal sinus rhythm with ventricular parasystole*
   Comment: *There is also a nonspecific ventricular conduction delay. The QRS width is prolonged, but the characteristic features of either RBBB or LBBB are not present.*

6. Atrial rate: *75 beats/min*   P-R interval: *0.16 s*   Axis: *Indeterminate*
   Ventricular rate: *75 beats/min*   QRS width: *0.08 s*
   Rhythm: *NSR*
   Interpretation: *True dextrocardia*
   Comment: *The P wave is negative in lead I. There are three possible explanations. This is not junctional rhythm because the P-R interval is normal. The QRS complexes in the frontal plane are not only negative, but they get smaller in the direction of lead V$_6$, suggesting that the electrode is moving farther away, rather than toward the left ventricle.*

7. Atrial rate: *86 beats/min*   P-R interval: *–*   Axis: *+90°*
   Ventricular rate: *66 beats/min*   QRS width: *0.15 s*
   Rhythm: *Ventricular pacing*
   Interpretation: *There is ventricular pacing throughout, with no instance of spontaneous activity and no failure to capture. The axis of +90° in the frontal plane suggests that the electrode tip is located in or near the right ventricular outflow tract, rather than in the apex of the right ventricle.*

8. Atrial rate: *120 beats/min*   P-R interval: *Variable*
   Ventricular rate: *80 beats/min*   QRS width: *0.08 s*
   Rhythm: *Sinus tachycardia with Wenckebach conduction. The first P wave of each group is clearly seen. The second P wave is immediately behind the T wave of the preceding beat, and the blocked P wave is on top of the T wave of the preceding beat, causing it to look distorted.*
   Interpretation: *Although a diagnosis should never be made from an isolated monitoring lead, the presence of Q waves, and especially the greatly elevated S-T segment, suggests an acute myocardial injury.*

9. Atrial rate: *72 beats/min*   P-R interval: *0.15 s*   Axis: *+30°*
   Ventricular rate: *72 beats/min*   QRS width: *0.08 s*   Q-T interval: *0.40 s*
   Rhythm: *NSR*
   Interpretation: *The conspicuous abnormality is the troughlike S-T segment and the apparent Q-T prolongation. Actually this apparent prolongation is probably due to the large U wave. This is best appreciated in lead V$_2$. The most likely diagnosis is pronounced hypokalemia. Administration of drugs such as quinidine may produce a similar effect.*

10. Atrial rate: *60 beats/min* P-R interval: *0.20 s* Axis: *0*
    Ventricular rate: *60 beats/min* QRS width: *0.08 s* Q-T interval: *0.50 s*
    Rhythm: *NSR*

    Interpretation: The outstanding feature of this tracing is the *pronounced inversion of T waves seen in most leads. This is accompanied by prolongation of the Q-T interval, the normal interval for this rate being 0.39 to 0.42 s. The alternative diagnoses compatible with this finding are: widespread myocardial ischemia, subendocardial infarction, or an intracranial problem, such as cerebrovascular accident, subdural hematoma.*

    Comment: *There are many instances in which precise interpretation of the ECG is not possible without some clinical information. In this instance, the patient was admitted for subdural hematoma. An ECG (Fig A-10a), obtained after burr holes were placed in the skull, shows marked improvement of the ECG, suggesting that the changes observed had, indeed, been due to increased intracranial pressure.*

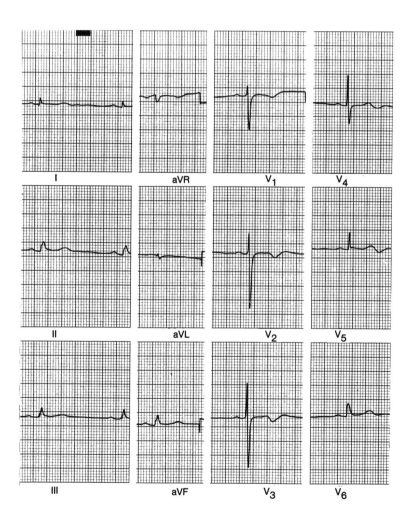

11. Atrial rate: *62 beats/min*   P-R interval: *0.14 s*   Axis: *+45°*
    Ventricular rate: *62 beats/min*   QRS width: *0.08 s*   Q-T interval: *0.37 s*
    Rhythm: *NSR*
    Interpretation: Normal ECG
    Comment: *There is a 1.5-mm elevation of the S-T segment in a number of leads, notably lead V₃, with elevation of the J point. This finding represents a normal variant frequently encountered in young, black males and attributed to vagotonia. In doubtful cases, examination of previous and/or follow-up tracings confirms that the pattern is benign and stable.*

12. Atrial rate: *100 beats/min*   P-R interval: *0.16 s*   Axis: *+30°*
    Ventricular rate: *100 beats/min*   QRS width: *0.09 s*   Q-T interval: *0.32 s*
    Rhythm: *Sinus tachycardia with occasional PVCs and PACs*
    Interpretation: *LVH with pronounced strain and myocardial ischemia*

13. Atrial rate: *170 beats/min*   P-R interval: *0.09 s*   Axis: *+30°*
    Ventricular rate: *170 beats/min*   QRS width: *0.08 s*   Q-T interval: *0.20 s*
    Rhythm: *Atrial tachycardia. The possibility of 2:1 atrial flutter may be considered; vagal maneuvers may confirm this diagnosis.*
    Interpretation: *LVH with strain and digitalis effect.*
    Comment: *This tracing was obtained from the same patient about 1 month after the tracing shown in Figure A-12. Although there has been some decrease in the voltages recorded, LVH is still present, as indicated because V₆ is greater than V₅. The presence of digitalis is reflected by the short Q-T interval (low normal limit for rate is 0.23 s). The previously seen strain pattern has been affected by the administration of digitalis: there is now minimal S-T segment depression, and the sagging T wave has a convex appearance in many leads.*

14. Atrial rate: *100 beats/min*   P-R interval: *0.22 s (conducted beats)*
    Ventricular rate: *Variable*   QRS width: *0.09 s*
    Rhythm: *High-degree AV block, with at least 3 s of ventricular asystole*
    Comment: *This is a monitoring lead, and the gain has been turned up until the complexes could be seen. This accounts for the unusual formation and height of the P waves. The tracing reflects a potentially extremely dangerous error. The monitoring system counted the tallest upright deflections, so the prolonged period of ventricular asystole did not trigger the alarm system, and the problem went unrecognized for some time.*

15. Atrial rate: *75 beats/min*   P-R interval: *0.28 s*   Axis: *+120°*
    Ventricular rate: *85 beats/min*   *(conducted beats)*   Q-T interval: *0.40 s*
                                          QRS width: *0.09 s*
    Rhythm: *Isorhythmic AV dissociation, with two captures. The independent atrial rhythm is best seen in lead V₁. The second beat in the frontal plane, as well as the second beat in the horizontal plane, which are slightly different, represent captures by the preceding sinus impulses. The other QRS complexes are of junctional origin.*
    Interpretation: *Hyperacute, extensive AWMI. The QRS complexes of the dominant rhythm show LPH.*

16. Atrial rate: ?   P-R interval: –   Axis: +30°
     Ventricular rate: *55 beats/min*   QRS width: *0.09 s*   Q-T interval: *0.36 s*
     Rhythm: *Atrial fibrillation with complete AV block and junctional rhythm*
     Interpretation: *LVH and digitalis effect. Probable digitalis toxicity.*

17. Atrial rate: *68 beats/min*   P-R interval: *0.16 s*   Axis: –30°
     Ventricular rate: *68 beats/min*   QRS width: *0.15 s*   Q-T interval: *0.44 s*
     Rhythm: *NSR with occasional PACs.*
     Interpretation: *Rate-related LBBB.*
     Comment: *Most of the beats show LBBB, except for the beats that follow the prolonged*
       pause after the PACs. This finding strongly suggests cardiac disease.

18. Atrial rate: *150 beats/min*   P-R interval: *Variable*   Axis: *Indeterminate*
     Ventricular rate: *150 beats/min*   QRS width: *0.08 s*   Q-T interval: *0.24 s*
     Rhythm: *Multifocal (chaotic) atrial tachycardia*
     Interpretation: *RVH, probably due to pulmonary disease*
     Comment: *The diagnosis of RVH is based on the positive R wave in lead V_1 in the*
       presence of the indeterminate axis. The diagnosis of pulmonary disease is based on
       the following findings: arrhythmia, RVH, low voltage, and a P axis of +90°.

19. Atrial rate: 88 beats/min   P-R interval: 0.18 s
     Ventricular rate: *70 beats/min*   QRS width: *0.12 s*
     Rhythm: *Sinus rhythm with 2° AV block (Mobitz II) and VVI pacing. The pacemaker is*
       set for an escape interval of 1200 ms, corresponding to a rate of 50 pulses/min.
     Comment: *The cause of the T wave abnormality and the Q-T interval prolongation*
       cannot be determined on the basis of the three leads shown.

20. Atrial rate: ?   P-R interval: –   Axis: 0
     Ventricular rate: *110 beats/min*   QRS width: *Variable*   Q-T interval: *Variable*
     Rhythm: *Atrial fibrillation*
     Interpretation: *LVH with strain and intermittent LBBB*

21. Atrial rate: *90 beats/min*   P-R interval: –   Axis: –75°
     Ventricular rate: *100 to 72 beats/min*   QRS width: *0.12 s*
     Rhythm: *Properly functioning CPI pacemaker*
     Comment: *During the first few beats, when the rate was 100 beats/min, a magnet was*
       applied, shutting off the sensing mechanism; for this reason the patient's spontane-
       ous beat was not sensed. When the magnet was removed, the pacer dropped to its
       fixed rate of 72 beats/min, and the spontaneous beat near the end of the strip was
       sensed, demonstrating appropriate VVI function.

22. Atrial rate: *100 beats/min*   P-R interval: –   Axis: –30°
     Ventricular rate: *70 beats/min*   QRS width: *0.08 to 0.16 s*   Q-T interval: *0.36 s*
     Rhythm: *Complete heart block, with accelerated junctional pacemaker*
     Interpretation: *Recent IWMI and LVH; every second beat shows LBBB.*

23. Atrial rate: *55 beats/min* P-R interval: *0.16 s* Axis: *+ 15°*
    Ventricular rate: *55 beats/min* QRS width: *0.08 s* Q-T interval: *0.44 s*
    Rhythm: *Sinus bradycardia*
    Interpretation: *Posterior wall ischemia*
    Comment: *There appears to be some depression of the S-T segment in leads II and aVF, with inversion of the T wave in leads III and aVF. Unfortunately this cannot be well identified due to an artifact caused by patient movement. The most striking feature of the tracing is the size of the T waves in leads V_1 to V_3. Figure A-23a, representing leads V_7 to V_9 of the same patient, reveals that these changes are the mirror image of posterior wall T wave inversion. It is possible that this seems unusual only because we do not generally look for it.*

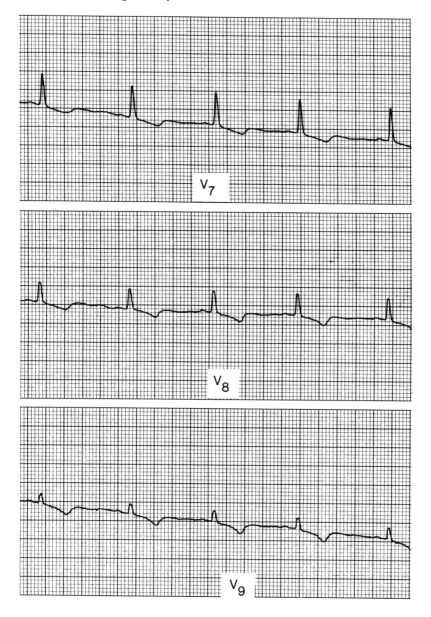

24. Atrial rate: *62 beats/min* P-R interval: *0.08 s* Axis: *−45°*
    Ventricular rate: *62 beats/min* QRS width: *0.12 s*
    Rhythm: *NSR*
    Interpretation: *WPW, type B*
    Comment: *The deflection that looks like part of the P wave (for example, in lead V₂) is the beginning of the delta wave. The latter can best be seen in leads V₅ and V₆. WPW frequently mimics IWMI and presents a source of erroneous diagnosis, unless one notices the P-R interval and the delta wave.*

25. Atrial rate: *64 beats/min* P-R interval: *−*
    Ventricular rate: *50 beats/min* QRS width: *0.16 s*
    Rhythm: *Sinus rhythm with complete heart block, ventricular pacemaker with intermittent failure to capture, and ventricular escape beat after an interval of more than 2 s.*

26. Atrial rate: 94 beats/min P-R interval: 0.16 s Axis: +90°
    Ventricular rate: *94 beats/min* QRS width: *0.07 s* Q-T interval: *0.32 s*
    Rhythm: *NSR with occasional PACs*
    Interpretation: *Pulmonary disease*
    Comment: *The configuration of P, QRS, and T waves in lead I is classically seen with chronic pulmonary disease. This is further supported by the P- pulmonale and the clockwise rotation of the precordial leads.*

27. Atrial rate: *75 to 80 beats/min* P-R interval: *0.24 s*
    Ventricular rate: *75 to 80 beats/min* QRS width: *0.08 s*
    Rhythm: *NSR with 1° AV block and short burst of VT, followed by two ventricular paced beats*
    Interpretation: *Recent IWMI with VVI pacing*

28. Atrial rate: *132 to 35 beats/min* P-R interval: *0.20 s*
    Ventricular rate: *132 to 25 beats/min* QRS width: *0.09 s*
    Rhythm: *Sick sinus syndrome*
    Comment: *The beginning of the continuous tracing shows sinus tachycardia. This comes to a sudden halt and is followed by a very slow and irregular sinus rhythm.*

29. Atrial rate: *90 beats/min* P-R interval: *0.20 s* Axis: *Indeterminate*
    Ventricular rate: *90 beats/min* QRS width: *0.08 s*
    Rhythm: *NSR with occasional PACs*
    Interpretation: *Inferoposteroapical myocardial infarction of indeterminate age*
    Comment: *The IWMI is revealed by the prominent Q waves in leads II, III, and aVF. The normal S-T segment and upright T waves suggest that this is not an acute lesion. The apical infarct is recognized by the Q waves and the apparent loss of voltage in leads V₅ and V₆. The appearance of these leads does not suggest acute injury. The tall R wave in V₁ is the mirror image of Q waves over the posterior wall. The S-T segment depression and T wave inversion in leads V₁ to V₄ probably represent S-T elevation over the posterior wall, so this lesion is probably recent. The findings may be confirmed by obtaining ECGs from leads V₇ to V₉ and by comparing serial tracings over several days.*

30. Atrial rate: *110 beats/min*   P-R interval: *0.13 s*   Axis: *+45°*
    Ventricular rate: *110 beats/min*   QRS width: *0.08 s*
    Rhythm: *Sinus tachycardia*
    Interpretation: *Acute, extensive anterolateral myocardial infarction*
    Comment: *Sinus tachycardia is an adverse rhythm in acute myocardial infarction, since it causes increased oxygen consumption. Persistent sinus tachycardia is an ominous finding in this situation, since it is generally a sign of decreased stroke volume.*

31. Atrial rate: *?*   P-R interval: *−*   Axis: *+60°*
    Ventricular rate: *70 beats/min*   QRS width: *0.08 s*   Q-T interval: *0.42 s*
    (average)
    Rhythm: *Atrial fibrillation*
    Interpretation: *LVH, myocardial ischemia, probable hypokalemia*

32. Atrial rate: *65 beats/min*   P-R interval: *0.12 s*
    Ventricular rate: *65 beats/min*   QRS width: *0.07 s*
    Rhythm: *NSR and VVI pacemaker with failure to capture*
    Comment: *Pacing spikes are present but do not produce ventricular depolarization. In the two instances when spontaneous beats occur outside the pacemaker's refractory period, the pacer's escape interval is reset, indicating that ventricular sensing is intact. The most likely explanation of this phenomenon is deviation of the electrode tip.*

33. Atrial rate: *70 to 35 beats/min*   P-R interval: 0.24 s
    Ventricular rate: *70 to 35 beats/min*   QRS width: *0.08 s*
    Interpretation: *Sinus rhythm with 1° AV block and 2:1 sinus exit block*
    Comment: *The first four beats represent sinus rhythm with 1° AV block. The long pauses in front of the last two P waves are equal to double the previous P-P interval. Therefore the P wave is missing due to sinus exit block.*

34. Atrial rate: *90 beats/min*   P-R interval: *−*   Axis: *Indeterminate*
    Ventricular rate: *126 beats/min*   QRS width: *0.13 s*
    Interpretation: *Ventricular tachycardia*
    Comment: *The tracing in Figure A-34 shows the following characteristics of ventricular tachycardia: regular ventricular rhythm with wide QRS complexes; independent atrial rhythm in lead V_1; indeterminate axis; and concordance of the precordial leads.*

35. Atrial rate: *−*   P-R interval: *−*   Axis: *+100°*
    Ventricular rate: *140 beats/min*   QRS width: *0.08 s*   Q-T interval: *0.29 s*
    Rhythm: *Atrial fibrillation*
    Interpretation: *RVH*
    Comment: *The diagnosis of RVH is supported by RAD, tall R wave in V_1, and T wave inversion in leads II, III, aVF, and V_1, which probably represent a right ventricular strain pattern. The size of the ventricular complexes in leads V_3 and V_4 suggests LVH as well. The length of the Q-T interval suggests the absence of a significant digitalis effect.*

Index